Challenges and Concerns in Multiple Pregnancy

Challenges and Concerns in Multiple Pregnancy

Editor: Sophie Roberts

MURPHY & MOORE
www.murphy-moorepublishing.com

www.murphy-moorepublishing.com

MURPHY & MOORE

Cataloging-in-Publication Data

Challenges and concerns in multiple pregnancy / edited by Sophie Roberts.
p. cm.
Includes bibliographical references and index.
ISBN 978-1-63987-102-5
1. Multiple pregnancy. 2. Multiple pregnancy--Complications. 3. Multiple birth. 4. Pregnancy. I. Roberts, Sophie.
RG567 .C43 2022
618.25--dc23

Murphy & Moore Publishing,
1 Rockefeller Plaza,
New York City, NY 10020, USA

ISBN 978-1-63987-102-5 (Hardback)

Contents

Preface

Multiple pregnancy is a pregnancy when the mother delivers two or more offspring. Multiple births can occur in most of the mammals and such births are named according to the number of offspring. It can occur as a result of either fertilization of multiple eggs creating fraternal fetuses or a result of a single fertilized egg that got divided, creating identical fetuses or maybe a combination of both factors. Multiple pregnancies which occur from a single zygote, double zygotes and more zygotes are termed as monozygotic, dizygotic and polyzygotic respectively. A few of the complications associated with multiple pregnancies are gestational hypertension, premature labor, fetal growth restriction and placenta abruption. This book includes some of the vital pieces of work being conducted across the world, on various topics related to multiple pregnancy. It provides comprehensive insights. This book will help new researchers by foregrounding their knowledge in this branch.

The researches compiled throughout the book are authentic and of high quality, combining several disciplines and from very diverse regions from around the world. Drawing on the contributions of many researchers from diverse countries, the book's objective is to provide the readers with the latest achievements in the area of research. This book will surely be a source of knowledge to all interested and researching the field.

In the end, I would like to express my deep sense of gratitude to all the authors for meeting the set deadlines in completing and submitting their research chapters. I would also like to thank the publisher for the support offered to us throughout the course of the book. Finally, I extend my sincere thanks to my family for being a constant source of inspiration and encouragement.

Editor

1

Early Pregnancy Ultrasound Assessment of Multiple Pregnancy

Panagiotis Antsaklis, Maria Papamichail,
Marianna Theodora, Michael Syndos and
George Daskalakis

Abstract

As the frequency of multiple pregnancies is increasing, every obstetrician has to know that the correct, accurate, and timely determination of gestational age, chorionicity, and amnionicity has significant importance in the management of a multiple pregnancy. Surveillance, complications, outcome, morbidity, and mortality are totally different in a monochorionic and a dichorionic pregnancy. In this chapter, we will present the sonographic figures that are visualized in the first trimester in a multiple pregnancy and help us define the gestational age, chorionicity, and amnionicity. We will classify them into two periods: the early first trimester, including the 10 first weeks of gestation and the late first trimester including the period between the 10th and 14th week of gestation. Finally, we will review some interesting, although infrequent, cases from the literature, showing that pitfalls in the determination of both chorionicity and amnionicity exist and highlighting the importance of being aware of their subsistence.

Keywords: multiple pregnancy, early ultrasound assessment, gestational age, chorionicity, amnionicity

1. Introduction

It is a well-established fact that multiple pregnancies occur more commonly nowadays than a few decades ago. The progress of reproductive technologies and *in vitro* fertilization has played a major role in this increase. In fact, twins comprise about 3% of all live births in the United States [1]. As we speak about history, the vast majority of multiple pregnancies that occurred in the past were diagnosed during the intrapartum period [2]. Today, as the use of ultrasound has become a routine in daily medical practice, multiple pregnancies are diagnosed in the initial ultrasound scan [3]. Beyond the diagnosis of early multiple pregnancy, ultrasound scan is more than necessary to define chorionicity, amnionicity, and gestational age [4].

In this chapter, we will present the ultrasound figures that help us determine gestational age, chorionicity, and amnionicity, focused on the 14 first weeks of gestation in multiple pregnancies. We will also focalize the discussion on twin pregnancies, as they comprise >98% of multiple pregnancies and the vast majority of studies today include twin pregnancies [4]. Nonetheless, we will review some cases from the literature that show that situations can be a little more complicated and may lead to a false diagnosis of chorionicity and amnionicity, in order to highlight that when we manage multiple pregnancies, we have to be alert about exceptions despite being infrequent [5].

A twin pregnancy can be either dizygotic (two-third of twin pregnancies), in which two different eggs are fertilized by two different sperms, and in this case, the pregnancy is always dichorionic-diamniotic or monozygotic. A monozygotic pregnancy occurs when an egg is fertilized by one sperm, producing one embryo, which can split any time, more commonly between day 2 and day 13 after fertilization. Chorionicity and amnionicity are differentiated by the timing of embryo splitting. **Table 1** presents this differentiation and the frequency of each type of a monozygotic pregnancy [3].

2. Defining gestational age

The accurate determination of gestational age is critical for pregnancy management as it shows wherever the measurements of the fetus are in line for the estimate gestational age [4]. In addition, a correct pregnancy dating is necessary not only for the appropriate timing for screening and diagnostic testing but also for optimal scheduling of delivery [6]. For women with regular cycles, the date of the last menstrual period is used to estimate gestational age, taking into account the biological variability and correct the cycle length. For IVF pregnancies, the date of the embryo transfer has been used to define pregnancy dating. The vast majority of authors embraced with multiple pregnancies agree that during the second trimester the evaluation of gestational age is more accurate and it is statistically superior to the second trimester [4]. Moreover, there is an agreement that the parameters and formulas that have been used for dating singleton pregnancies are also accurate for dating multiple pregnancies, since studies in this area include a combination of singleton and multiple pregnancies [7–9].

Time of embryo splitting (in days)	Chorionicity	Amnionicity	Frequency (%)
2–3	Dichorionic	Diamniotic	30
3–8	Monochorionic	Diamniotic	70
8–13	Monochorionic	Monoamniotic	<1

Table 1. How the chorionicity and amnionicity are differentiated by the timing of the embryo splitting in monozygotic twins (Table is modified from Simpson L, 2015 [6]).

In the first trimester—before the 14th week of gestation—crown-rump length (CRL) is the parameter that is used in order to estimate gestational age with 5–7 days of deviation [7–9]. If there is a doubt about the reliability of the menstrual cycle or if the woman is administrated late for care, a repeat scan in 3–4 weeks can be helpful to determine pregnancy dating [10].

Modest size discordance is very common in multiple pregnancies [4]. Some studies suggest that pregnancy dating must be defined by using the mean of the fetuses [11]. However, more recent studies agreed that if the gestational age is based on the CRL of the larger twin, the possibility of missing a fetus that might develop intrauterine fetal growth restriction (IUGR) is decreased [12]. Salomon et al. [13] suggested that the CRL of the smallest fetus can estimate more accurately the gestational age, if the intertwin CRL discrepancy is less than the 95th percentile, using charts from studies. An interesting finding is that if the intertwin discordance in CRL is higher than 10%, the possibility of pregnancy loss, aneuploidy, or congenital anomalies is increased [3, 14, 15].

In the second trimester, a combination of parameters is used to define pregnancy dating such as abdominal circumference, femur length, and biparietal diameter [8]. Further discussion about calculating gestational age in second trimester is beyond the scope of this chapter.

3. Defining chorionicity and amnionicity

Early and accurate definition of chorionicity and amnionicity has an undeniably determinant role in the management of multiple pregnancies, since chorionicity plays a key role in the appearance of complications: monochorionic-monoamniotic twins present the highest mortality and morbidity. There is no doubt that the continuous surveillance and the timely intervention can optimize the outcome of the pregnancy [4].

The determination of chorionicity and amnionicity is better to be done in the first trimester [4]. If chorionicity is defined in the first trimester, accuracy is extremely close to 100% and if the definition is carried out in the second trimester, correct assignment decreases to 90% [16, 17].

At this point, we will classify the determination based on gestational age, separated in two periods: the first before the 10th week of gestation and the second that includes the period from week 10 to week 14.

3.1. Before 10 weeks of gestation

Three ultrasound findings can help in the detection of chorionicity: These are (1) the number of observable gestational sacs, (2) the number of amniotic sacs within the chorionic cavity, and (3) the number of yolk sacs [4].

3.1.1. Number of observable gestational sacs

The number of the gestational sacs and the number of fetal heartbeats in early multiple pregnancy scan are strongly related with chorionicity: each gestational sac will form a distinct placenta and chorion. Therefore, visualization of a single gestational sac with two visible heart beats indicates a monochorionic twin pregnancy, while the presentation of two distinctive gestational sacs implies a dichorionic pregnancy (**Picture 1**) [18]. The number of gestational sacs is the parameter with the highest accuracy to define chorionicity which is extremely close to 100% [16].

3.1.2. Number of amniotic sacs within the chorionic cavity

Identification of the number of amniotic sacs present in a single gestational sac helps define amnionicity in a monochorionic pregnancy. Prior to the 10th week of gestation, the amnions grow outward from the embryonic disk and at that age are not big enough to contact each other and create the intertwin septum [4]. As a result, separate and distinct amnions indicate a diamniotic twin pregnancy (**Pictures 2a**, **b** and **3a**, **b**). The evaluation of the amnion should be done diligently via transvaginal ultrasound since the intertwin membrane is extremely thin and it may be invisible via transabdominal ultrasound. Even when the separate amnions cannot be visualized via the transvaginal ultrasound, their absence can be confirmed by demonstrating umbilical cord enlargement by using pulsed wave Doppler and identifying two distinct heart rates [3]. In addition, the impossible visualization of the intertwin membrane may be technical: if the membrane is parallel to the ultrasound beam or because the ultrasound gain is low, the membrane may be hard to evaluate. This problem can be solved by changing the angle of insonation and increasing gain facilitates visualization [5]. Another way to confirm amnionicity, wherever there is any doubt about the presence of the intertwin membrane, is to suggest a small chain of repeat scans [4].

However, is evaluation of intertwin membrane always that simple? There are two rare yet important situations that may lead to a false diagnosis of monoamniotic twins. The first case

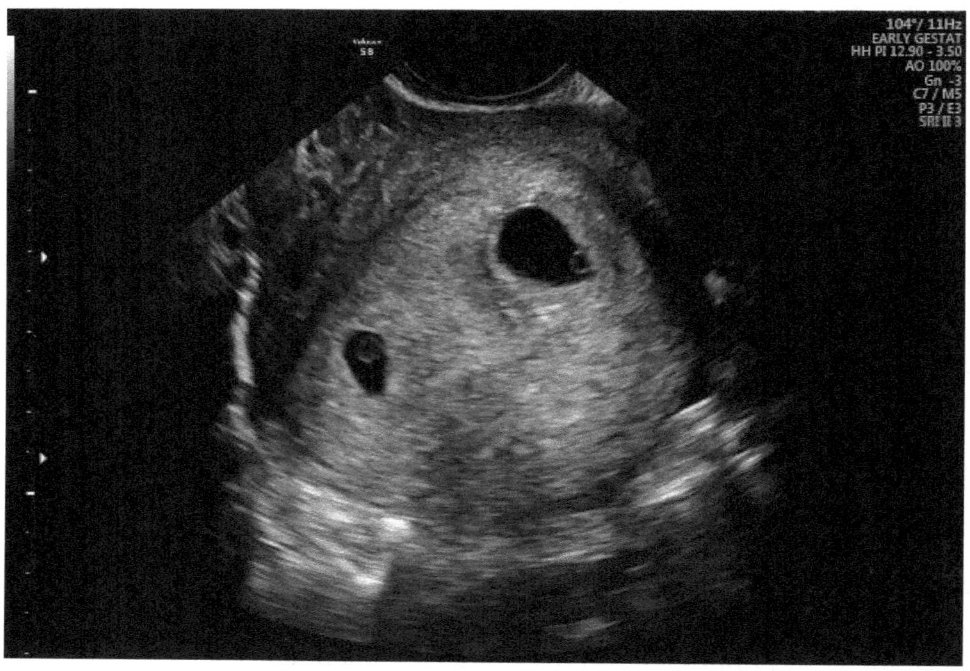

Picture 1. Dichorionic diamniotic pregnancy at 5 weeks of gestation. The two separate gestational sacs with one yolk sac each are visible and a thick septum separates them.

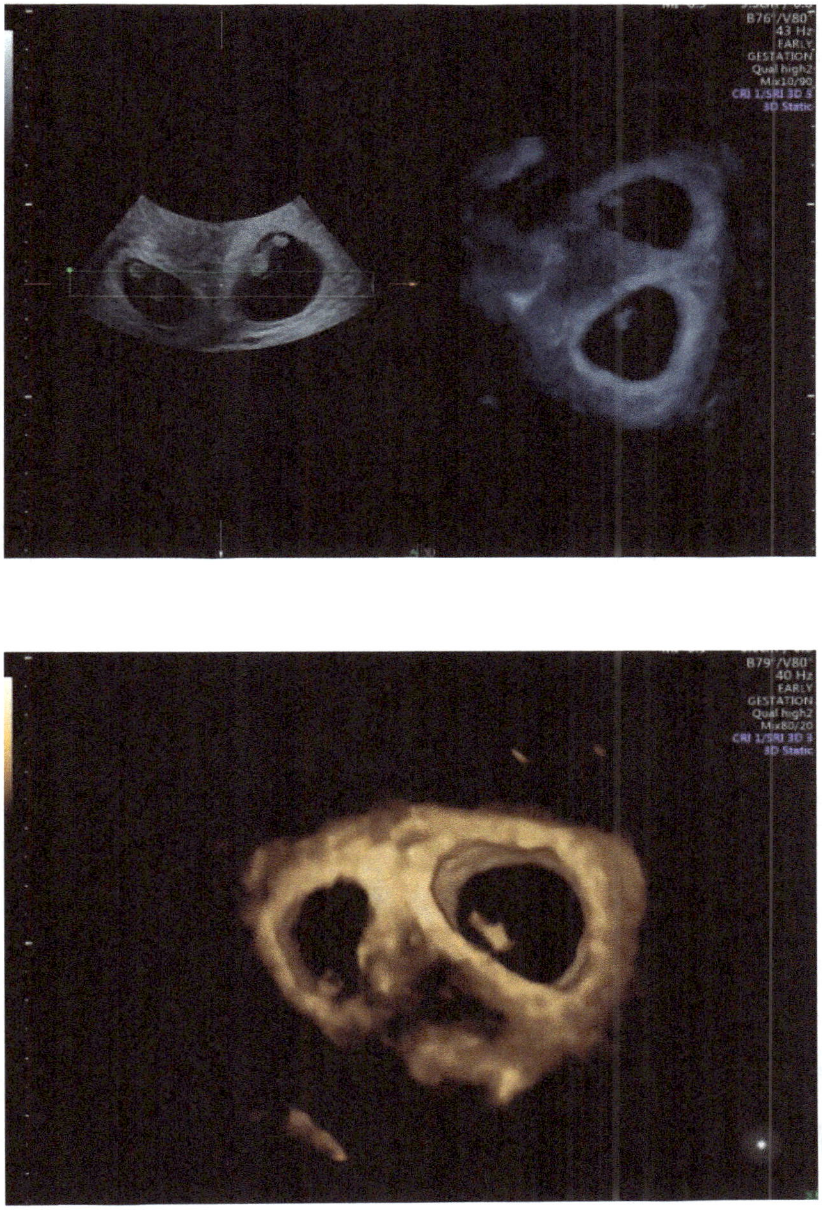

Picture 2. (a) 3D imaging of dichorionic diamniotic pregnancy at 6 weeks of gestation. (b) 3D imaging of dichorionic diamniotic pregnancy at 6 weeks of gestation.

is when the monochorionic-diamniotic twins are complicated with twin-to-twin transfusion syndrome (TTTS) the donor twin has severe oligohydramnios or anhydramnios, and the intertwin membrane collapses resulting in wrapping the donor twin. The collapse of the membrane can be overtaken if we evaluate extremely carefully the wrapping membrane around the limbs of the donor twin. A possible rupture of the intertwine membrane is another case that may lead to "pseudo-MA" twins. Rupture of the membrane may occur spontaneously, but more often is a complication of invasive *in utero* procedures. Discontinuity of the membrane and cord enlargement can be visualized on the ultrasound scan. Other facts helping

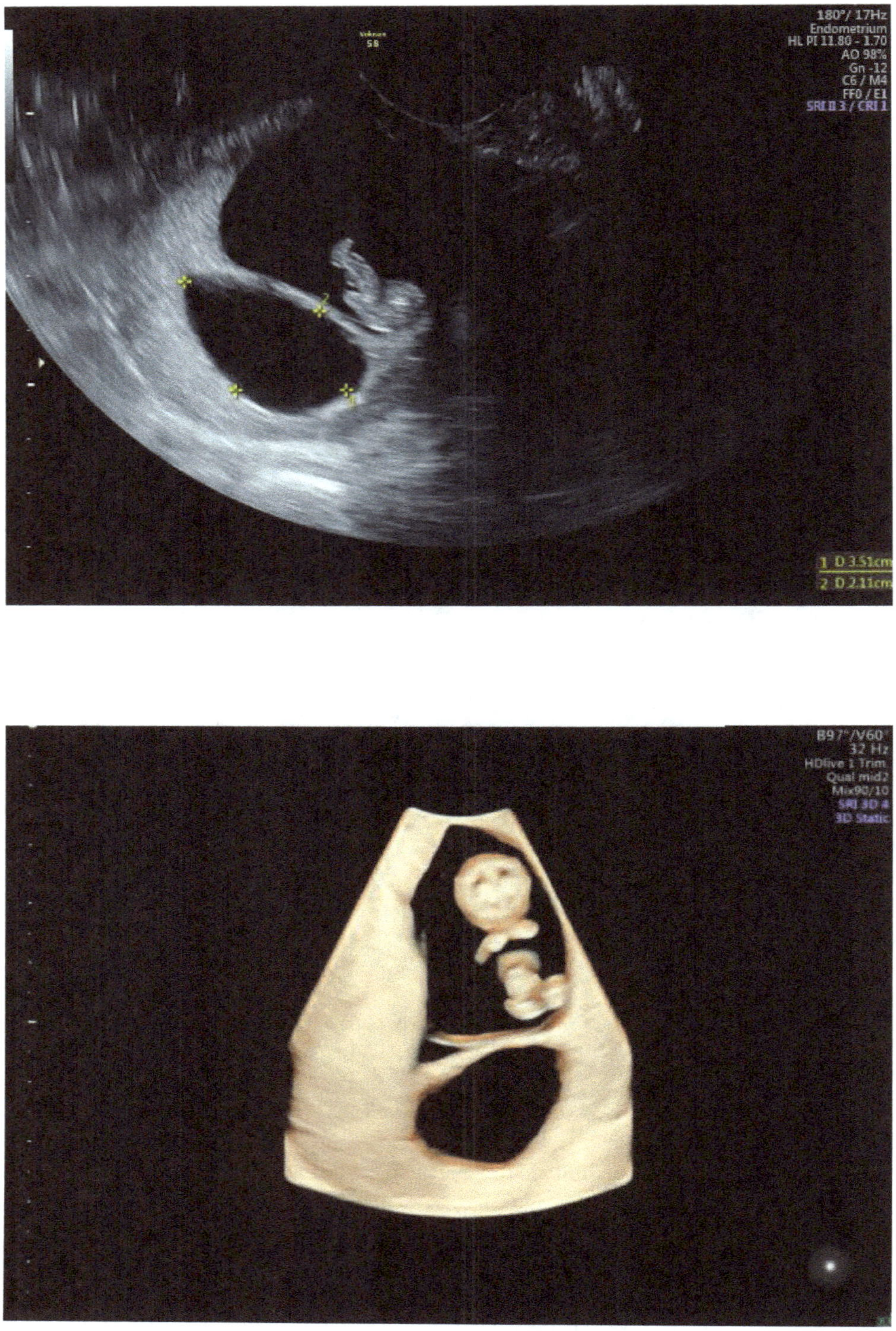

Picture 3. (a) Dichorionic diamniotic pregnancy with one of the pregnancies having miscarried. The size of the empty sac has been measured. (b) 3D imaging of DCDA pregnancy in which one of the sacs appears "empty" due to miscarriage.

in the identification of the membrane rupture are the location of the fetuses in the same side of the warped membrane, the equal quantity of amniotic fluid in both sides of the dividing membrane in a pregnancy, which was complicated with TTTS, and of course a previous diagnosis of a monochorionic-diamniotic twin pregnancy [5].

3.1.3. *Number of yolk sacs*

Over the past few years, there is an uncertainty regarding the relation between the number of yolk sacs and amnionicity. If there are two yolk sacs present in the extraembryonic coelom, the pregnancy will be regarded as diamniotic. However, a single yolk sac cannot set the definitive diagnosis of a monoamniotic pregnancy. This is well-established since it is known that the differentiation of a yolk sac and an amnion occur very close to each other in time, around 6–8 days after fertilization [5]. If a single yolk sac is detected, a repeat first trimester scan is undertaken, or a refer to a tertiary center with advanced experience in multiple pregnancies can be helpful [3, 4].

3.2. 10th–14th week of gestation

As the pregnancy continues, the ultrasound signs that help in the determination of chorionicity and amnionicity are changing: gestational sacs are now fused and the intertwin membrane is formed. As a result, four other ultrasound figures set the diagnosis of chorionicity and amnionicity. These are: (1) sex discordance, (2) distinct placentas number, (3) intertwin membrane characteristics and (4) chorionic peak sign—'λ' sign.

3.2.1. *Sex discordance*

If a male and a female fetus are identified in the late first or early second trimester, a dichorionic twin pregnancy is the rule. However, gender discordance is the biggest pitfall for the diagnosis of chorionicity. Discordant fetal sex phenotype can be present in monochorionic twins, leading to a false diagnosis of dichorionic twins.

A false diagnosis of dichorionic twins might be the result of a postzygotic sex chromosome aneuploidy. For instance, there is a 46,XY zygote which splits, but a postzygotic anaphase lag can cause the loss of the Y chromosome in one of the twins. The karyotype of one of the fetuses will be 46,XY which corresponds to a normal male fetus, while the other karyotype will be 45,XO which is a female fetus with Turner syndrome (**Figure 1**). If we want to take our example a step forward, postzygotic nondisjunction after the anaphase lag can lead to mosaicism in the monozygotic twins leading to two embryos with a variety of proportion of 45,XO and 46,XY cells. The phenotype of this individual will correspond to the amount of cells having the abnormal karyotype (**Figure 2**) [19, 20].

A sex discordance in monozygotic twins can also be caused by a trisomic 47,XXY zygote. A process known as trisomy rescue can lead to either the production of a normal 46,XY male fetus (loss of X chromosome) or a normal 46,XX female fetus (loss of Y chromosome) Hence, this mechanism causes the production of two euploids fetuses from a trisomic zygote (**Figure 3**) [21]. In addition, confusion might be caused if a 46,XY zygote splits with nondisjunction of the Y chromosome, producing a male fetus with a 47,XYY karyotype and a female fetus with a 45,XO karyotype, Turner syndrome, and female sex phenotype (**Figure 4**) [22].

Beyond sex chromosome abnormalities, sex discordance may be the result of epigenetic single gene defects in only one of the monoygotic twins, effecting testis-determining genes such as SOX9 which inhibits the expression of SRY gene [23, 24].

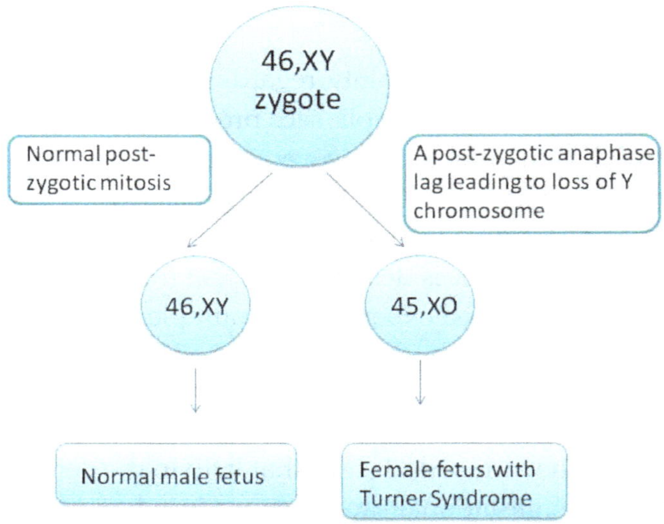

Figure 1. Postzygotic anaphase lag causing sex discordance due to loss of Y chromosome in one of the fetuses.

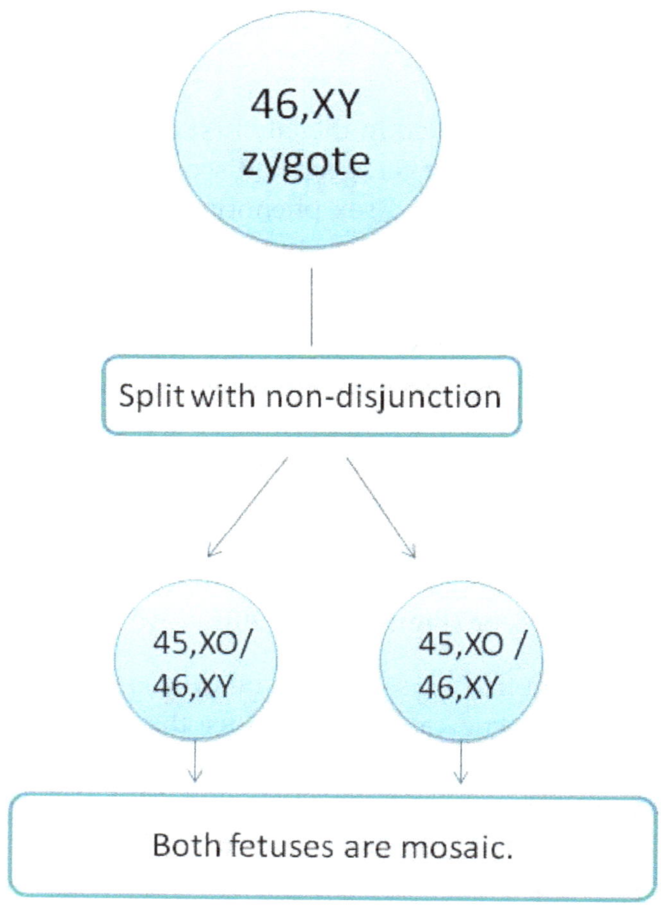

Figure 2. Postzygotic nondisjunction leading to both fetuses with gonadal mosaicism.

Nonetheless, sex discordance may be caused by malformed genitalia unrelated to chromosomal or genetic disorders. It is well established that a monochorionic twin pregnancy is complicated frequently with selective growth restriction [25], and hypospadias is a known complication of

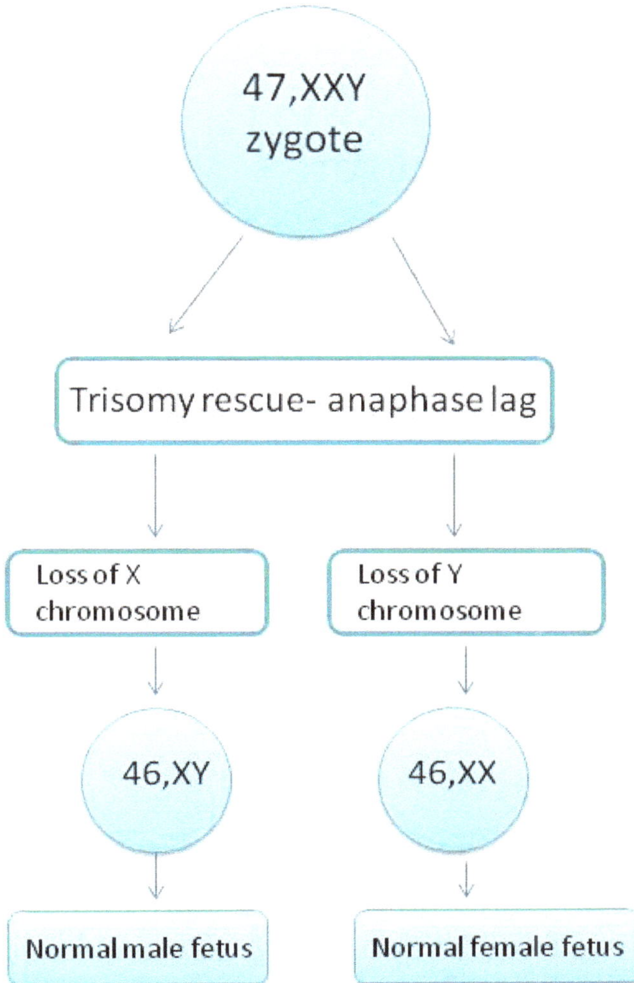

Figure 3. Trisomy rescue.

IUGR [26, 27]. As hypospadias might lead to female sex phenotype, confusion about chorionicity is expected, as the IUCR male fetus will present with female external genitalia, while the normally developing twin will be present as a normal male fetus. Cloacal malformation in one of the female fetuses (karyotype 46,XX) leads to phallus-like structure, causing phenotypically male external genitalia. The outcome is again confusion of chorionicity [28].

A very rare mechanism can cause the transverse situation: a dizygotic twin pregnancy is been diagnosed as monochorionic because of the fusion of the trophoblasts. Two distinct blastocysts produce two distinctive trophoblasts. If these trophoblasts fuse before the implantation, the result is the creation of a placental mass. The fused placenta will form vascular anastomoses, and the twins can exchange blood cells. As a result, blood chimerism of two populations of blood cells will be present in both fetuses [29, 30]. This mechanism is present more frequently in pregnancies carried out from ART because of the disruption of the zona pellucida and spatial proximity of multiple embryos [29, 31]. Dizygotic twins forming a monochorionic placenta have significant importance because these twins are genetically and phenotypically normal and they have to be distinguished from the pathological sex discordance [5].

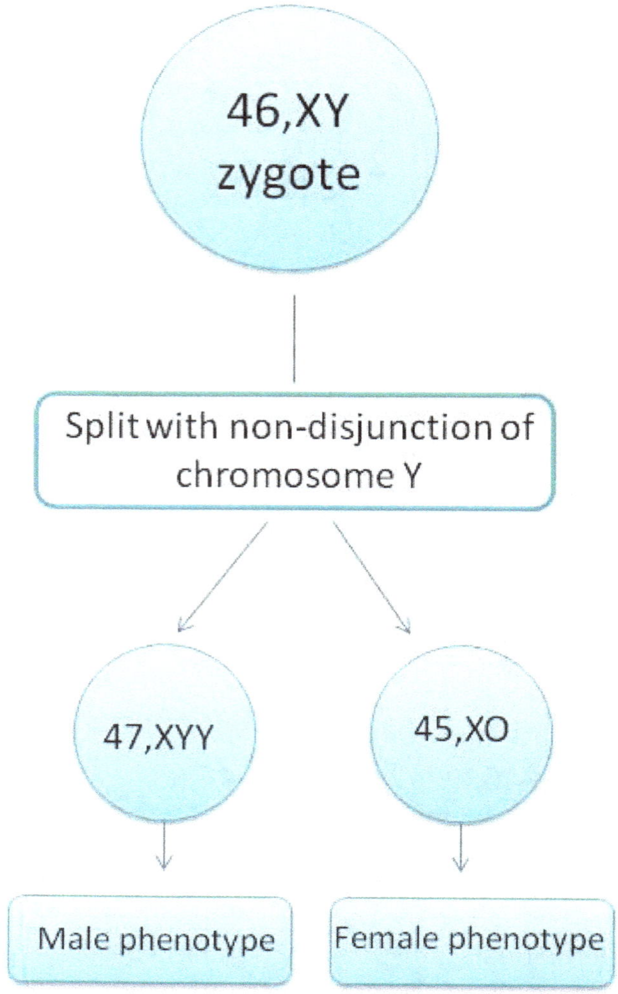

Figure 4. Nondisjunction of chromosome Y.

3.2.2. Number of distinct placentas

It is logical that the visualization of two separate placental masses confirms dichorionicity as a single placenta identifies monochorionicity [4]. Careful ultrasound evaluation has to be done in order to define the presence of a single placenta or two placentas in abutment.

As the pattern above, monochorionic twins may form a bipartite placenta. This sonographic finding is visible in 3% of monochorionic twin pregnancies. As a result, two separated placental masses are present with two nearly equal-sized placental lobes, which can be totally separated or connected by chorion laeve. Things can be more complicated when each placental mass has its own umbilical cord connection. Bipartite placenta can be distinguished from the dichorionic placental masses by using color Doppler and identifying vascular anastomoses that are present between the two lobes. Thus, this leads to the conclusion that if an ostensibly dichorionic pregnancy is complicated with TTTS, the diagnosis of a monochorionic pregnancy with bipartite placenta has to be considered [32–35].

3.2.3. *Intertwin membrane characteristics*

The intertwin membrane of a dichorionic pregnancy comprises three layers of three membranes: amnion-chorion-amnion, as the monochorionic pregnancy consists only two layers of amnion. Therefore, intertwin membrane in a dichorionic pregnancy is thicker and more echogenic than the intertwin membrane in monochorionic pregnancies. Measuring the thickness of the membrane can help us define chorionicity: a membrane thicker than 2 mm indicates dichorionicity (positive predictive value: 95%), and if the membrane is thinner than 2 mm, the possibility of monochorionic pregnancy is about 90% [4].

The intertwin membrane has to be carefully detected and if it cannot be visualized, a transvaginal ultrasound scan has to be performed, to set the definitive diagnosis of monoamniotic pregnancy [4]. When a single placental mass is visualized and chorionicity is identified as monochorionic, evaluation of the intertwin membrane characteristics is the key to determine amnionicity. The most significant sonographic figure that demonstrates monoamniocity is the demonstration of cord enlargement from the placental or umbilical origin and it is identified easier via color Doppler. Other important findings intimating monoamnionicity are the entanglement of limbs or observation of a limb circumscribing the other, the failure to find the membrane between the two cord insertions in the placenta [4], and the short intercord distance [5].

However, intertwin membrane thickness difference between monochorionic and dichorionic pregnancy decreases during gestation [36]. In addition, the measurement of the thickness of the membrane is not widely accepted since this parameter can be affected by many factors such as the position and the quality of the probe, and as a result, it has poor reproducibility [37]. A rare but significant pitfall may lead to a wrong determination of a monochorionic pregnancy as dichorionic is the intrauterine synechiae in twin pregnancy with a fetus with anencephaly. Intrauterine synechiae can mimic the thick dichorionic membrane [38]. This septum is not the intertwin membrane and does not include the layer of chorion between the layers of amnion.

3.2.4. *The chorionic peak sign—the "λ" sign*

The chorionic peak sign or the "λ" sign supports strongly dichorionicity, with an accuracy of 99% [5]. It shows a projecting zone of tissue which is as echogenic as the placenta; it has a triangular shape in cross-section; and it is wider at the chorionic surface of the placenta, extending into, and tapering to a point within, the intertwin membrane [39, 40]. The absence of the "λ" sign or the presence of "T" sign indicates monochorionicity. The "T" sign represents the two opposing amnions "standing" at the base of the intertwin membrane [10].

The chorionic peak sign is ideally evaluated during the late first trimester or the very early second trimester, as in second trimester, it is more difficult to be visualized and it might be disappeared at 16–20 weeks of gestation, leading to a false negative "λ" sign. As a result, the impossible depiction of the "λ" sign in late second trimester cannot exclude dichorionicity [41, 42]. Nonetheless, a false positive "λ" sign might also exist. This can be due to umbilical cord insertion into the intertwin membrane or because of the visualization of a hematoma presented along the insertion of the membrane. Another interesting reason that may lead to a false positive "λ" sign is the presence of an echogenic retrograded yolk sac of the placental junction of the intertwin membrane in a monochorionic-diamniotic twin gestation. The sonographic finding that succors determinate the true "λ" sign is that the true "λ" has been seen along with the whole insertion area, in contrast to the false "λ" sign, which appears in only a small region of the intertwin membrane [43, 44]. Finally, in very rare instances, the placentation may be both monochorionic and dichorionic, and each chorionicity is presented in different regions of the intertwin membrane. Therefore, the same intertwin membrane has parts with two layers of amnions and parts with three layers: amnion-chorion-amnion [45–47]. This situation shows the importance of scanning the whole insertion of the intertwin membrane in early ultrasound assessment of multiple pregnancy.

In some cases and despite the best possible ultrasound assessment, chorionicity is impossible to be defined. In these situations, the pregnancy has to be considered as monochorionic. Therefore, surveillance has to be as close as in monochorionic pregnancies [45], and this is discussed below.

4. Surveillance

Surveillance in multiple pregnancies has a significant importance, as it plays the major role in the detection of complications that are associated with a high-risk pregnancy, and it is well known that multiple pregnancy is a classic example of a high-risk pregnancy. However, the appropriate frequency of the ultrasound assessment in both dichorionic and monochorionic pregnancies, which provides the best balance between cost and effectiveness, is not be established and worldwide accepted [3].

4.1. Dichorionic pregnancies

Finberg et al. [46] suggested repeat scans every 4–6 weeks for noncomplicated dichorionic pregnancies. However, in current daily medical routine, surveillance is closer: follow-up ultrasound assessments are performed every 3–4 weeks [4, 47]. But, if a complication is suspected, and more specifically when CRL, estimated fetal weight or amniotic fluid volume are different between the two fetuses, routine scans have to be repeated every 2 weeks, or within a week [48].

4.2. Monochorionic pregnancies

It is a well-established fact that surveillance in monochorionic pregnancies has to be closer in relation to a dichorionic pregnancy. Finberg et al. [46] recommended ultrasound monitoring for noncomplicated monochorionic twins every 3–4 weeks. As the pattern mentioned previously, nowadays, routine scans are performed more frequently: they are performed every 2–3 weeks, starting from the gestational age of 16 weeks. Finally, in some cases, surveillance is even closer: a follow-up scan can be repeated every 2 weeks.

The parameters that are necessary to be evaluated in these follow-up scans are estimated fetal weight and fetal biometry, amniotic fluid volume, and Doppler assessment of the umbilical artery [49].

5. Conclusion

There is no doubt that multiple pregnancies are now more frequent than a few years before, due to the spreading of artificial reproductive technologies. Determination of gestational age, chorionicity, and amnionicity has to be done as soon as possible and ideally in the first trimester of the pregnancy, as the accuracy of the determining sonographic figures is extremely close to 100%, in contrast to the definition in the second trimester whose accuracy is slightly decreased. Last but not least, timely determination of both chorionicity and amnionicity can optimize the outcome of the pregnancy, as the correct and early intervention or a refer to a tertiary center could be really valuable.

Acknowledgements

We would like to thank Kyriaki Savva, PhD student of Cyprus Institute of Neurology and Genetics, for her comments that greatly improved the manuscript.

Author details

Panagiotis Antsaklis[1]*, Maria Papamichail[2], Marianna Theodora[1], Michael Syndos[3] and George Daskalakis[1]

*Address all correspondence to: panosant@gmail.com

1 Alexandra Maternity Hospital, University of Athens, Athens, Greece

2 University of Athens, Athens, Greece

3 Obstetrics and Gynecology, Alexandra Maternity Hospital, Athens, Greece

References

[1] Martin JA, Hamilton BE, Osterman MJ. Three decades of twin births in the United States, 1980-2009. NCHS Data Brief. 2012;**80**:1-8

[2] Kurtz GR, Keating WJ, Loftus JB. Twin pregnancy and delivery: Analysis of 500 twin pregnancies. Obstetrics and Gynecology. 1995;**6**:370-378

[3] Glanc P, Nyberg DA, Khati NJ, Deshmukh SP, Dudiak KM, Henrichsen TL, Poder L, Shipp TD, Simpson L, Weber TM, Zelop CM. ACR Appropriateness Criteria® Multiple Gestations. Journal of American College of Radiology. 2017;**14**(11):S476-S489

[4] Morin L, Lim K. Ultrasound in twin pregnancies. Journal of Obstetrics and Gynaecology Canada. 2011;**33**(6):643-656

[5] Lu J, Cheng YKY, Ting YH, Law KM, Leung TY. Pitfalls in assessing chorioamnionicity: Novel observations and literature review. American Journal of Obstetrics and Gynecology. 2018;**219**(3):242-254. DOI: 10.1016/j.ajog.2018.02.010

[6] Simpson L. What you need to know when managing twins: 10 key facts. Obstetrics and Gynecology Clinics of North America. 2015;**42**(2):225-239

[7] Kalish RB, Thaler HT, Chasen ST, Gupta M, Berman SJ, Rosenwaks Z, et al. First- and second-trimester ultrasound assessment of gestational age. American Journal of Obstetrics and Gynecology. 2004;**191**:975-978

[8] Tunón K, Eik-Nes SH, Grøttum P, Von Düring V, Kahn JA. Gestational age in pregnancies conceived after in vitro fertilization: A comparison between age assessed from oocyte retrieval, crown-rump length and biparietal diameter. Ultrasound in Obstetrics & Gynecology. 2000;**15**:41-46

[9] Wisser J, Dirschedl P, Krone S. Estimation of gestational age by transvaginal sonographic measurement of greatest embryonic length in dated human embryos. Ultrasound in Obstetrics & Gynecology. 1994;**4**:457-462

[10] Simpson L. Ultrasound in Twins: Dichorionic and Monochorionic. Seminars in Perinatology; 2013;**37**(5):348-358

[11] Chervenak FA, Skupski DW, Romero R, Myers MK, Smith-Levitin M, Rosenwaks Z, et al. How accurate is fetal biometry in the assessment of fetal age? American Journal of Obstetrics and Gynecology. 1998;**178**:678-687

[12] Sebire NJ, D'Ercole C, Soares W, Nayar R, Nicolaides KH. Intertwin disparity in fetal size in monochorionic and dichorionic pregnancies. Obstetrics and Gynecology. 1998;**91**:82-85

[13] Salomon LJ, Cavicchioni O, Bernard JP, Duyme M, Ville Y. Growth discrepancy in twins in the first trimester of pregnancy. Ultrasound in Obstetrics & Gynecology. 2005;**26**: 512-516

[14] D'Antonio F, Khalil A, Pagani G, Papageorghiou AT, Bhide A, Thilaganathan B. Crown-rump length discordance and adverse perinatal outcome in twin pregnancies: Systematic review and metaanalysis. Ultrasound in Obstetrics & Gynecology. 2014;**44**:138-146

[15] Kalish RB, Gupta M, Perni SC, Berman S, Chasen ST. Clinical significance of first trimester crown-rump length disparity in dichorionic twin gestations. American Journal of Obstetrics and Gynecology. 2004;**191**:1437-1440

[16] Carroll SG, Soothill PW, Abdel-Fattah SA, et al. Prediction of chorionicity in twin pregnancies at 10-14 weeks gestation. BJOG. 2002;**109**:182-186

[17] Lee YM, Cleary-Goldman J, Thanker HM, et al. Antenatal sonographic prediction of twin chorionicity. American Journal of Obstetrics and Gynecology. 2006;**195**:863-867

[18] Monteagudo A, Roman AS. Ultrasound in multiple gestations: Twins and other multifetal pregnancies. Clinics in Perinatology. 2005;**32**:329-354, vi

[19] Perlman EJ, Stetten G, Tuck-miiller CM, et al. Sexual discordance in monozygotic twins. American Journal of Medical Genetics. 1990;**37**:551-557

[20] Nieuwint A, Zalen-Sprock R Van, Hummel P, et al. Identical twins with discordant karyotypes. Prenatal Diagnosis. 1999;**19**:72-76

[21] Zech NH, Wisser J, Natalucci G, Riegel M, Baumer A, Schinzel A. Monochorionic-diamniotic twins discordant in gender from a naturally conceived pregnancy through postzygotic sex chromosome loss in a 47,XXY zygote. Prenatal Diagnosis. 2008;**28**:759-763

[22] Bohec C, Douet-Guilbert N, Basinko A, et al. Difficult diagnosis and management of an heterokaryotypic monochorionic twin pregnancy with discordant fetal sex and 45,X/47,XYY karyotypes. Fetal and Pediatric Pathology. 2010;**29**:424-430

[23] Prior HM, Walter MA. SOX genes: Architects of development. Molecular Medicine. 1996;**2**: 405-412

[24] Wolf U. Reorganization of the sex-determining pathway with the evolution of placentation. Human Genetics. 1999;**105**:288-292

[25] De Paepe ME, Shapiro S, Young L, Luks FI. Placental characteristics of selective birth weight discordance in diamniotic-monochorionic twin gestations. Placenta. 2010;**31**: 380-386

[26] Chen M, Macias CG, Gunn SK, Dietrich JE, Roth DR, Schlomer BJ. Intrauterine growth restriction and hypospadias: Is there a connection? International Journal of Pediatric Endocrinology. 2014;**2014**:20

[27] Toufaily MH, Roberts DJ, Westgate M, Hunt A, Holmes LB. Hypospadias, intrauterine growth restriction, and abnormalities of the placenta. Birth Defects Research Journal. 2017;**29**:1-6

[28] Chitrit Y, Vuillard E, Khung S, et al. Cloaca in discordant monoamniotic twins: Prenatal diagnosis and consequence for fetal lung development. American Journal of Perinatology. 2014;**4**:33-36

[29] Mcnamara HC, Kane SC, Craig JM, Short RV, Umstad MP. A review of 21 the mechanisms and evidence for typical and atypical twinning. American Journal of Obstetrics and Gynecology. 2016;**214**:172-191

[30] Souter VL, Kapur RP, Nyholt DR, et al. A report of dizygous monochorionic twins. The New England Journal of Medicine. 2003;**349**:154-158

[31] Miura KNN. Do monochorionic dizygotic twins increase after pregnancy by assisted reproductive technology? Journal of Human Genetics. 2005;**50**:1-6

[32] Lopriore E, Sueters M, Middeldorp JM, Klumper F, Oepkes D, Vandenbussche FP. Twin pregnancies with two separate placental masses can still be monochorionic and have vascular anastomoses. American Journal of Obstetrics and Gynaecology. 2006;**194**:804-808

[33] Kim K, Lage JM. Bipartite diamnionic monochorionic twin placenta with 6 superficial vascular anastomoses: Report of a case. Human Pathology. 1991;**22**:501-503

[34] Altshuler G, Hyde S. Placental pathology casebook: A bidiscoid, monochorionic placenta. Journal of Perinatology. 1993;**13**:492-493

[35] Walsh CA, Wilkinson M, Downey P, Mooney EE, Carroll S. "False" lambda sign in monochorionic twin pregnancy. Ultrasound in Obstetrics & Gynecology. 2015;**46**:376-377

[36] Townsend RR, Simpson GF, Filly RA. Membrane thickness in ultrasound prediction of chorionicity of twin gestations. Journal of Ultrasound in Medicine. 1988;**7**:327-332

[37] Stagiannis KD, Sepulveda W, Southwell D, Price DA, Fisk NM. Ultrasonographic measurement of the dividing membrane in twin pregnancy during the second and third trimesters: A reproducibility study. American Journal of Obstetrics and Gynecology. 1995;**173**:1546-1550

[38] Machin G. Non-identical monozygotic twins, intermediate twin types, zygosity testing, and the non-random nature of monozygotic twinning: A review. American Journal of Medical Genetics. Part C, Seminars in Medical Genetics. 2009;**151C**:110-127

[39] Stenhouse E, Hardwick C, Maharaj S, Webb J, Kelly T, Mackenzie FM. Chorionicity determination in twin pregnancies: How accurate are we? Ultrasound in Obstetrics & Gynecology. 2002;**19**:350-352

[40] Wood SL, St. Onge R, Connors G, Elliot PD. Evaluation of the twin peak or lambda sign in determining chorionicity in multiple pregnancy. Obstetrics and Gynecology. 1996;**88**:6-9

[41] Scardo JA, Ellings JM, Newman RB. Prospective determination of chorionicity, amnionicity, and zygosity in twin gestations. American Journal of Obstetrics and Gynecology. 1995;**173**:1376-1380

[42] Sepulveda W. Chorionicity determination in twin pregnancies: Double trouble. Ultrasound in Obstetrics & Gynecology. 1997;**10**:79-81

[43] Dias T, Arcangeli T, Bhide A, Napolitano R, Mahsud-Dornan S, Thilaganathan B. First-trimester ultrasound determination of chorionicity in twin pregnancy. Ultrasound in Obstetrics & Gynecology. 2011;**38**:530-532

[44] Gueneuc A, Spaggiari E, Bonniere M, Hajal NJ, Ville Y, Salomon LJ. Pitfall in the diagnosis of chorionicity in twin pregnancy at first trimester. Ultrasound in Obstetrics & Gynecology. 2017;**49**:277-278

[45] D'Antonio F, Bhide A. Early pregnancy assessment in multiple pregnancies. Best Practice & Research. Clinical Obstetrics & Gynaecology. 2014;**28**(2):201-214

[46] Finberg H, Mendelson E, Bohm-Velez M, et al. Evaluation of Multiple Gestations. American College of Radiology. 2000;**215**(Suppl):903-914

[47] Vayssiere C, Favre R, Audibert F, et al. Cervical length and funneling at 22 and 27 weeks to predict spontaneous birth before 32 weeks in twin pregnancies: A French prospective multicenter study. American Journal of Obstetrics and Gynecology. 2002;**187**:1596-1604

[48] Modena AB, Berghella V. Antepartum management of multifetal pregnancies. Clinics in Perinatology. 2005;**32**:443-454, vii

[49] Lodeiro JG, Vintzileos AM, Feinstein SJ, Campbell WA, Nochimson DJ. Fetal biophysical profile in twin gestations. Obstetrics and Gynecology. 1986;**67**:824-827

2

Particularities of Oxidative Stress in Newborns

Melinda Mátyás and Gabriela Zaharie

Abstract

The oxidative stress at newborns is augmented by different conditions like preterm birth, asphyxia, respiratory distress, and intraventricular hemorrhage. Preterm neonates associate a more pronounced oxidative stress than healthy term newborns. Several neonatal conditions like respiratory distress (RDS), asphyxia, intraventricular hemorrhage, bronchopulmonary dysplasia, retinopathy, and necrotizing enterocolitis will increase the oxidative stress. The harmful effects of free radicals are linked to their capacity to react with polyunsaturated fatty acids of cell membranes, proteins, and nucleic acids. Free radicals will produce protein alteration with function loss and lipid peroxidation.

Keywords: oxidative stress, new born, prematurity

1. Introduction

Oxidative stress represents all injuries caused by reactive oxygen species (ROS) on biomolecules, inducing the destruction of membranes, enzymes, receptors, as well as alteration of cell function. The consequence of oxidative stress is a disruption of the physiological balance between pro-oxidants and antioxidants [1, 2].

Newborn possesses defense mechanisms such us molecules protection, limitation of ROS production, and mechanisms for repair and adaptation to endogenous and exogenous ROS overproduction.

Reactive oxygen species are involved in physiological processes such as physical exercise, hyperbarism, regulation of vascular tone, stimulation of cell growth and proliferation, stimulation of erythropoietin secretion, the learning and memory process, as well as in pathological processes: inflammation, aging, carcinogenesis [1–3].

In neonatal pathology, there are multiple circumstances that are associated with oxidative stress. An excess of reactive oxygen species in the context of immature, deficient antioxidant defense mechanisms may cause multisystemic diseases [2, 3].

1.1. Effects of reactive oxygen species on biomolecules

Reactive oxygen species will act on molecules, inducing their deterioration as follows:

- DNA lesions—action on the bases in the DNA structure—thymine, cytosine, adenine, guanine, deoxyribose, followed by cell damage and mutations
- Alteration of NADPH—inhibition of the nucleotide coenzyme activity
- Lipids and proteins—action on the covalent bond in their structure
- Glycoproteins—action on hyaluronic acid in their structure
- Lipid peroxidation—structural and functional changes in cell membranes

1.1.1. Effects of oxidative stress on proteins and amino acids

Reactive oxygen species (ROS) act on the side chain of amino acids. Through oxidation of amino acids in the structure of proteins, the following changes are induced: protein fragmentation, aggregation, and proteolytic degradation. Aldehydes resulting from lipid peroxidation and glycosylation will also act on proteins. The consequence will be the functional alteration of proteins, with the loss of their contractile, enzymatic, and transport function.

1.1.2. Effects of oxidative stress on lipids

The most extensively studied action on lipids is their cellular and extracellular peroxidation. Lipids and lipoproteins are involved, particularly those mainly composed of polyunsaturated fatty acids (PUFA) such as linoleic and arachidonic acids, abundantly in cholesterol esters, lecithin, and erythrocytic phospholipids. Lipoproteins can be oxidized by two pathways:

- Specific enzymatic oxidation—with the formation of prostaglandins, thromboxane, prostacyclin, leukotrienes, and isoprostanes
- Nonspecific enzymatic oxidation—a peroxidation process with the formation of products with a damaging effect.

As a result of lipid peroxidation, a disorganization of the cell structure occurs, lipids being part of the membrane structure. A more rigid membrane will develop, with implications on essential membrane proteins, such as Na^+-K^+-dependent ATPase. Thus, a change in the ion pump rate will occur.

Lipid peroxides alter the properties of cellular, mitochondrial, and lysosomal membranes, with the disappearance of osmotic, chemical, and electrical gradients. Thus, cell excitability and metabolic processes are disturbed, and morphological lesions occur. In the nerve fiber, the myelin sheath is attacked. At pulmonary level, there is an alteration of endothelial membrane permeability, with the movement of lipids from the vascular space to the extravascular (interstitial) and intracellular space, and the development of pulmonary edema.

1.1.3. Effects of oxidative stress on carbohydrates

Glucose and monosaccharide oxidation leads to the formation of activated molecules that may interact with other molecules, generating new compounds. By polysaccharide oxidation, structural changes in deoxyribonucleic acid (DNA) may occur.

1.1.4. Effects of oxidative stress on nucleic acids

The number of oxidative attacks on DNA in humans is 10,000/cell. Thus, chromosome fragmentation occurs. Double-chain DNA is much more vulnerable than single-chain DNA. Altered fragments are eliminated as purine and pyrimidine bases by urinary excretion and they can be dosed. Oxidative DNA lesions accumulate with age. Aging and carcinogenesis are explained by incomplete DNA repair after oxidative attacks.

The superoxide anion resulting from the xanthine/xanthine oxidase system induces DNA breaks. The hydroxyl radical through its instantaneous reaction with nucleic acids also causes DNA breaks. These breaks should be normally repaired by cell enzymes, but due to their low fidelity, the repair process is inadequate through the inclusion of inappropriate bases in the DNA structure.

Oxygenated water also has effects on DNA. Through its reaction with DNA-bound metal ions, oxygenated water will induce the formation of hydroxyl radical, which will immediately fragment the DNA molecule.

2. Oxidative stress in newborns

The literature currently speaks about free radical disease in newborns, a term introduced by Sullivan [2], which includes the following pathogenic conditions: bronchopulmonary dysplasia (BPD), retinopathy of prematurity (ROP), intra-periventricular hemorrhage (IPVH), necrotizing enterocolitis (NEC), and renal failure [1]. Premature newborns with a gestational age of less than 30 weeks and a weight of less than 1500 g, respectively, have a major risk to develop these disorders. At cerebral level, there is a predisposition to oxidative stress, due to the high amount of polyunsaturated fatty acids in the immature brain, particularly in neuronal membranes, but also due to the relatively high amount of protein-unbound iron [41]. Immaturity associated with premature birth and also oxygen therapy used for the treatment of respiratory distress significantly increase oxidative stress in premature newborns. The knowledge of oxygen toxicity mechanisms is important both for their prevention and to ensure a harmonious development of newborns in general and premature newborns in particular, given their low antioxidant defense capacity [1, 3].

2.1. Implication of oxidative stress in pulmonary disorders

Respiratory distress due to surfactant deficiency is one of the most frequent disorders in premature newborns. The higher the degree of prematurity, the higher is the incidence and severity of this disease. Due to the immature lung structure, surfactant deficiency, pulmonary fluid retention, and poorly developed bone and muscle structures, there is an increased susceptibility of the premature to pulmonary lesions. The mechanism of these pulmonary lesions is based on alveolar instability and pulmonary atelectasis.

Mechanical ventilation, in addition to its role of ensuring an adequate oxygen supply to the body, also has undesired effects. Thus, it interferes with inflammatory cell metabolism and pulmonary mediators. Pulmonary vascularization is supplied from the heart but is also a reservoir of neutrophils—1/3 of the total number of neutrophils outside the bone marrow is found in the lungs [38].

Animal experiments have evidenced that in the context of mechanical ventilation, the number of neutrophils and the level of mediators, platelet activating factors, thromboxane B2 in pulmonary lavage fluid, and TNF-alpha in alveolar macrophages increase [11]. In premature animals with RDS, mechanical ventilation will cause an increase in pulmonary inflammation mediators, an increase in granulocytes, and cytokine activation [8]. Ventilatory support may affect the alveolar-capillary barrier and induces a release of inflammation mediators from the alveolar space into the circulation. The translocation of endotoxins from the aerial space to the circulatory space will generate a systemic inflammatory response [8, 9].

Mechanical ventilation along with oxygen supplementation will generate oxidative stress, with protein oxidation under the action of ROS. The carbonyl group of proteins will react with 2,4-dinitrophenylhydrazine, and 2,4-dinitrophenyl-hydrazone will form, which is measured by spectrophotometry [16]. Prematures who develop bronchopulmonary dysplasia (BPD) have significantly higher levels of protein carbonyls during the first week of life [1, 16].

Newborns requiring mechanical ventilation are more exposed to free radical production as a result of oxygen therapy exposure, inflammatory response, and ischemia reperfusion [10, 49].

Experimentally, it has been demonstrated on animals that the synthesis of enzymatic and consequently, antioxidant systems occurs at the end of gestation. Hemolysis after birth associated with a low level of iron-binding antioxidants can favor protein damage [5].

Protein carbonylation in the tracheobronchial fluid is a marker of oxidative stress at pulmonary level, while the exhalation of lipid peroxidation products (ethane, pentane) is a marker of lipid peroxidation in the entire body. As a result, a high level of exhaled peroxidation products is associated with extrapulmonary morbidity [9, 10].

Enzymes protecting against oxidant agents in the lungs, such as catalase, can be the target of oxidative attack inducing their inactivation. Liposoluble free radical scavengers such as tocopherol or beta-carotene have a protective effect against oxidative attack on lipids, but not on proteins. At the end of the first week of life, a depletion of these scavengers occurs as a result of the rapid increase in ROS production under the action of pulmonary inflammatory response. Thus, lipid peroxidation products are released through oxidation of polyunsaturated fatty acids. During the first 3–4 days of life, pulmonary proteins are the first target of free radicals. In the context of RDS, edema develops as a result of increased membrane permeability. Due to its high protein content, its presence in the lung will make it the ideal target for the initiation of oxidative attack by ROS [30, 31]. The inactivation of α_1-proteases under the action of oxidative attack will disrupt the balance of the pulmonary protease-antiprotease system. In infants with RDS, ROS will interact with the surfactant as well as with other proteins and lipid structures, delaying the normalization of pulmonary function [2, 5, 38].

Patients with respiratory distress have high levels of hydrogen peroxide in the pulmonary condensate. Oxidized glutathione and the altered alpha-1 protein also show high levels in the pulmonary fluid. In addition, the antioxidant proteins catalase and ferritin are elevated, which could represent a compensatory response. Oxidative stress markers are also increased in patients with sepsis, in those infected with HIV [40].

With the increase in the survival rate of newborns with extreme prematurity, the incidence of chronic pulmonary disorders has also increased, not only as an undesired consequence of RDS, but also of mechanical ventilation used for its treatment. The most frequent chronic pulmonary disease of premature infants with RDS and a history of mechanical ventilation is bronchopulmonary dysplasia. This is a chronic lung disease developing in newborns treated with oxygen and mechanical ventilation for a primary pulmonary disease. It affects between 20 and 60% of prematures, but it may also occur in term infants with severe respiratory distress [8].

Its etiopathogeny is complex. There is the hypothesis that bronchopulmonary dysplasia might start as an acute inflammation, which subsequently turns into a chronic lung disease under the action of free radicals [2, 5].

Preliminary studies have shown that pulmonary lesions can be improved by administration of antioxidants such as superoxide dismutase (SOD). The function of SOD is to convert the extremely toxic superoxide radical to less toxic hydrogen peroxide and water. Superoxide dismutase is also present naturally, but not as synthetic surfactant. Genetic engineering has demonstrated that in alveolar cells, SOD survives for a longer time period. An experimental animal with an SOD gene disrupted by genetic engineering, exposed to hyperoxia, will survive for a shorter time and will have more pulmonary lesions than an animal with an intact gene. Superoxide dismutase plays a major role in the prevention of pulmonary lesions in the context of hyperoxia. If SOD activity is increased in the newborn lung, inflammatory changes and pulmonary lesions can be prevented [9, 20, 21].

The incidence of bronchopulmonary dysplasia has increased not only with the extensive use of positive pressure ventilation for the treatment of neonatal respiratory distress, but also due to the increase of the survival rate by modern intensive care techniques in newborns with extreme prematurity. The Neonatal Research Network reported a 68% incidence of BPD in prematures with a gestational age of 22–28 WA.

Today, it is known that barotrauma, particularly at high inspiratory pressures, is a key factor in the development of pulmonary lesions independently of any other lesions generated by oxygen therapy. Epithelial alterations in the airways occur, as well as with an increase in capillary permeability with extravasation of protein substances. In addition to the implication of high inspiratory pressure in the genesis of pulmonary lesions, increased tidal volume also plays an important role. High but also significantly decreased tidal volume may generate an accumulation of neutrophils and a release of toxic agents such as proteases and free radicals, as well as proinflammatory cytokines. An analysis of pathological anatomy data has allowed to evidence a correlation between the incidence of interstitial emphysema during the first week of life and the incidence of interstitial fibrosis or proliferation in newborns with bronchopulmonary dysplasia surviving for more than 28 days [22, 24].

Another factor that plays a role in the development of BPD is inflammation. Proinflammatory cytokines were detected in the tracheal aspiration fluid during the first 1–2 weeks of life in newborns who subsequently developed BPD. Recently, it has been demonstrated that amnionitis and fetal infection are risk factors for BPD; consequently, inflammation, even prenatal, plays a role in its genesis [3].

Premature infants, due to their pulmonary immaturity, have a high risk for BPD, because they require additional oxygen supply for a longer time period in the treatment of the lung disease, their intracellular antioxidant defense capacity is affected, and they have an increased susceptibility to infections.

Studies have demonstrated the presence of a high level of lipid peroxidation products on days 1–2 of life in newborns who develop BPD. The presence of a high level of protein peroxidation products in the tracheal aspirate of infants weighing less than 1500 g compared to those with a higher weight has also been demonstrated. This confirms the fact that antioxidant defense decreases with the increase of immaturity [9, 15, 16].

There is also a close correlation between the protein oxidation level and activated neutrophils. This supports the presence of a relationship among neutrophil accumulation, oxidative stress, and the development of BPD [1].

In randomized trials for the study of STOP-ROP, some authors monitored oxygen exposure and the evolution of retrolental fibroplasia and BPD [36]. Thus, in groups with 89–94% O_2 Sat, compared to those with 96–99% O_2 Sat, the influence of saturation on the progression of retrolental fibroplasia was not significant. In contrast, in the group with higher saturation, the BPD progression rate was higher (13.2%) compared to subjects exposed to lower saturation levels (8.5%) [23, 39].

Exposure to a FiO_2 of 100% on the first day practically doubles the risk of BPD. Excessive oxygen administration and/or barotrauma may increase the risk of BPD. However, a high PaO_2 is a cofactor, not a causal agent in the development of BPD [36].

Preterm birth associates vitamin A deficiency, which is important in pulmonary epithelial lesion repair. A number of studies have evidenced a significant reduction in the incidence of bronchopulmonary dysplasia under conditions of vitamin A administration (Shenai et al.) [34, 37], but there are also studies that could not demonstrate this fact (Perason et al.) [32, 33].

Selenium deficiency can also be considered in association with low glutathione levels. Darlow et al. found a significant relationship between plasma selenium levels and the incidence of bronchopulmonary dysplasia at the age of 28 days, but could not clarify whether these were a cause or an effect of BPD.

A study conducted in our department, which assessed lipid peroxidation by measuring malondialdehyde (MDA) levels on the first and third days of life found that MDA values in newborns with respiratory distress increased with the increase in the severity of respiratory distress (**Table 1**).

MDA values in the mentioned study tended to decrease on day 3 compared to day 1, but without a statistically significant difference.

Also, the lipid peroxidation process was more intense in the study group-newborns with different pathologies generating oxidative stress compared with the control group of healthy term newborns, without any oxidative-stress inducing disorders (**Figures 1** and **2**).

In the same study, we also monitored protein peroxidation in newborns with respiratory distress, and we found the presence of a significant correlation between protein carbonyl values on the third day of life and respiratory distress ($r = 0.56$; $p < 0.05$). For the evaluation of protein peroxidation in the mentioned study, we measured protein carbonyls on the first and third days of life using the Reznick spectrophotometric method with dinitrophenylhydrazine. The protein substrate in the lung is an optimal target for the action of ROS and the triggering of oxidation reactions of these proteins. In fact, it was demonstrated that in newborns with RDS, this protein oxidation process under the action of ROS also contributes to the pathogenesis of BPD. Under the action of reactive oxygen species, peroxidation of proteins and other lipid and protein structures occurs. Thus, the normalization of pulmonary function is delayed. Surfactant administration before the initiation of mechanical ventilation limits oxidative injury induced by mechanical ventilation.

2.2. Effects of oxidative stress at endothelial level

The effects of ROS at endothelial level during the neonatal period are found in the following morbid conditions: septic shock, systemic inflammation, acute ischemia, inducing considerable oxidative stress [5]. Reactive oxygen species contribute to the development of ischemic and inflammatory vascular lesions by an important efflux of oxidants to the ischemic tissue and the induction of new lesions in tissues and organs in the next reperfusion stage [29].

		RankSum1	RankSum2	U	p	n1	n2
RDS mild vs. severe	MDA DOL 1	255.0	273.0	84.0	0.1159	18	14
	MDA DOL 3	281.0	247.0	110.0	0.5611	18	14
RDS mild vs. moderate	MDA DOL 1	307.5	638.5	136.5	0.0283	18	25
	MDA DOL 3	379.0	567.0	208.0	0.6877	18	25
RDS severe vs. moderate	MDA DOL 1	75.5	114.5	23.5	0.1740	6	13
	MDA DOL 3	79.0	111.0	20.0	0.0956	6	13
MV yes vs. no	MDA DOL 1	376.5	1453.5	285.5	0.7229	13	47
	MDA DOL 3	407.5	1422.5	294.5	0.8454	13	47

RDS = respiratory distress syndrome, MV = mechanical ventilation, RankSum = rank sum, p = test sign, and n = group size.

Table 1. MDA values according to RDS severity.

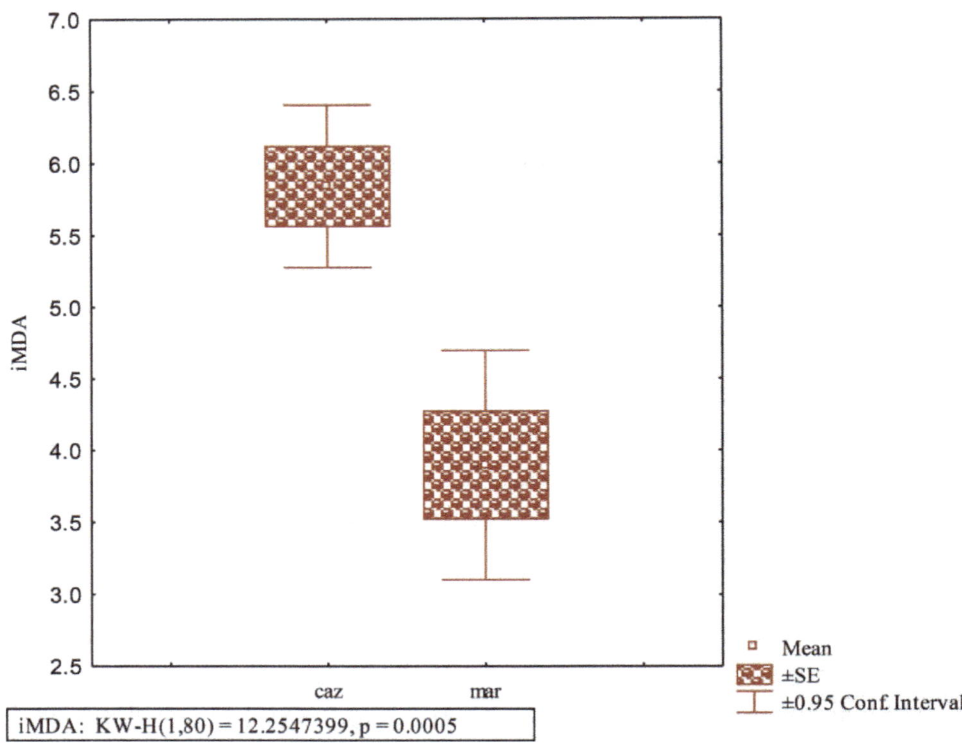

Figure 1. MDA values of case group DOL 1 vs. control group (caz = case, mar = control).

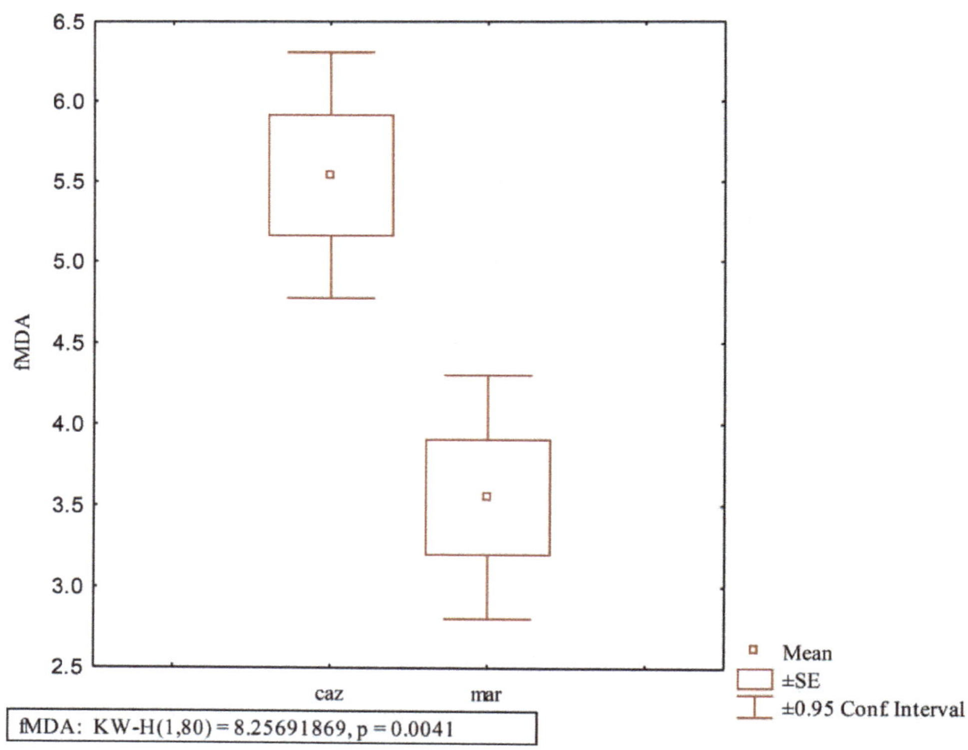

Figure 2. MDA values of case group DOL 3 vs. control group (caz = case, mar = control).

The vascular surface has the role to control critical processes for the functioning of organs. During inflammatory processes, the endothelium is exposed to oxidation [25]. It has been demonstrated that TNF-alpha stimulates the release of oxygenated water at the contact area between neutrophils and the endothelial cell, inducing endothelial cell retraction.

The exposure of endothelial cells to significant concentrations of exogenous oxidants will cause specific physiological effects. Endogenous oxidants have been recognized as a physiological signal component, probably triggered by lung injury, with the release of TNF-alpha, interleukin, growth factor β, and platelet growth factors. These will stimulate tyrosine phosphorylation, with the activation of ERK, extracellular signal-regulated kinase. DNA synthesis will occur accompanied by an increase in hydrogen peroxide levels. Oxidants mediate the effects of growth factors β and insulin, which will stimulate mitogen-activated proteins [27–28].

2.2.1. Oxidative stress in retinopathy of prematurity

The harmful effects of ROS at endothelial level also manifest in ROP [10, 23]. In the pathogenesis of ROP, the following factors are involved: self-regulation, which is absent in newborns, hyperoxygenation of the retina, which is frequent because antioxidant defense is reduced, particularly in the premature. Hyperoxygenation induces peroxidation of vasoactive isoprostanes. Vasoconstriction and vascular cell toxicity with ischemia and vascular proliferation occur [4, 7].

Glutathione is the most important intracellular antioxidant; however, its synthesis is reduced during intrauterine life and in prematures. In the vitreous fluid of the premature at risk for retinopathy, there is a high level of hypoxanthine with a role in the formation of free radicals [1, 12]. Papp et al. [6] found that the oxidized glutathione/reduced glutathione ratio is more than double in prematures with retinopathy compared to those without this disease. This is why the problem of using this ratio as a screening method for the detection of ocular involvement in premature infants was posed. The same authors found that in infants with active disease aged less than 3 months, reduced glutathione values were lower, and those of oxidized glutathione were higher, the greatest decrease in reduced glutathione occurring after the in vitro alteration of oxidative status.

2.2.2. Effects of oxidative stress in ulceronecrotic enterocolitis

In ulceronecrotic enterocolitis, there are multiple pathogenic mechanisms. One of the pathogenic links is hypoxic ischemic injury. Hypoxic ischemic injury in the mesentery is followed by a cascade of events, with intestinal mucosal reperfusion injury. Cytotoxic damage of vascular endothelial cells occurs, which in turn will cause ischemia and new cytotoxic effects through the formation of free radicals [41].

The regulation of mesenteric blood flow includes a reflex self-regulation mechanism. The peripheral autonomic nervous system plays a role in the regulation of mesenteric blood flow.

The initiated ischemia will induce transcapillary fluid passage and local edema. Reperfusion will exacerbate transcapillary fluid production and induce tissue destruction. This event is mediated by factors released from the ischemic intestine, including endotoxins, histamine, prostaglandins, and superoxide anion, which result from oxygen metabolization. Superoxide will induce lipid peroxidation with the disruption of the integrity of capillaries and epithelial cells. Mucosal lesions characterized by edema, hemorrhage, ulceration, and necrosis may be induced experimentally by a combination of oxidants (hypoxanthine and xanthine oxidase) [14]. Superoxide dismutase can experimentally prevent or attenuate the described lesions. The protective effect of SOD was experimentally observed in animals with superior mesenteric artery occlusion. The sequential development of intestinal enzymes: SOD and xanthine oxidase can be a determining factor of neonatal intestinal susceptibility to ischemic mucosal injury [13, 45]. Regarding NEC prevention, many studies performed on animals show the beneficial effect of melatonin in preventing oxidative stress involved in the development of NEC lesions. Melatonin acts by reducing the level of inflammatory cytokines and by stimulating the activity of antioxidant enzymes. A decrease in TNF-α and IL-1β levels was found in animals treated with melatonin. Melatonin also counteracts the reduction of intestinal motility generated by lipopolysaccharides. Melatonin is an indolamine produced by the pineal gland, having serotonin as a precursor. It is synthesized by serotonin-rich enterochromaffin cells in the digestive tract. This synthesis takes place postprandially in the digestive tube and its level is 100 times higher than blood levels [45, 46].

The pathophysiological mechanism of NEC is based on a hypoxic-ischemic process similar to that found in postasphyxia brain injury. A number of studies have demonstrated that the association of melatonin with misoprostol, a gastric mucosal protective agent, is more beneficial than melatonin therapy alone. These studies on animals found that the administration of 10 mg/kg body weight melatonin for 3 days to animals with induced NEC-like lesions significantly reduced the severity of the disease by decreasing cytokine levels and stimulating antioxidant enzyme activity [45, 48].

2.2.3. Effects of oxidative stress in neonatal asphyxia and hypoxic ischemic encephalopathy

In the brain, there are some particularities that increase the vulnerability of this tissue to oxidative stress: cell membranes are rich in polyunsaturated fatty acids, the brain is poor in catalase and SOD, and there are some brain areas rich in iron. Nerve cell injury in the context of asphyxia will induce iron release [13]. Given the low antioxidant defense, the release of low molecular mass iron will allow the formation of hydroxyl radical and lipid peroxidation. By lipid peroxidation, free radicals induce molecular damage, including endothelial factor destruction. The low level of antioxidants in the serum seems to be directly involved in the genesis of cerebral hemorrhage [17]. Transferrin and ceruloplasmin levels can be indicators of the risk of cerebral hemorrhage in newborns with asphyxia at birth [17, 18]. In prematures with asphyxia, a decrease in these enzymes will precede cerebral hemorrhage. Ceruloplasmin acts as a strong ferroxidase, catalyzing iron oxidation to less reactive ions. The antioxidant defense capacity can be exceeded, making transferrin inadequate for binding, with the release of low molecular mass iron, which will subsequently induce lipid peroxidation. In case of iron overloading or severe oxidative stress, the antioxidant defense capacity is exceeded, making nontransferrin bonds available, with the release of low molecular mass iron, followed by lipid peroxidation. This may occur even if transferrin is not completely iron saturated [42].

Hypoxic ischemic brain injury is a long process that starts with the occurrence of the insult and continues during the recovery period, after reperfusion. This reperfusion process represents a paradoxical tissue response: the appearance of oxidative lesions in a hypoxic tissue, poorly perfused after circulatory stabilization, at the time of its perfusion with oxygenated blood. This stage of reperfusion will cause an excessive production of free radicals generating new lesions after the initial oxidative attack. In the premature, an increased risk of cerebral ischemia persists postnatally, during the first week of life [19, 26, 27].

In the reperfusion stage, ROS with a cell damaging effect are produced, in the first place by the conversion of xanthine dehydrogenase to xanthine oxidase. This process will result in the formation of thiol groups or proteolysis by activation of proteases in energetically depressed cells. In the reoxygenation stage, hypoxanthine is converted to uric acid under the action of xanthine oxidase, and superoxide and peroxide are released through the mediation of xanthine oxidase by molecular oxygen binding. Hydroxyl radical generated through the Fenton reaction will also be released, due to the catalytic effect of metals such as iron [42]. Perinatal hypoxic stress is a frequent cause of morbidity, mortality, and neurological damage in survivors. In the perinatal hypoxic context, several factors play a role in the pathogenesis of lesions: hypoxia with initial ROS formation, followed by ischemia-reperfusion, a stage at which arachidonic acid and phagocytes will be activated under the action of inflammation mediators. Thus, a vicious circle is created. ROS will be formed, followed by tissue lesions and the genesis of new free radicals [42, 43].

At CNS level, under asphyxia conditions, encephalopathy lesions are induced by activation of leukocytes or glial cells and release of new free radicals. Hypoxic lesions will be perpetuated by release of protein-unbound iron. Endothelial lesions, hemostasis abnormalities, and inflammatory lesions occur, as well as with an increase in anaerobic metabolism, lactic acid levels, brain damage as a result of oligodendroglial vulnerability, astrocyte dysfunction, N-methyl-D-aspartate receptor abnormalities, and synaptic damage [28, 29].

Mitochondrial DNA damage induces changes in respiratory chain proteins, with the formation of new free radicals and subsequent cell lesions. Neonatal cerebral hypoxia stimulates activin secretion, which in turn stimulates erythropoietin, resulting in the production of nucleated red blood cells [35, 43].

The types of lesions that occur in the brain as a result of hypoxia are variable. In the extremely immature brain, preoligodendrocytes and cell precursors of oligodendrocytes are affected. As the brain matures, the resistance of oligodendrocytes to oxidative stress increases due to an increase in antioxidant defense, as well as to the protein structure involved in programmed cell death.

After the hypoxic episode, there is an increase in the density of glutamate receptors, and mitochondrial calcium accumulation occurs, which will trigger apoptosis. Caspase 6 and, subsequently, caspase 3 are activated. NMDA receptor activation depresses the mitochondrial respiratory process and induces apoptosis—a process which is not found in adults, known as the NMDA paradox [41, 48].

Studies conducted by Peeters and Schulte regarding the activity of glutathione peroxidase in the cerebrospinal fluid of newborns with asphyxia and the neuron-specific enolase value evidenced a correlation between the glutathione peroxidase value and gestational age, as well as between the neuronal enolase value and the neurological evolution of perinatal asphyxia cases. The influence of the genetic factor on postischemic evolution was also demonstrated, as well as on the presence of a correlation with patient's sex, males being more predisposed to develop lesions compared to females.

With the stabilization of newborns with asphyxia at birth, in the reoxygenation stage, the exposure of the diseased cell to a new oxidative attack follows. The use of 100% oxygen in resuscitation is an important source for the formation of ROS. Hyperoxia causes an increase in the activity of antioxidant enzymes such as catalase or superoxide dismutase, as well as an activation of enzymes in the glutathione reductase cycle: GSH-reductase and GSH-S-transferase. Some studies demonstrated that the urinary level of N-acetyl-glucosaminidase is correlated with the value of oxidized glutathione and is higher in newborns exposed to a FiO_2 of 100%. Based on these findings, resuscitation guidelines were changed in 2010, indicating to start neonatal resuscitation with atmospheric air, followed by an increase by titration in the FiO_2 value depending on the improvement of blood oxygen saturation [1, 3, 43].

In the study conducted in our unit, we found that lipid peroxidation in newborns with asphyxia was maintained at a high level on the third day compared to the first day of life, without a statistically significant difference. This high plateau value on day 3 was attributed to perinatal hypoxic stress and to the reoxygenation-reperfusion process. None of the newborns with asphyxia received hypothermia treatment, because at the time of the study, this therapeutic method was not available in our unit. The analysis of lipid peroxidation after neonatal asphyxia by gestational age groups evidenced more intense peroxidation in premature infants compared to term infants with asphyxia. We explained this process by the association of neonatal asphyxia with respiratory distress in the case of prematures, which involved oxygen therapy and respiratory support for its treatment, factors that increased oxidative stress and implicitly, malondialdehyde values. Regarding protein peroxidation, its markers are found in high amounts in the plasma of prematures with asphyxia. Their high values are maintained until the seventh day of life [43]. In newborns with hypoxic ischemic encephalopathy in our study, protein peroxidation was more intense compared to the other newborns. Hypoxic injury is aggravated by protein-unbound iron release. In its presence, as part of the Fenton reaction, hydroxyl radicals are released, which will exert a strong toxic effect on the brain. ROS toxicity in newborns is enhanced by the increased production of ROS, their rapid tissue growth, and impaired antioxidant defense. In the developing brain, endothelial lesions, hemostasis abnormalities, inflammatory reaction, an increase of anaerobic metabolism occur, which are followed by lactic acid accumulation. Oligodendroglial injury, astrocyte dysfunction, and synaptic abnormalities will result [43, 44].

Oxidative stress markers have an important predictive value for neuronal injury in newborns at risk. The correlation between the values of oxidative stress markers and imaging electrophysiological brain changes, near-infrared spectroscopy (NIRS) aspects, and the degree of neurological impairment is not currently described in the literature. This is why further studies are required in this respect. Also, research on therapies protecting against cerebral oxidative stress after perinatal asphyxia has not reported a clearly beneficial medication at this stage of knowledge. The only therapy currently applied with positive, beneficial results in perinatal asphyxia is controlled hypothermia. In the near future, studies are needed which should attempt to identify free radical scavengers that can be administered to newborns and could be useful in limiting oxidative stress, particularly in prematures, in whom antioxidant defense is impaired due to the end of pregnancy before term [44, 47].

3. Conclusion

Oxidative stress at newborns has role in pathogenesis of different neonatal diseases. The oxidative stress is more severe in preterm than in term neonates. The antioxidant defense of preterm less developed than in term neonates, mainly the enzymatic antioxidant defense.

In the near future, studies are needed which should attempt to identify free radical scavengers that can be administered to newborns and could be useful in limiting oxidative stress, particularly in prematures, in whom antioxidant defense is impaired due to the end of pregnancy before term.

Author details

Melinda Mátyás* and Gabriela Zaharie

*Address all correspondence to: melimatyas@yahoo.com

Department of Neonatology, University of Medicine and Pharmacy, Cluj-Napoca, Romania

References

[1] Saugstad OD. Update on oxygen radical disease in neonatology. Current Opinion in Obstetrics & Gynecology. 2001;**13**:147-153

[2] Sullivan JL. Iron, plasma antioxidants, and the oxygen radical disease of prematurity. American Journal of Diseases of Children. 1988;**142**:1341-1344

[3] Saugstad OD. Chronic lung disease: The role of oxidative stress. Biologia Neonatorum. 1998;**74**:21-28

[4] Raju TN, Langenberg P, Bhutani V, Quinn GE. Vitamin E prophylaxis to reduce rethinopaty of prematurity; a reappraisal of published trials. Journal of Pediatrics. 1997; **131**:844850

[5] Luukkainen P, Aejmelaeus R, Alho H, et al. Plasma chain–breaking antioxidants in preterm infants with good and poor short term outcome. Free Radical Research. 1999; (3):189-197

[6] Papp A, Nemeth I, Karg E, Papp E. Gluthatione status in retinopathy of prematurity. Free Radical Biology & Medicine. 1999;**27**:738-743

[7] Silverman WA. Rethinopaty of prematurity: Oxigen dogma challenged? Archives of Disease in Childhood. 1982;**57**:731-733

[8] Northway WHJ, Rosan RC, Porter DY. Pulmonary disease following respiartor therapy of hyaline-membrane disease. The New England Journal of Medicine. 1967;**276**:357-368

[9] Buss IH, Darlow BA, Winterbourn CC. Elevated lipid carbonyls and lipid peroxidation products correlating with myeloperoxidase in tracheal aspirates from premature infants. Pediatric Research. 2000;**47**:640-645

[10] Winterbourn CC, Chan T, Buss IH, Inder TE, Mogridge N, Darlow BA. Protein carbonyls and lipid peroxidation products as oxidation markers in preterm infant plasma: Association with chronic lung disease and rethinopaty and effects of selenium supplimentation. Pediatric Research. 2000;**48**:84-90

[11] Yu XQ, Medbo S, Saugstad OD. Sodium nitroprusside prevents oxygen-free-radical-included pulmonary vasoconstriction in newborn piglets. Biology of the Neonate. 1999; **75**:319-326

[12] Hardy P, Dumont I, Bhattacharya M, et al. Oxidants, nitric oxide and prostanoids in the developing ocular vasculature: A basis for ischemic retinopathy. Cardiovascular Research. 2000;**47**:489-509

[13] Saugstad OD. Hypoxanthine as a measurement of hypoxia. Pediatric Research. 1975; **9**:158-161

[14] Supnet MC, David-Cu R, Walther FJ. Plasma xanthine oxidase and lipid hydroperoxide levels in the preterm infants. Pediatric Research. 1994;**36**:283-287

[15] Rogers S, Witz G, Anwar M, et al. Antioxidant capacity and oxygen radical disease in the preterm newborn. Archives of Pediatrics & Adolescent Medicine. 2000;**154**:544-548

[16] Buonocore G, Perrone S, Longini M, et al. Total hydroperoxide and advanced oxidation protein products in preterm hypoxidic babies. Pediatric Research. 2000;**47**:221-224

[17] Domergues MA, Gallego J, Evrard P, Gressens P. Iron supplementation aggravates periventricular cystic white matter lesions in newborn mice. European Journal of Pediatric Neurology. 1998;**2**:313-318

[18] Palmer C, Menzies SL, Roberts RL, et al. Changes in iron histochemistry after hypoxic-ischemic brain injury in the neonatal rat. Journal of Neuroscience Research. 1999;**56**:60-71

[19] Vento M, Garcia-Sala F, Vina J, et al. The use of room air ventilation enhances the establishment of a sustained spontaneous respiratory pattern after perinatal asphyxia. Pediatric Research. 2000;**47**:438

[20] Rosenfeld WN, Davis JM, Parton L, Richter SE, Price A, Flaster E, Kassem N. Safety and pharmacokinetics of human recombinant superoxide dismutase administered intratracheally to premature neonates with respiratory distress syndrome. Pediatrics. 1996;**97**:811-817

[21] Davis JM, Rosenfeld WN, Richter SE, Price A, Parad R, Gewolb IH, Spitzer AR, et al. Safety and pharmacokinetics of recombinant human CuZn superoxide dismutase administered intratracheally to premature neonates with respiratory distress syndrome. Pediatrics. 1997;**100**:24-30

[22] Carlo WA, Stark AR, BAUer C, et al. Effects of minimal ventilation in multicenter randomized controlled trial of ventilatory support and early corticosteroid therapy in extremely low birth weight infants. Pediatric Research. 2000;**47**:2310A

[23] Tin W, Milligan DW, Pennefather P, Hey E. Pulse oximetry, severe retinopathy and outcome at one year in babies of less than 28 weeks gestation. Archives of Disease in Childhood. Fetal and Neonatal. 2001;**84**:F106-F110

[24] Wispe JR, Warner BB, Clark JC, et al. Human Mn-superoxide dismutase in pulmonary epithelial cells of transgenic mice confers protection from oxygen injury. Journal of Biological Chemistry. 1992;**267**:2393-2397

[25] Lance S. Terada. Oxidative stress and endothelial activation. Critical Care Medicine; 2002 Vol.30, No.5 suppl:S186-S191

[26] Rosenberg AA, Murdaugh E, White CW. The role of oxygen free radicals in postasphyxia cerebral hypoperfusion in newborn lambs. Pediatric Research. 1989;**26**:215-219

[27] Liu TH, Beckman JS, Freeman BA, Hogan EL, Hsu CY. Polyethylene glycol –conjugated superoxide dismutase and catalase reduce ischemic brain injury. The American Journal of Physiology. 1989;**256**:H589-H593

[28] Carney J, Starke-Reed P, Oliver C, Landum RW, Cheng MS, Wu JF, a. Reversal of age-related increase in brain protein oxidation, descrease in enzyme activity, and loss in temporal and spatial memory by chronic administration of the spin-trapping compound N-tert-butyl-alpha-phenilnitron. Proceedings of the National Academy of Sciences of the United States of America. 1991;**88**:3633-3636

[29] Mishra OP, Delivoria-Papadopoulos M. Cellular mechanism of hypoxic injury in the developing brain. Brain Research Bulletin. 1998;**48**:233-238

[30] Davis JM, Rosenfeld WN, Parad R, et al. Improved pulmonary outcome at one year corrected age in premature neonates treated with recombinant human superoxide dismutase. Pediatric Research. 2000;**47**:395A

[31] Robbins CG, Horowitz S, Merritt TA, Kheiter A, Tierney J, Narula P, Davis JM. Recombinant human superoxide dismutase reduces lung injury caused by inhaled nitric oxide and hyperoxia. The American Journal of Physiology. 1997;**272**:L903-L907

[32] Dani C, Cecchi A, Bertini G. Role of oxidative stress as physiopathologic factor in the preterm infant. Minerva Pediatrica. 2004;**56**(4):381-394

[33] Pitcanen OM, Hallman M. Evidence for increased oxidative stress in preterm infants eventually developing chronic lung disease. Seminars in Neonatology. 1998;**2**:199-2005

[34] Saugstad OD. Bronchopulmonary dysplasia – Oxidative stress and antioxidants. Seminars in Neonatology. 2003;**8**:39-49

[35] Szabo M, Vasarhelyi B, Balla G, Szabo T, Machay T, Tulassay T. Acute postnatal increase of extracellular antioxidant defence of neonates: The role of iron metabolism. Acta Paediatrica. 2001;**90**:1167-1170

[36] The STOP-ROP Multicenter Study Group. Supplemental therapeutic oxygen for Prethreshold retinopathy of prematurity (STOP-ROP), a randomized, controlled trial. I: Primary outcomes. Pediatrics. 2000;**105**:295-310

[37] Allen RG, Tresini M. Oxidative stress and gene regulation. Free Radical Biology and Medicine. 2000;**28**:463-499

[38] Gitto E, Reiter RJ, Xian-Tan D, Barberi I. Respiratory distress syndrome in the newborn: Role of oxidative stress. Intensive Care Medicine. 2001;**27**:1116-1123

[39] Grobben DJH, Lindeman E, Houdkamp RM, Moison JT, Berger WHM. Markers of oxidative stress and antioxidant activity in plasma and erythrocytes in neonates with respiratory distress syndrome. Acta Paediatrica. 1997;**86**(12):1356-1362

[40] Sola A, Rodigo MR, Deulofeut R. Oxygen as a neonatal health hazard: Call for détente in clinical practice. Acta Paediatrica. 2007 jun;**96**(6):801-812

[41] Perrone S, Tataranno ML, Negro S, Longini M, Marzocchi B, Proietti F, Iacoponi F, Capitani S, Buonocore G. Early identification of the risk for free radical-related diseases in preterm newborns. Early Human Development. 2010;**86**:241-244

[42] Torres-Cuevasa I, Parra-Llorcaa A, S-Illanaa A, Nuñez-Ramiroa A. Oxygen and oxidative stress in the perinatal period. Redox Biology. 2017;**12**:674-681

[43] Buonocore G, Groenendaal F. Anti-oxidant strategies. Seminars in Fetal & Neonatal Medicine. 2007;**12**:287-295

[44] Tataranno ML, Perrone S, Buonocore G. Plasma biomarkers of oxidative stress in neonatal brain injury. Clinics in Perinatology. 2015 sept;**42**:529-539

[45] Marseglia et al. Oxidative stress and necrotizing Enterocolitis. American Journal of Perinatology 2015;**32**:905-909

[46] Thor PJ, Krolczyk G, Gil K, Zurowski D, Nowak L. Melatonin and serotonin effects on gastrointestinal motility. Journal of Physiology and Pharmacology. 2007;**58**(Suppl 6): 97-103

[47] Guven A, Uysal B, Gundogdu G, Oztas E, Ozturk H, Korkmaz A. Melatonin ameliorates necrotizing enterocolitis in a neonatal ratmodel. Journal of Pediatric Surgery. 2011; **46**(11):2101-2107

[48] Negi R, Pande D, Karki R, Kumar A, Khanna RS, Khanna HD. A Novel approach to study oxidative stress in neonatal respiratory distress syndrome. BBA Clinical, 2015;**3**: 65-69

3

Time and Mode of Delivery in Twin Pregnancies

Eduardo Félix Martins Santana, Vivian Melo Corrêa,
Isabela Bottura and José Pedro Parise Filho

Abstract

There are many suitable recommendations for twin gestation term in the literature. In many protocols, resolution is recommended for dichorionic pregnancies around 38 weeks, at 36 weeks for monochorionic (devoid of complications) and at 32–34 weeks in cases of single amniotic chamber. The main risk associated with vaginal delivery is connected to the possibility of anoxia of the second twin. However, a cesarean delivery performed by non-cephalic presentation of the second twin is associated with increased maternal morbidity without improved neonatal outcome. The most important factors in the decision of the delivery mode include the presentation of the fetus, gestational age, and weight or the weight difference between the fetuses.

Keywords: twin pregnancy, delivery, labor

1. Introduction

It is known that multiple pregnancy presents morbidity and mortality rates about 3–7 times greater than single pregnancies, and these are often determined in delivery care [1].

Among the difficulties in twin birth, we highlight: prematurity, non-cephalic presentations, dystocia, funicular prolapse, placental abruption, increased operative incidence, postpartum hemorrhages, perinatal anoxia and tocotraumatism [2].

In this chapter we will review the main aspects related to the time and mode of delivery in multiple pregnancies and issues related to fetal weight assessment.

2. Risk of fetal death in the third trimester for twin pregnancies

Multiple pregnancies have high rates of mortality and morbidity when compared to single pregnancies. This is mainly due to prematurity, complications close to delivery, and placental insufficiency [1].

In fact, this risk is related to chorionicity. The monochorionic (MC) pregnancies present a higher incidence of perinatal mortality, higher admission in neonatal intensive care unit and low birth weight [3]. It is possible that the single placental mass shared between pairs originates from an imbalance in placental anastomoses, may be overloaded in the third trimester [4].

A large Dutch cohort with 1407 multiple pregnancies showed that after 32 weeks' gestation, mortality was 11.6% in MC and 5% in dichorionic (DC) [5]. The risk of uterine death was significantly higher in MC than in DC (hazard ratio 8.8, 95% CI 2.7–28.9), and in most cases no change in fetal status was observed. The authors concluded that fetal vitality control was not sufficient to prevent adverse events and delivery should be planned up to the 37th week for MC.

A study with 94,170 multiple deliveries showed that the risk of fetal death increased significantly between 37 and 38 weeks of gestation in twin pregnancies. This risk was higher between 34 and 37 weeks of gestation in triplet pregnancies. The risk of child death after delivery gradually declined as pregnancies neared full term. This group recommended increased fetal surveillance after 34 weeks of gestation in multiple pregnancies [6].

3. Time of delivery in dichorionic pregnancies

The American College of Obstetricians and Gynecologists (ACOG) suggests that delivery be performed between 38 + 0 and 38 + 6 weeks in uncomplicated twin dichorionic pregnancies [7]. Depending on complications such as fetal growth restriction, termination of pregnancy is recommended before 38 weeks.

In 2016, a systematic review included 32 studies (29,685 dichorionic, 5486 monochorionic pregnancies) and showed that in dichorionic pregnancies beyond 34 weeks (15 studies, 17,830 pregnancies), the weekly risk of stillbirths due to expectant management and the risk of neonatal death were balanced at the 37th week of gestation. When delivery was delayed for 1 week (up to 38 weeks) led to an additional 8.8 perinatal deaths per 1000 pregnancies [8].

4. Time of delivery in monochorionic pregnancies

The same review showed that monochorionic pregnancies beyond 34 weeks (13 studies, 2149 pregnancies), had a tendency for an increase in stillbirths compared to neonatal deaths after 36 weeks, with an additional 2.5 per 1000 perinatal deaths, which was not significant [8].

Just like DC gestations, there are no high-quality studies to respond with great certainty the right time for terminate monochorionic pregnancies. Most specialists in large reference centers recommend delivery of monochorionic/diamniotic twins between 36 + 0 and 36 + 6 weeks. This may be the point of balance between the already reduced risk of prematurity and the risk of fetal death [9].

There is still a lot of divergence between medical societies for the correct time of delivery. ACOG suggests delivery of monochorionic twins between 34 + 0 to 37 + 6 weeks of gestation [7] and the North American Fetal Therapy Network suggests delivery at 36 + 0 to 37 + 6 weeks of gestation [9]. However, others delegate delivery at 32 weeks of gestation [10]. It is clear that in cases of Twin-Twin Transfusion Syndrome, most of deliveries are performed earlier and this depends on the degree of complication that is present.

On the other hand, in monoamniotic pregnancies, most specialized centers in the world recommend delivery between 32 and 34 weeks. This fact is justified by the high rate of perinatal mortality in the third trimester (30–70%) and has as main motive the umbilical cords entanglement in the same amniotic chamber [4, 11, 12].

5. Delivery mode: vaginal delivery vs. cesarean section

The mode of delivery in twin pregnancy depends on multiple factors and is very controversial in the literature. The most important factors to be considered on deciding the delivery mode are the fetus presentation, especially the first twin, fetal weight, weight difference between the fetuses, gestational weight and maternal clinical conditions. Women's parity is also a condition with high influence in mode of delivery in a twin pregnancy, as nulliparous usually result in less success when attempting a vaginal delivery [13].

The decision on either performing an elective cesarean delivery must consider the best neonatal and maternal outcomes, to reduce neonatal morbidity and mortality, maternal complications and preserving the women's reproductive future. The biggest risk in a vaginal delivery is for the second twin, as complications can occur after the delivery of the first twin, including placental abruption, cord prolapse and long delivery intervals [14].

It is important to consider that conditions that would indicate a cesarean section in singleton pregnancies should also be applied in multiple pregnancies.

5.1. Fetus presentation

Determining fetal presentation is fundamental in the decision of the mode of delivery. The presentation of twin pairs in a term twin pregnancy is 40% of the times cephalic/cephalic, 35–40% cephalic/non-cephalic and only 20% with the first twin non-cephalic [15]. It is a general consensus that, when both fetuses are in cephalic presentation, a vaginal delivery should be attempted [13–15]. However, it is important to notice that the second twin change its presentation in about 20% of the time, after the first one is born [15].

When the second twin is in a non-cephalic presentation, vaginal delivery is controversial. Some studies say that neonatal morbidity is higher for the second twin in those cases and an elective cesarean section should be planned [16, 17]. However, both a systematic review and meta-analysis [14] and a recent published prospective cohort study [18] support that cesarean deliveries neither add neonatal morbidity nor mortality. Therefore, a vaginal delivery is a safe option. In those cases, the second twin can either be delivered by breech extraction or an external cephalic version can be attempted [19].

Finally, when the first twin is non-cephalic, the safest delivery mode is the cesarean section. A randomized multicenter trial, The Breech Trial, showed that a planned cesarean delivery decreases significantly perinatal mortality and neonatal serious morbidity, when compared with a planned vaginal delivery in pregnancies with a non-cephalic presenting twin [20].

5.2. Fetal weight estimation in twin pregnancies

Twin pregnancies are more likely to show deviations in fetal growth curve. Conditions such as prematurity, intrauterine growth restriction and fetal malformations are common in multiple gestations, raising the risk of mortality and perinatal morbidity to 3–7 times when compared to single pregnancies [21]. Prematurity is present in approximately 55% of twin pregnancies, with adverse consequences even in short and long term [22].

When comparing the weights of fetuses from twin pregnancies to those of single pregnancies, it is observed that fetuses of twin pregnancies have a lower weight than fetuses of single pregnancies, especially from the end of the second trimester. It is known that this variation between the weights starts at around 28 weeks and at 38 weeks the 50th percentile for a twin pregnancy corresponds to the 10th percentile for a single pregnancy [23], but this difference does not seem to increase neonatal mortality. Therefore, it is argued that the lower weight of twin fetuses, when compared to that of single pregnancies, may be physiological of this condition.

Accuracy in the estimation of fetal weight is of paramount importance for the proper follow-up of prenatal care and ultrasonography study has been the main tool for this evaluation.

Currently fetal weight estimation by ultrasonography is most commonly performed by the formula of Hadlock et al. [24], which uses two-dimensional measures of cephalic pole, abdominal circumference and femur length. However, studies have shown that formulas using two-dimensional parameters can generate variations of up to 15% in relation to the real weight of the fetus [25].

New methods have been sought to improve the accuracy of fetal weight estimation such as three-dimensional ultrasonography. In the early 2000s, Lee et al. [26] introduced a new sonographic parameter, the fraction limb volume. This parameter is based on evaluation of 50% of bone diaphysis length (arm and thigh).

This method has the advantage of reducing the time spent to perform the test, maintaining a good accuracy for the estimation fetal weight.

In general, the accuracy of estimation weight in twin pregnancies is worse than single pregnancies. Biometric measurement of these fetuses in the third trimester is greatly impaired due to the technical difficulty of examination. When using 33 formulas to assess the accuracy of estimation weight by two-dimensional ultrasonography, 25 of these formulas present a weight variation of less than 10% for single pregnancies, but only 3 of these formulas present the same result for twin pregnancies [27].

An ongoing study that has been developed in multiple pregnancy unit of Federal University of São Paulo has shown that the use of fraction limb volume in twin pregnancies can improve the accuracy of estimation weight in these pregnancies, as well as reduce the time of the examination.

Although evaluation of fetal body volume through the use of magnetic resonance imaging is still considered an expensive method, there is good accuracy in fetal weight estimation, besides being a good predictor in the diagnoses of small fetuses for gestational age when compared to two-dimensional ultrasonography [28].

Estimating weight in twin pregnancies remains a challenge. New research needs to be conducted in search for new methods in order to improve accuracy.

Fetal weight should not be considered when both fetuses are cephalic. In those cases, regardless the fetal weight, a vaginal delivery can be attempted. However, in cephalic/non-cephalic twin pregnancies, the influence of weight on mode of delivery is controversial. Most studies showed worst perinatal outcomes for vaginal deliveries when the second twin was non-cephalic and under 1500 g [29, 30].

Weight difference is related to worst neonatal outcomes, regardless the delivery mode [31], and also to unsuccessful attempt of labor [32]. Furthermore, a weight difference above 40% has been associated with higher neonatal mortality rates in vaginal deliveries, regardless fetal presentation, in a retrospective study in 2005 [33].

5.3. Previous C-section

A previous cesarean delivery is considered a risk factor for an emergency C-section after attempting a vaginal delivery in twin pregnancies [34]. Regardless, a caution trial of labor can be a safe option in those patients, when the first twin is cephalic [35].

On the other hand, patients with two or more previous cesarean sections should not attempt a vaginal delivery due to higher risk of uterine rupture.

5.4. Preterm pairs

There is limited existing evidence to determine the safest mode of delivery for extremely preterm twins. Therefore, it is important to consider the fetal presentation and weight when deciding the delivery mode, regardless gestational age.

A recently published meta-analysis showed no significant difference in neonatal death and severe brain injury by mode of delivery for cephalic/non-cephalic twins with a gestational age under 28 weeks [36]. This study found higher rates of maternal complications in growth-discordant twins.

5.5. Maternal conditions

Higher rates of maternal morbidities are found in multiple gestations, compared to singletons. There is a higher risk of pre-eclampsia, diabetes and post-partum complications, as uterine atony and postpartum hemorrhage. Regardless, maternal conditions are rarely an indication of a cesarean section. An elective cesarean delivery can be performed after maternal request, after exposing the risks of the procedure, as longer maternal hospital stay, increased risk of the newborn going to the ICU due to respiratory problems and increased risks for subsequent pregnancies, as placenta previa and uterine rupture [37]. In those cases, the surgery should be planned to the appropriate gestational age, considering chorionicity and amnionicity.

6. Exceptional situations

Although the data about triplet pregnancies are still limited, and the monoamniotic and diamniotic triplets should be delivered between 32 + 0 and 32 + 6 weeks [38], most studies and guidelines suggest delivery time at no later than 36 weeks, even in uncomplicated triamniotic triplets [6, 39, 40]. The preferred delivery route is the cesarean section because vaginal delivery is associated with an increased risk of adverse outcomes if compared with the cesarean [41, 42].

In conjoined twins, the data available is based in small case report studies and expert opinion, but what is suggested is the delivery time and mode of the viable ones must be near term cesarean section after confirming lung maturity. In selected cases an EXIT procedure can be performed in order to stabilize the fetuses with cardiac union to examine and close the vessel communication safely [43].

7. Twin-to-twin delivery time intervals

Another controversial subject about delivery in twins is the time interval between fetuses in vaginal delivery.

New guidelines such as the American College of Obstetricians and Gynecologists do not recommend an upper limit to the time interval between fetuses, if the fetal heart rate is reassuring, as some studies also suggests [44–47]. However, there are studies that provide evidence of an association, but not necessarily causality, between longer twin-to-twin time interval and poor second twin outcome, such as lower apgar grades and decreasing pH in umbilical arterial blood gas [48–50]. This lack of strong evidence leaves space for different approach and expectant management [51].

A very specific approach can be performed in the case of a dichorionic twin pregnancy with spontaneous preterm delivery <24 weeks and never above 28 weeks, which is called delayed interval delivery when the second twin do not have an indication for labor such as infection among other complications. Several techniques and interventions are described but the evidence is not strong, but the main goal is to provide a better outcome for the second twin, and success rates of these particular cases are good according to a systematic review of 2016 [52].

8. Associated risks: vaginal and cesarean delivery

During the last few years, a lot of studies were performed trying to elucidate the question about the best delivery route for twins, according to the associated risks and benefits of planned cesarean section or planned attempt vaginal delivery.

The twin birth study, showed that planned cesarean section was not superior to planned vaginal delivery regarding maternal risk or neonatal mortality or morbidity [53], and ever since some society guidelines suggest attempt to vaginal delivery to diamniotic twin pregnancies if the first twin is in cephalic presentation [54].

The concern about the risks includes the possibility of combined delivery, which involves an unplanned cesarean after attempt of vaginal delivery and is associated with higher second twin morbidity [14] and may be an increased risk of neonatal and/or maternal infection probably because the exposure to labor and rupture of membranes are higher than in a planned cesarean delivery.

Cesarean delivery can expose mothers to short-term risks such as endometritis, wound complications, surgical injuries, hemorrhage [55], although maternal outcomes past 3 month and long-term risks, including abnormal placentation, are similar both ways cesarean an vaginal planned delivery [56, 57].

Newborns delivered by planned cesarean present a higher risk in developing allergic disorders [58–60].

9. Adverse neonatal outcome

The twin birth study did not found statistically significant difference in morbidity and fetal or neonatal mortality between planned cesarean or planned vaginal delivery [14, 53], and a 2-year follow up after delivery found no difference in neurodevelopment and death in both groups [61].

A retrospective study with 1070 twin pregnancies attempted trial of labor between 2003 and 2015 showed that in planned cesarean, the first twin has a lower blood pH and base excess than in vaginal delivery, but the study was unpowered for neonatal outcome assessment [13].

10. Conclusion

The time of delivery in twin pregnancies is around 38 weeks for dichorionic pairs, 36 weeks for monochorionic and 32 weeks for monoamniotic. When both fetuses are on cephalic presentation at delivery, the vaginal route is preferable regardless of weight. Being the first twin in non-cephalic presentation, cesarean section is the best choice. When the first twin is in cephalic presentation and the second non-cephalic, cesarean section is indicated if the fetus weight is less than 1,500g. However, vaginal delivery is possible if the fetus' weight is above

1,500g. In those cases, the second twin can either be delivered by breech extraction or an external cephalic version can be attempted.

Author details

Eduardo Félix Martins Santana[1,2]*, Vivian Melo Corrêa[1], Isabela Bottura[2] and José Pedro Parise Filho[2]

*Address all correspondence to: dudes.felix@gmail.com

1 Department of Obstetrics, Paulista School of Medicine, Federal University of São Paulo (EPM-UNIFESP), São Paulo, SP, Brazil

2 Department of Perinatology, Albert Einstein Hospital, São Paulo, SP, Brazil

References

[1] Sherer DM. Adverse perinatal outcome of twin pregnancies according to chorionicity: Review of the literature. American Journal of Perinatology. 2001;**18**:23-37

[2] Hatkar PA, Bhide AG. Perinatal outcome of twins in relation to chorionicity. Journal of Postgraduate Medicine. 1999;**45**:33-37

[3] Sebire NJ, Snijders RJ, Hughes K, Sepulveda W, Nicolaides KH. The hidden mortality of monochorionic twin pregnancies. British Journal of Obstetrics and Gynaecology. 1997;**104**:1203-1207

[4] Elito Junior J, Santana EFM, Nardini GC. Monochorionic twin pregnancy: Potencial risks and perinatal outcomes. In: Obstetric and Gynecologic Practice in 2014. 67th ed. Europe: InTech; 2014. pp. 203-234

[5] Hack KE, Derks JB, Elias SG, Franx A, Roos EJ, Voerman SK, et al. Increased perinatal mortality and morbidity in monochorionic versus dichorionic twin pregnancies: Clinical implications of a large Dutch cohort study. BJOG: An International Journal of Obstetrics and Gynaecology. 2008;**115**(1):58-67

[6] Ko HS, Choi SK, Wie JH, Park IY, Park YG, Shin JC. Optimal timing of delivery based on the risk of stillbirth and infant death associated with each additional week of expectant management in multiple pregnancies: A National Cohort Study of Koreans. Journal of Korean Medical Science. 2018;**33**(10):e80

[7] Committee on Practice Bulletins—Obstetrics, society for maternal–fetal medicine. Practice bulletin no. 169: Multifetal gestations: Twin, triplet, and higher-order multifetal pregnancies. Obstetrics and Gynecology. 2016;**128**:e131

[8] Cheong-See F, Schuit E, Arroyo-Manzano D, et al. Prospective risk of stillbirth and neonatal complications in twin pregnancies: Systematic review and meta-analysis. BMJ. 2016;**354**:i4353

[9] Emery SP, Bahtiyar MO, Dashe JS, et al. The north American fetal therapy network consensus statement: Prenatal management of uncomplicated monochorionic gestations. Obstetrics and Gynecology. 2015;**125**:1236

[10] Simões T, Amaral N, Lerman R, et al. Prospective risk of intrauterine death of monochorionic-diamniotic twins. American Journal of Obstetrics and Gynecology. 2006;**195**:134

[11] Beasley E, Megerian G, Gerson A, Roberts NS. Monoamniotic twins: Case series and proposal for antenatal management. Obstetrics and Gynecology. 1999;**93**:130

[12] Rodis JF, McIlveen PF, Egan JF, et al. Monoamniotic twins: Improved perinatal survival with accurate prenatal diagnosis and antenatal fetal surveillance. American Journal of Obstetrics and Gynecology. 1997;**177**:1046

[13] Schachter-Safrai N, Karavani G, Haj-Yahya R, Ofek Shlomai N, Porat S. Risk factors for cesarean delivery and adverse neonatal outcome in twin pregnancies attempting vaginal delivery. Acta Obstetricia et Gynecologica Scandinavica. Jul 2018;**97**(7):845-851

[14] Rossi A, Mullin P, Chmait R. Neonatal outcomes of twins according to birth order, presentation and mode of delivery: A systematic review and meta-analysis. BJOG. 2011;**118**:523-532

[15] Bibbo C, Robinson JN. Management of twins: Vaginal or cesarean delivery? Clinical Obstetrics and Gynecology. 2015;**58**(2):294-308

[16] Yang Q, Wen SW, Chen Y, Krewski D, Fung KFK, Walker M. Neonatal death and morbidity in vertex-nonvertex second twins according to mode of delivery and birth weight. American Journal of Obstetrics and Gynecology. 2005;**192**:840-847

[17] Grisaru D, Fuchs S, Kupferminc MJ, Har-Toov J, Niv J, Lessing JB. Outcome of 306 twin deliveries according to first twin presentation and method of delivery. American Journal of Perinatology. 2000;**17**:303-307

[18] Schmitz T, Korb D, Battie C, et al. Neonatal morbidity associated with vaginal delivery of noncephalic second twins. American Journal of Obstetrics and Gynecology. 2018;**4**:449.e1-449.e13

[19] Chervenak FA, Johnson RE, Berkowitz RL, et al. Intrapartum external version of the second twin. Obstetrics and Gynecology. 1983;**62**:160-165

[20] Hannah ME, Hannah WJ, Hewson SA, et al. Planned caesarean section versus planned vaginal birth for breech presentation at term: A randomised multicentre trial. Term Breech Trial Collaborative Group. Lancet. 2000;**356**:1375-1383

[21] Hack KE, Derks JB, Elias SG, et al. Increased perinatal mortality and morbidity in monochorionic versus dichorionic twin pregnancies: Clinical implications of a large Dutch cohort study. BJOG. 2008;**115**:58-67

[22] Elliott JP. High-order multiple gestations. Seminars in Perinatology. 2005;**29**:305-311

[23] Alexander GR, Kogan M, Martin J, Papiernik E. What are the fetal growth patterns of sigletons, twins and triplets in the United States? Clinical Obstetrics and Gynecology. 1998;**41**(1):114-125

[24] Hadlock FP, Harrist RB, Sharman RS, Deter RL, Park SK. Estimation of fetal weight with the use of head, body and femur measurements. A prospective study. American Journal of Obstetrics and Gynecology. 1985;**151**(3):333-337

[25] Dudley NJ. A systematic review of ultrassound estimation of fetal weight. Ultrasound in Obstetrics & Gynecology. 2005;**25**(1):80-89

[26] Lee W, Deter RL, Ebersole JD, Huang R, Blarchart K, Romero R. Birth weight prediction by three-dimensional ultrassonography fractional limb volume. Journal of Ultrasound in Medicine. 2001;**20**:1283-1292

[27] Khalil A, D'Antonio F, Dias T, Cooper D, Thilaganathan B, Southwest Thames Obstetric Research Collaborative (STORK). Ultrasound estimation of birth weight in twin pregnancy: Comparison of biometry algorithms in the STORK multiple pregnancy cohort. Ultrasound in Obstetrics & Gynecology. 2014;**44**:210-220

[28] Kadji C, Bevilaqua E, Hurtado I, et al. Comparison of conventional 2D ultrassound to magnetic resonance imaging for prenatal estimation of birthweight in twin pregnancy. American Journal of Obstetrics and Gynecology. 2018;**218**(1):128.e1-128.e11

[29] Barrett JM, Staggs SM, Van Hooydonk JE, et al. The effect of type of delivery upon neonatal outcome in premature twins. American Journal of Obstetrics and Gynecology. 1982;**143**:360-367

[30] Zhang J, Bowes WA, Grey TW, et al. Twin delivery and neonatal and infant mortality: A population-based study. Obstetrics and Gynecology. 1996;**88**:593-598

[31] D'Antonio F, Khalil A, Dias T, et al. Weight discordance and perinatal mortality in twins: Analysis of the Southwest Thames Obstetric Research Collaborative (STORK) multiple pregnancy cohort. Ultrasound in Obstetrics & Gynecology. 2013;**41**:643-648

[32] Ko HJ, Jun JK. Clinical factors associated with failed trials of labor in late preterm and term twin pregnancies. Journal of Perinatal Medicine. 2014;**42**(4):449-455

[33] Kontopoulos EV, Ananth CV, Smulian JC, et al. The influence of mode of delivery on twin neonatal mortality in the US: Variance by birth weight discordance. American Journal of Obstetrics and Gynecology. 2005;**192**:252-256

[34] Spiegel E, Kessous R, Sergienko R, Sheiner E. Risk factors predicting an emergency cesarean delivery for the second twin after vaginal delivery of the first twin. Archives of Gynecology and Obstetrics. 2015;**292**(3):531-536

[35] Delaney T, Young DC. Trial of labour compared to elective caesarean in twin gestations with a previous caesarean delivery. Journal of Obstetrics and Gynaecology Canada. 2003;**25**(4):289-292

[36] Dagenais C, Lewis-Mikhael AM, Grabovac M, et al. What is the safest mode of delivery for extremely preterm cephalic/non-cephalic twin pairs? A systematic review and meta-analyses. BMC Pregnancy Childbirth. 2017;**17**:397

[37] American College of Obstetricians and Gynecologists. ACOG committee opinion no. 559: Cesarean delivery on maternal request. Obstetrics and Gynecology. 2013;**121**(4):904-907

[38] Van Mieghem T, De Heus R, Lewi L, et al. Prenatal management of monoamniotic twin pregnancies. Obstetrics and Gynecology. 2014;**124**:498.65

[39] Kahn B, Lumey LH, Zybert PA, Lorenz JM, Cleary-Goldman J, D'Alton ME, et al. Prospective risk of fetal death in singleton, twin, and triplet gestations: Implications for practice. Obstetrics and Gynecology. 2003;**102**(4):685-692

[40] National Collaborating Centre for Women's and Children's Health (GB). Multiple Pregnancy: The Management of Twin and Triplet Pregnancies in the Antenatal Period. London, United Kingdom: RCOG Press; 2011

[41] Vintzileos AM, Ananth CV, Kontopoulos E, Smulian JC. Mode of delivery and risk of stillbirth and infant mortality in triplet gestations: United States, 1995 through 1998. American Journal of Obstetrics and Gynecology. 2005;**192**:464

[42] Lappen JR, Hackney DN, Bailit JL. Maternal and neonatal outcomes of attempted vaginal compared with planned cesarean delivery in triplet gestations. American Journal of Obstetrics and Gynecology. 2016;**215**:493.e1

[43] Mackenzie TC, Crombleholme TM, Johnson MP, et al. The natural history of prenatally diagnosed conjoined twins. Journal of Pediatric Surgery. 2002;**37**:303

[44] Stein W, Misselwitz B, Schmidt S. Twin-to-twin delivery time interval: Influencing factors and effect on short-term outcome of the second twin. Acta Obstetricia et Gynecologica Scandinavica. 2008;**87**(3):346-353

[45] McGrail CD, Bryant DR. Intertwin time interval: How it affects the immediate neonatal outcome of the second twin. American Journal of Obstetrics and Gynecology. 2005;**192**(5):1420-1422

[46] Rayburn WF, Lavin JPJ, Miodovnik M, Varner MW. Multiple gestation: Time interval between delivery of the first and second twins. Obstetrics and Gynecology. 1984;**63**(4): 502-506

[47] Committee on Practice B-O, Society for Maternal-Fetal M. Practice bulletin no. 169: Multifetal gestations: Twin, triplet, and higher-order multifetal pregnancies. Obstetrics and Gynecology. 2016;**128**(4):e131-e146

[48] Leung TY, Tam WH, Leung TN, Lok IH, Lau TK. Effect of twin-to-twin delivery interval on umbilical cord blood gas in the second twins. BJOG: An International Journal of Obstetrics and Gynaecology. 2002;**109**(1):63-67

[49] Hjorto S, Nickelsen C, Petersen J, Secher NJ. The effect of chorionicity and twin-to-twin delivery time interval on short-term outcome of the second twin. The Journal of Maternal-Fetal & Neonatal Medicine. 2014;**27**(1):42-47

[50] Lindroos L, Elfvin A, Ladfors L, Wennerholm UB. The effect of twin-to-twin delivery time intervals on neonatal outcome for second twins. BMC Pregnancy and Childbirth. 2018;**18**:36

[51] Rydhström H, Ingemarsson I. Interval between birth of the first and the second twin and its impact on second twin perinatal mortality. Journal of Perinatal Medicine. 1990;**18**:449

[52] Feys S, Jacquemyn Y. Delayed-interval delivery can save the second twin: Evidence from a systematic review. Facts, Views & Vision in ObGyn. 2016;**8**:223

[53] Barrett JF, Hannah ME, Hutton EK, et al. A randomized trial of planned cesarean or vaginal delivery for twin pregnancy. The New England Journal of Medicine. 2013;**369**:1295

[54] American College of Obstetricians and Gynecologists, Society for Maternal-Fetal Medicine. Obstetric care consensus no. 1: Safe prevention of the primary cesarean delivery. Obstetrics and Gynecology. 2014;**123**:693-711

[55] Hammad IA, Chauhan SP, Magann EF, Abuhamad AZ. Peripartum complications with cesarean delivery: A review of maternal-fetal medicine units network publications. The Journal of Maternal-Fetal & Neonatal Medicine. 2014;**27**:463

[56] Hutton EK, Hannah ME, Ross S, et al. Maternal outcomes at 3 months after planned caesarean section versus planned vaginal birth for twin pregnancies in the twin birth study: A randomised controlled trial. BJOG. 2015;**122**:1653

[57] Marshall NE, Fu R, Guise JM. Impact of multiple cesarean deliveries on maternal morbidity: A systematic review. American Journal of Obstetrics and Gynecology. 2011;**205**:262.e1

[58] Moore HC, de Klerk N, Holt P, et al. Hospitalisation for bronchiolitis in infants is more common after elective caesarean delivery. Archives of Disease in Childhood. 2012;**97**:410

[59] Black M, Bhattacharya S, Philip S, et al. Planned cesarean delivery at term and adverse outcomes in childhood health. JAMA. 2015;**314**:2271

[60] Bager P, Wohlfahrt J, Westergaard T. Caesarean delivery and risk of atopy and allergic disease: Meta-analyses. Clinical and Experimental Allergy. 2008;**38**:634

[61] Asztalos EV, Hannah ME, Hutton EK, et al. Twin birth study: 2-year neurodevelopmental follow-up of the randomized trial of planned cesarean or planned vaginal delivery for twin pregnancy. American Journal of Obstetrics and Gynecology. 2016;**214**:371.e1

4

Historical Studies of Hellin's Law

Johan Fellman

Abstract

Theorems, proofs, laws and rules are commonly named according to the presumed discoverer, but often earlier investigators have contributed substantially to the findings. One example of this is Hellin's law, which was named after Hellin, although he was not the first to derive it. In research on twinning and higher multiple maternities, the law has played a central role because it is approximately correct, despite showing discrepancies that are difficult to explain or eliminate. However, most studies are based on empirical rates of multiple maternities. Such studies can only serve to identify errors too large to be characterized as random. It has been mathematically proven that Hellin's law does not hold as a general rule. Consequently, improvements to this law have been proposed.

Keywords: twinning rates, triplet rates, quadruplet rates, Stigler's law, maternal age, temporal trends

1. Introduction

During the history of research on multiple maternities, Hellin's law has been applied as a rule of thumb. Consequently, the law contributes to the description of the twinning models. In this paper, we consider how Hellin's law can be tested and used. It is of particular interest to determine why the rates of higher multiple maternities are sometimes too high or too low when Hellin's law is used as a benchmark. The analysis of Fellman and Eriksson [1] of triplet and quadruplet rates indicated that triplet rates are closer to Hellin's law than quadruplet rates. According to the analyses by Fellman and Eriksson [2] of the twinning rate and the transformed triplet rate and quadruplet rate for Sweden (1751–2000), both triplet and quadruplet rates showed excesses after the 1960s. This is mainly caused by the influence of the artificial reproduction technologies, particularly the use of fertility-enhancing drugs. Fellman and Eriksson [2] introduced measures of concordance between triplet rates with Hellin's law.

Regression analyses of twinning and triplet rates yield rather good fits with respect to Hellin's law, but deficiencies in the triplet rates are commonly present. According to Hellin's law, historical data show deficiencies in triplet rates, but recent data reveal excesses, especially among older mothers. The excesses obtained are in good agreement with other studies of recent data. Here, we pay special attention to the use of Hellin's law in investigations of multiple maternities.

2. Prerequisites for twinning research

In the nineteenth century, a series of statistical congresses, most notable in Brussels in 1853 and in St. Petersburg in 1872, was important for the start of demographic research and especially twinning research [3]. Levi [4] gave a detailed presentation of the suggestions accepted at the congress in Brussels.

> *[T]here ought to be an annual registry of population, exhibiting the births by sex, by age of both parents, legitimate and illegitimate, number of twins, stillborn, marriages and divorces, by months. The deaths, by sex, by age, and by months, distinguishing among dead children, till three years of age, the legitimate from the illegitimate. The deaths by month, with the causes of death, and the profession of the deceased; marriages, with the age of the parties, their condition, profession, and number of children, distinguishing the legitimate and those acknowledged as such. Considering the extreme importance of a uniform nomenclature of diseases equally applicable to all countries, the attention of learned men is to be called to the question for further consideration at some future congress.*

According to Brown [5], the principal discussion at the St. Petersburg congress centred around facts relating to the movement of the population and the mode in which they should be registered. Among the facts to be registered were in multiple maternities the sex and number of the children, stillborn or born alive, whether legitimate or not and the age and parity of the mother on the birth date.

Westergaard [6] has devoted a whole chapter in his history of statistics to the presentations of the statistical congresses in the middle of the nineteenth century and their importance [1]. The first congress was held in Brussels in 1853. Brussels was chosen as the first meeting place because the Belgian Central Commission undertook the great preparatory work. The congress was held under the presidency of Adolphe Quetelet. The aim of the congress being chiefly a practical one, there was no room for lectures on special scientific problems. During congresses after Brussels, discordance increased among the European countries, and thus, the International Statistical Congress came to an end.

Recently, Droesbeke [7] gave a short but detailed presentation of the planning and findings of the Brussels congress and subsequent international statistical congresses. His text agrees the ideas of Westergaard [6]. A commission was created in March 1841 as a first step towards the realization of the congress. The president of the Central Commission of Statistics, Adolphe Quetelet, played a central role in the planning process. Quetelet was held in high esteem in London since 1833, when he had taken part in the congress of the British Association for the

Advancement of Science, at the end of which he had contributed to the creation of a section devoted to statistics. The idea to organize a congress, the main objective of which was to lay down a common foundation for statistical data to enable international comparisons, was presented by Quetelet 1851. He offered to

> *bring together at a congress in Brussels the persons, who in various countries, are dealing specifically with statistics, in order to give their works a common impulse, and to adopt, for the computations, uniform grounds which will allow for comparison of observations and results. (Bulletin of the Commission, 1853, p. 106).*

Furthermore, Droesbeke describes the congress programme and stressed the content of the congress according to Quetelet's words:

> *It is to be hoped that the works which belongs to this science will now be taken on, in every State, following the bases which have been laid down during the Congress of Brussels. It is not any more a theoretical wish, to see the states adopt uniform bases for scientific works in order to make the results comparable; the opportunity of implementation of the idea has been proclaimed; the framework has been chosen and the reading of the report [...] will demonstrate what is allowed to expect from the wisdom, maturity, perfect intelligence and good harmony which presided over the deliberations of the Congress.*

Finally, Droesbeke listed the Statistical Congresses during the nineteenth century that followed the first one in Brussels.

Recently, Randeraad [8] directed attention to and even criticism of the international statistical congresses in the second half of the nineteenth century. He stated that it would be overly simplistic to assume that they were an outright success. In fact, no more congresses were held after 1876. Furthermore, he stressed that:

> *More importantly, by then it was clear that the aspirations of the early congresses had been too high. International uniformity in statistics was evidently not a goal that could be reached overnight. Much of this failure to bring about rapid change can be explained by the difficulties in realizing effective knowledge transfers, in other words effective communication, in an age that was not fully prepared for truly international activities. It has been shown that the second half of the nineteenth century was a period of numerous experiments in internationalism, but at the same time rampant nationalism nipped many initiatives in the bud.*

In most countries, the registers were deemed lacking in essential facts; those of Belgium and Sweden were perhaps the most detailed for scientific inquiries [3]. Arosenius [9] presented a detailed study of the emergence of the official statistics of Sweden. His presentation shows just how difficult the development of the process is until an official statistics of modern proficiency is born.

Already in the eighteenth century, Wargentin published demographic data for Sweden. However, he did not pay any attention to twinning and higher multiple maternities [10]. Berg [11] published a comprehensive study of multiple maternities. He analyzed the rates of multiple maternities in Sweden from 1776 to 1878. He also presented corresponding data for several

European countries and analyzed the sex combinations of twin, triplet and quadruplet sets in Sweden from 1869 to 1878. His study was published in Swedish, and thus, few scientists were aware of this paper. Since Swedish is the native language of our group, Berg's results have been of great value in our studies [1, 12–14].

During the second half of the nineteenth century, Statistics Sweden published in the journal Statistisk Tidskrift an extensive time series of demographic data. The data were given separately for different counties of Sweden and contained the size of the population, the number of births (live and stillborn) and twin, triplet and quadruplet sets. A list of these data was given in **Table 1** in [1], indicating that Sweden has overall the oldest continuous population statistics worldwide. Our group has used these data in different studies [1, 15].

County (Län)	Period	Reference
Stockholm city	1749–1858	ST, 1860–62:43–47
Stockholm county	1749–1773, 1795–1858	ST, 1860–62:134–141
Uppsala	1749–1773, 1795–1859	ST, 1860–62:280–288
Södermanland	1749–1773, 1795–1859	ST, 1860–62:317–324
Östergötland	1749–1773, 1795–1860	ST, 1863–65:164–171
Jönköping	1749–1773, 1795–1862	ST, 1863–65:266–273
Kronoberg	1749–1773, 1795–1862	ST, 1863–65:274–281
Kalmar	1749–1773, 1795–1868	ST, 1870:211–220
Gotland	1759–1869	ST, 1870:27:221–231
Blekinge	1749–1773, 1795–1869	ST, 1870:232–240
Kristianstad	1749–1773, 1795–1871	ST, 1873:133–142
Malmöhus	1749–1773, 1795–1871	ST, 1873:143–152
Halland	1749–1773, 1795–1871	ST, 1873:153–162
Göteborg and Bohus	1749–1773, 1795–1859	ST, 1860–62:388–400
Älvsborg	1749–1773, 1795–1874	ST, 1875:127–136
Skaraborg	1749–1773, 1795–1876	ST, 1877:156–168
Värmland	1795–1865	ST, 1877:170–176
Örebro (Närke)	1749–1773	ST, 1877:166–169
Västmanland	1749–1773, 1795–1887	ST, 1888:159–170
Kopparberg	1749–1773, 1795–1887	ST, 1888:171–182
Gävleborg	1749–1773, 1795–1887	ST, 1888:161–172
Västernorrland	1792–1888	ST, 1888:173–184
Jämtland	1792–1888	ST, 1888:185–196
Västerbotten	1802–1860	ST, 1863–65:50–57
Norrbotten	1802–1860	ST, 1863–65:44–49

Table 1. The Division of Sweden into 25 counties for regional data concerning population size, births and multiple maternities, 1749–1888 (ST = Statistisk Tidskrift) [1].

3. Genesis of Hellin's law

The Veit data set from Prussia (1826–1849), presented by Fellman and Eriksson [1] in **Table 2**, consists of 13,360,557 maternities, including 13,208,868 single, 149,964 twin, 1689 triplet and 36 quadruplet maternities [16]. Veit analyzed the temporal trend in the twinning rate (TWR) and noted very small variations, but during the first half of the period, the annual TWRs were almost constantly higher than during the last half of the period (except for the year 1849). The trend may be seen elsewhere ([1], **Table 2** and **Figure 1**). For the total data set, Veit noted the following rates: for twin pairs 1:89, for triplet sets 1:7910 and for quadruplet sets 1:371126. He did not give the relations between TWR, triplet rate (TRR) and quadruplet rate (QUR), that is,

			Maternities		
Year	**All**	**Single**	**Twin**	**Triplet**	**Quadruplet**
1826	519,633	513,727	5824	80	2
1827	485,165	479,724	5374	65	2
1828	493,749	488,060	5620	69	0
1829	489,604	483,796	5738	69	1
1830	491,659	486,141	5455	62	1
1831	484,889	479,281	5543	65	0
1832	476,035	470,175	5783	76	1
1833	530,954	524,525	6340	87	2
1834	549,750	542,947	6717	83	3
1835	527,148	521,156	5918	73	1
1836	544,177	537,805	6301	69	2
1837	551,450	545,084	6289	77	0
1838	560,086	553,837	6186	61	2
1839	568,487	562,065	6360	59	3
1840	580,747	574,293	6381	72	1
1841	585,085	578,738	6277	67	3
1842	616,845	610,058	6716	71	0
1843	597,912	591,420	6426	64	2
1844	616,287	609,452	6771	59	5
1845	640,214	633,123	7029	60	2
1846	619,727	613,101	6556	69	1
1847	577,007	570,766	6183	58	0
1848	570,737	564,633	6030	73	1
1849	683,210	674,961	8147	101	1
Total	13,360,557	13,208,868	149,964	1689	36

Table 2. Data from Prussia, 1826–1849, according to Veit (1855) [16].

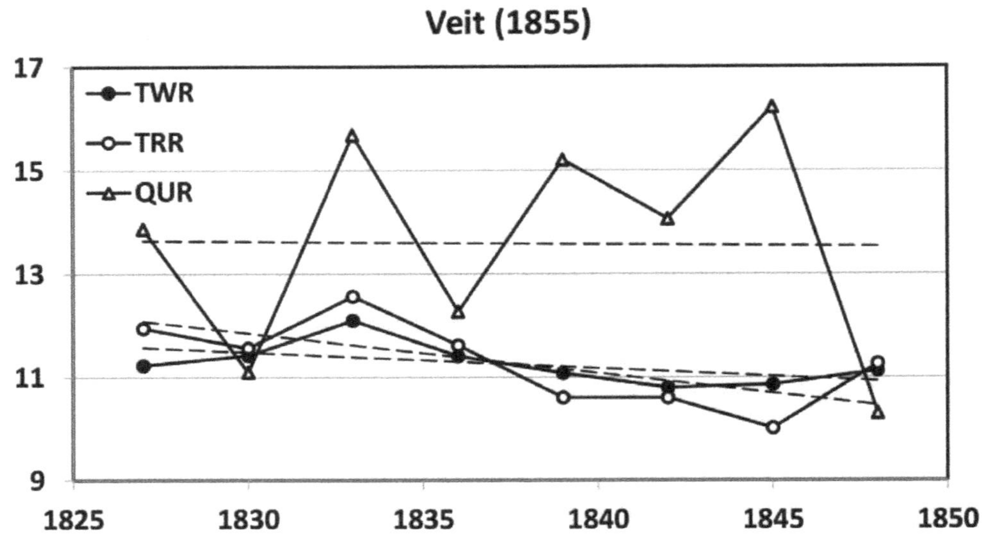

Figure 1. Temporal trends in TWR and transformed TRR and QUR per 10^3 for the Prussian data presented in [16]. Note the excess among QUR.

Hellin's law. He also presented the sex compositions within the twin, triplet and quadruplet sets and noted a lower sex ratio (males to females) among multiple births than among singleton births [1].

The Wappäus data set was collected from different European countries and comprised 19,698,322 maternities, including 226,807 twin and 2623 triplet maternities [1]. Wappäus [17] presented the rates of multiple maternities, but did not discuss the relation between the number of twin, triplet and quadruplet maternities [1].

Bertillon [18] foresaw Hellin's law. He considered multiple maternity data from different countries in central Europe. In his study, he presented the number of triplet maternities per year and per one million total maternities. He also presented the number of total maternities per one triplet maternity and the number of twin maternities per one triplet maternity, i.e., he considered the relation between twin and triplet rates. However, he did not relate the number of total maternities to one twin maternity. Fellman and Eriksson [1] presented a translated version of his table ([18], page 285) and included in columns calculations of the number of total maternities in relation to one twin maternity and the annual mean number of maternities. They believed that had Bertillon included the first of their columns in his table, he would have discovered Hellin's law [1].

Shortly after the congresses in Brussels and St. Petersburg, Neefe [19] published his classical work. He emphasized how important the abovementioned statistical congresses were for the standardization of the demographic registers in different countries, and he used the new possibilities that the improved birth registers offered. Although other contemporaneous studies were published, Fellman and Eriksson [1] stressed that the history of twinning research starts with this publication. Neefe analyzed a long series of problems connected to twinning; these problems have been shown to be central in later studies. He considered inter alia:

1. The rates of twin and higher multiple maternities.
2. The crude birth rates among single and multiple maternities.
3. The regional and seasonal variations in TWRs.
4. The rates of live and stillbirths among twins.
5. The sex composition of sets of multiple maternities.
6. The sex ratio among single and multiple maternities.
7. The effect on the number of multiple maternities of the age of the parents, the marital status and confession of faith of mothers, the residence in urban and rural regions, and the seasonality of the birth.

In addition, he considered weight and prematurity among multiples and mortality among multiples and mothers. This list indicates clearly that Neefe introduced a thorough research programme for twinning studies. It is noteworthy that Neefe did not comment on the relation between the rates of multiple maternities, and consequently, he did not explicitly foretell Hellin's law [1].

Strassmann [20] noted the findings in [16, 17] and concluded, using Veit's total data set, that there is one twin maternity per 89^1 and one triplet maternity per 89^2 total maternities. Strassmann related the number of multiple maternities to the number of all maternities, in contrast to Hellin [21], who related the number of multiple maternities to the number of single maternities. However, both used the same relation, 1:89 [1]. While in the literature authors generally refer to Hellin, they formulate the law according to Strassmann's version. While in the literature authors generally refer to Hellin, the law was already formulated by Strassmann in 1889. Hellin's law has played a central role in the history of research on multiple maternities [3].

Drejer [22] was apparently unaware of Hellin but referred to Strassmann, stating that he had noted the relation between the rates of twin and triplet maternities. Drejer was dubious about the regularity between the rates. He stressed that under such circumstances the rule had to hold also for higher multiple maternities, but he could not find any clear indication of this being the case [1].

Particularly important scientific observations are often associated with a person, but historians of science have, however, noted that often the person associated with a particular finding was not its original discoverer. Scientific observations and results are frequently associated with people who have high visibility and social status, and the results are named long after the discovery. Based on his studies on the history of statistics, Stigler [23] proposed his own *Stigler's law of eponymy*. In brief, the law says: "No scientific discovery is named after its original discoverer". Stigler himself attributes the discovery of Stigler's law to Merton [24], which makes the law self-referencing. Consequently, in this study, one must bear in mind Stigler's law [1].

4. Investigations of Hellin's law

Hellin's law has played a central role in the history of research on multiple maternities. The interest in Hellin's law is mainly the result of its being mathematically simple and approximately correct, but it shows discrepancies that are difficult to explain or eliminate. Statistical studies on empirical rates of multiple maternities can never confirm the law but serve only to identify errors too large to be characterized as random. It is of particular interest to ask why the rates of higher orders of multiple maternities are sometimes too high and sometimes too low when Hellin's law is used as a benchmark [32].

Usually, the arguments for Hellin's law are based on stochastic models for multiple fertilizations and fissions of fertilized eggs. The influence of both multiple fertilizations and fissions of fertilized eggs has inspired scientists to associate the rates of higher multiple maternities with both monozygotic (MZ) and dizygotic (DZ) TWRs (e.g., [25–30]). The contributions by Zeleny [25] have resulted in the law also being known as the Hellin-Zeleny law.

Peller [31] was the first, at least indirectly, to connect Hellin's law to interindividual variation in mothers' chances for multiple maternities. Later, Eriksson [12] considered recurrent twin maternities in families on the Åland Islands (Finland) and presented a modified model (in the paper, the law was called Fellman's law). When Eriksson applied this law to his Åland data, he obtained better congruence with Hellin's law than if Peller's version had been applied. Fellman and Eriksson [1] reviewed papers where the genesis of Hellin's law was traced and where the strengths and weaknesses of the law were analyzed and improvements suggested [32].

Hellin's law presupposes strong correlations between TWR and TRR, but even strong correlations do not prove Hellin's law, establishing only a linear relationship. Fellman and Eriksson [30] considered the correlation between the TWR and the square root of the TRR in Sweden. After elimination of influential temporal factors, they found that the correlation was positive, but not very strong. This finding indicates that, in general, Hellin's law cannot be exact. One application of Hellin's law is to compare TWR and the square root of TRR, the cubic root of QUR and so on [14, 32, 33].

In the following, we consider formulae applicable in the statistical analysis of Hellin's law. Let the theoretical TRR be r. One has different possibilities to study the random errors of the TRR and particularly of the square root of the TRR. The first one is to estimate the standard deviations (SDs) of the TRR and construct confidence intervals (CIs) for r [32].

Let the observed TRR be $\widehat{r}$, then SD $\widehat{r} = \sqrt{\frac{r(1-r)}{n}}$, and the observed standard CI of r is

$$\left(\widehat{r} - \mathrm{k}\sqrt{\frac{\widehat{r}(1-\widehat{r})}{n}},\ \widehat{r} + \mathrm{k}\sqrt{\frac{\widehat{r}(1-\widehat{r})}{n}}\right) \tag{1}$$

where the factor k defines the confidence level. The Hellin-transformed TRR is $\sqrt{\widehat{r}}$. The variance of $\sqrt{\widehat{r}}$ is

$$\mathrm{Var}\left(\sqrt{\widehat{r}}\right) = \left(\frac{d}{dr}\left(\sqrt{r}\right)\right)^2 \mathrm{Var}\left(\widehat{r}\right) = \left(\frac{1}{2\sqrt{r}}\right)^2 \frac{r(1-r)}{n} = \left(\frac{1}{4r}\right)\frac{r(1-r)}{n} = \left(\frac{1-r}{4n}\right) \tag{2}$$

Fellman and Eriksson [34] proposed an alternative transformation $\arcsin(\sqrt{r})$. For small values of r, the difference between the two transformations is minute. The variance of $\arcsin\left(\sqrt{\hat{r}}\right)$ is

$$\mathrm{Var}\left(\arcsin\left(\sqrt{\hat{r}}\right)\right) = \left(\frac{\mathrm{d}}{\mathrm{dr}}\arcsin\left(\sqrt{r}\right)\right)^2 \mathrm{Var}\left(\hat{r}\right) =$$

$$\left(\frac{1}{2\sqrt{r}\sqrt{1-r}}\right)^2 \frac{r(1-r)}{n} = \left(\frac{1}{4r(1-r)}\right)\frac{r(1-r)}{n} = \left(\frac{1}{4n}\right) \tag{3}$$

The variance of $\arcsin\left(\sqrt{\hat{r}}\right)$ is slightly larger than the variance of $\sqrt{\hat{r}}$, but it is simpler and does not depend on r. Consider the difference

$$\arcsin\left(\sqrt{r}\right) - \sqrt{r} = \sqrt{r} + \frac{1}{2}\frac{r^{\frac{3}{2}}}{3} + \frac{1\times 2}{3\times 4}\frac{r^{\frac{5}{2}}}{5} + \ldots - \sqrt{r} = \frac{1}{2}\frac{r^{\frac{3}{2}}}{3} + \frac{1\times 2}{3\times 4}\frac{r^{\frac{5}{2}}}{5} + \ldots \approx \frac{1}{6}r\sqrt{r} \tag{4}$$

and $\frac{\arcsin(\sqrt{r})-\sqrt{r}}{\sqrt{r}} \approx \frac{r}{6}$. This relative difference between the transformed variables is of the dimension 10^{-4}. The square root is a monotone-increasing function, and consequently, one can construct the CI for $\sqrt{r}$ by a square root transformation of the limits of the CI for r. Hence, for $\sqrt{r}$ the corresponding transformed CI is

$$\left(\sqrt{\hat{r}} - \mathrm{k}\sqrt{\frac{1-\hat{r}}{4n}},\ \sqrt{\hat{r}} + \mathrm{k}\sqrt{\frac{1-\hat{r}}{4n}}\right) \tag{5}$$

Fellman and Eriksson [34] gave a mathematical proof that Hellin's law cannot hold in general. If one aggregates heterogeneous data, the fluctuations are smoothed out, but according to Hellin's law, the relation between the TWR and the TRR is not linear, and consequently, the aggregated and disaggregated data cannot simultaneously satisfy Hellin's law [1].

Jenkins [26, 35], Jenkins and Gwin [27], Bulmer [29] and later Fellman and Eriksson [30] have tried to modify the law in order to improve it. Using linear curves is the best method for identifying discrepancies from a presumptive model because graphs containing linear curves are easy to interpret. There are two possibilities for checking Hellin's law with linear curves. One is to use graphs with TWR^2 as abscissa and TRR as ordinate, that is, to use the model $\mathrm{TRR} = \alpha + \beta\mathrm{TWR}^2$. An alternative is graphs with TWR as abscissa and $\sqrt{\mathrm{TRR}}$ as ordinate. Now, the model is $\sqrt{\mathrm{TRR}} = \alpha + \beta\mathrm{TWR}$ [1].

Jenkins and Gwin [27] considered US data for the periods 1923–1924 and 1927–1936. They used TWR^2 as abscissa and TRR as ordinate. From their figure, they obtained the linear relation $\mathrm{TRR} = 0.000013 + 0.656\mathrm{TWR}^2$. The intercept indicated that the line did not pass through the origin and the parameter estimate was markedly below the value one, indicating a deficit in triplet sets. When Fellman and Eriksson [32] applied a regression model to the same data set, they obtained the slightly different result: $\mathrm{TRR} = 0.000039 + 0.584\mathrm{TWR}^2$. The coefficient of determination is $R^2 = 0.842$, indicating a rather good fit. They obtained a deficit in the TRR when they tested the parameter estimate against one with a one-sided t test. The $\mathrm{SE}\left(\widehat{\beta}\right) = 0.113$ yielded $t = -3.7$, and the estimate was significantly below one [1]. As an alternative model, Fellman and Eriksson used TWR as abscissa and $\sqrt{\mathrm{TRR}}$ as ordinate. The estimated model was $\sqrt{\mathrm{TRR}} = 0.0029 + 0.679\mathrm{TWR}$ and $R^2 = 0.844$, $\mathrm{SE}\left(\widehat{\beta}\right) = 0.130$ and $t = -2.5$, and the obtained estimate is significantly below one. Both alternatives indicate deficits in the TRR. The parameter estimates are slightly higher for the first model, but the goodness of fit for both models is comparable. Their analyses confirm the results given in [27].

Jenkins and Gwin [27] also considered data from Finland (1878–1916). They used the data given by Dahlberg [36]. However, Fellman and Eriksson [32] performed a check based on Finnish official registers and confirmed their suspicion that Dahlberg's data contained a misprint for the maternal age group 35 to 40 years. In the analyses, they used the corrected data and present the results in **Figure 7** in [32]. When they applied the linear model to the Finnish data, they obtained the results $\mathrm{TRR} = 0.00003 + 0.742\mathrm{TWR}^2$ and $R^2 = 0.930$. The $SE\left(\widehat{\beta}\right) = 0.091$, $t = -2.8$, and the obtained estimate is significantly below one. The linear relation between $\sqrt{\mathrm{TRR}}$ and TWR is $\sqrt{\mathrm{TRR}} = 0.0026 + 0.768\mathrm{TWR}$ with $R^2 = 0.906$. The $\mathrm{SE}\left(\widehat{\beta}\right) = 0.111$ and $t = -2.1$, and the obtained estimate is significantly below one. All of these results indicate good fit but deficits in triplet maternities [32].

The discrepancies between the results concerning Finnish data given by Fellman and Eriksson and Jenkins and Gwin were mainly caused by two facts; Jenkins and Gwin did not use regression models, but a geometric attempt, and they excluded in their analyses the extreme TRR for the age group 45+ years. In addition, they did not perform any statistical tests. Fellman and Eriksson [32] introduced measures to check both Hellin's law and Jenkins' [35] model in formula (6). They introduced the ratio $\mathrm{HR} = \mathrm{TRR}/\mathrm{TWR}^2$ named Hellin's ratio and assumed that it is a measure of the agreement with respect to Hellin's law. If $\mathrm{HR} > 1$, there is an excess, but if $\mathrm{HR} < 1$, there is a deficit in the TRR. An alternative measure is based on Jenkins' model [32]:

$$\mathrm{J} = \mathrm{TRR} = \frac{1}{n}\sum_{\mathrm{i}} \mathrm{TWR}_{\mathrm{i}}^2 n_{\mathrm{i}} \tag{6}$$

Fellman and Eriksson [29] defined Jenkins' ratio as $JR = \mathrm{TRR}/\mathrm{J}$, where TRR is the total triplet rate. If $\mathrm{JR} > 1$, there are excesses, and if $\mathrm{JR} < 1$, there are deficits in the TRRs. Hellin's ratio can be defined for both age-specific and total rates, but Jenkins' ratio applies only to total rates. In addition, Eq. (6) indicates that JR can be calculated only for data grouped according to maternal age. Based on Schwarz's inequality, a comparison between HR for the total set of maternities and JR yields [32].

$$(\mathrm{TWR})^2 = \left(\frac{1}{n}\sum_{i}(\mathrm{TWR}_{\mathrm{i}})n_{\mathrm{i}}\right)^2 \le \frac{1}{n}\sum_{i}\left(\mathrm{TWR}_{\mathrm{i}}{}^2 n_i\right)\frac{1}{n}\sum_{i} n_{\mathrm{i}} = \mathrm{J}.$$

Equality is obtained if and only if

$$\frac{\mathrm{TWR_i}\sqrt{n_\mathrm{i}}}{\sqrt{n_\mathrm{i}}} = \mathrm{TWR_i}$$

for all i. Consequently,

$$\mathrm{HR} = \frac{\mathrm{TRR}}{(\mathrm{TWR})^2} \geq \frac{\mathrm{TRR}}{\mathrm{J}} = \mathrm{JR}.$$

The following step is a simple analysis of the data to show that the transformations may cause excesses in the transformed TRRs and QURs. Fellman and Eriksson [29] simplified their studies by ignoring any random effects. Assume that after the fertilization and any fissions of the fertilized egg, the twinning rate is w_0, the triplet rate is r_0 and the quadruplet rate is q_0, and assume that Hellin's law holds for these rates [32]. Consequently, $r_0 = w_0^2$ and $q_0 = w_0^3$. During pregnancy the rates may decrease, and let the relative reductions be c_w, c_r and c_q for the twinning, triplet and quadruplet rates, respectively. An obvious assumption is that $c_\mathrm{w} \leq c_\mathrm{r} \leq c_\mathrm{q}$. At birth, the observed rates are.

$w = w_0(1 - c_\mathrm{w})$, $r = w_0^2(1 - c_\mathrm{r})$ and $q = w_0^3(1 - c_\mathrm{q})$,

and the variables w, r and q do not satisfy Hellin's law. A fundamental question is whether excesses in the transformed rates of triplets and quadruplets are possible. Compare $w = w_0(1 - c_\mathrm{w})$ and the transformed rates $\sqrt{r} = w_0\sqrt{(1 - c_\mathrm{r})}$ and $\sqrt[3]{q} = w_0\sqrt[3]{(1 - c_\mathrm{q})}$.

An excess for the triplet rate is obtained if $\sqrt{(1 - c_\mathrm{r})} > (1 - c_\mathrm{w})$,

that is, $c_\mathrm{r} < 2c_\mathrm{w} - c_\mathrm{w}^2 \approx 2c_\mathrm{w}$.

An excess for the quadruplet rate is obtained if $\sqrt[3]{(1 - c_\mathrm{q})} > (1 - c_\mathrm{w})$,

that is, $c_\mathrm{q} < 3c_\mathrm{w} - 3c_\mathrm{w}^2 + c_\mathrm{w}^3 \approx 3c_\mathrm{w}$.

These conditions are conceivable, and if the relative reductions in the triplet and quadruplet rates are not too strong, excesses are possible. If one speculates about these results, the extreme excesses observed for transformed quadruplet rates compared with triplet rates, would be explained by the fact that $c_\mathrm{q} < 3c_\mathrm{w}$ is more likely than $c_\mathrm{r} < 2c_\mathrm{w}$ [32]. Consequently, the transformations should be applied with caution and used only for descriptive purposes and not for comparisons between the levels of twinning, triplet and quadruplet rates.

5. Studies including the use of Hellin's law

Fellman and Eriksson [1, 2, 32] presented the temporal trends in TWR, the square root of TRR and the cubic root of QUR obtained from the Veit data [16]. Note that their figure shows stronger fluctuations in TRR than in TWR. However, the confidence bands included indicate that the TWR and the transformed TRR show good agreement for the whole period. The transformed QUR is too high for almost the whole period [32]. In **Figure 1**, we present a new version of the TWR, the transformed TRR and QUR per 10^3 for the Prussian data presented in [16]. In this figure and later, the transformed TRR and QUR per 10^3 are denoted by the initial untransformed names TRR and QUR. Note that the transformed QUR shows a marked excess compared with the TWR and the transformed TRR. This excess can be connected to the comparisons presented above between the rates from conceptions to deliveries. Furthermore, one can observe that all rates show slightly decreasing trends.

In this study, we investigate the temporal trends in TWR, TRR and QUR. The TRRs and QURs are in all figures transformed according to Hellin's law in order to show the association between TWR, TRR and QUR. In the figures, the transformed variables are still denoted TRR and QUR. The trends show variations during different periods and for different countries, but for different countries, one can observe similar patterns. During the eighteenth and nineteenth centuries, the rates are rather similar, but during the first half of the nineteenth century, there is a deficit in the TRR. During the second half of the twentieth century, the TRR shows an excess, and this finding is mainly caused by the influence of the artificial reproduction technologies, particularly the use of fertility-enhancing drugs. Below, we present graphs for different countries, and similar patterns can be noted.

The temporal trends in the TWR and the transformed TRR in Finland 1751–2000 show variations during different periods. During 1750–1900 the rates are rather similar, but during the period 1900–1970, there is a deficit in the TRR. After 1970, the TRR shows an excess, and this finding is mainly caused by the influence of the artificial reproduction technologies, particularly the use of fertility-enhancing drugs (**Figure 2**).

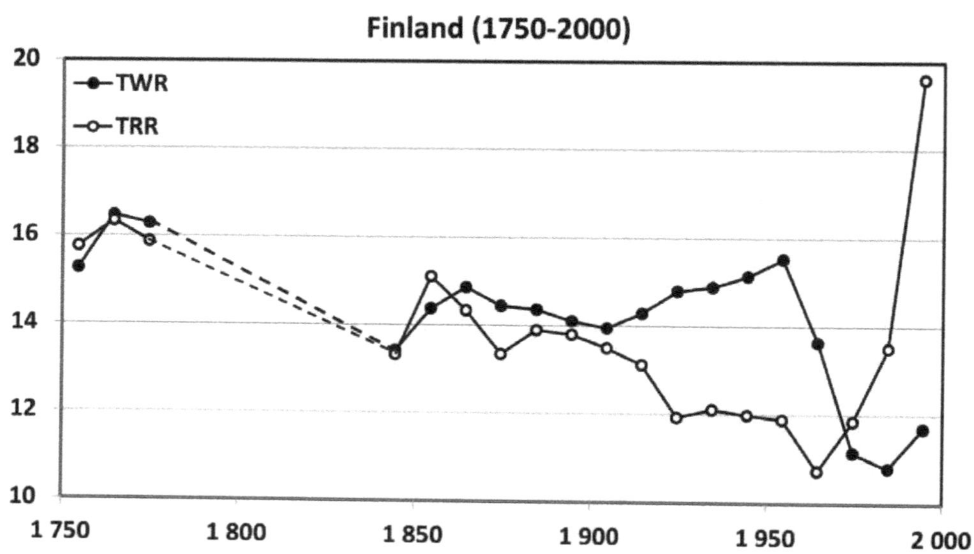

Figure 2. Temporal trends in TWR and transformed TRR in Finland (1751–2000).

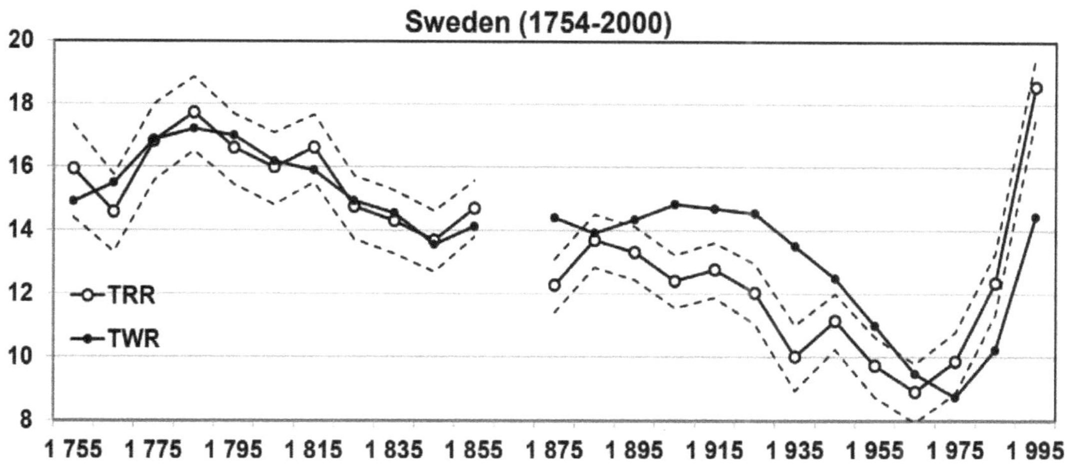

Figure 3. Temporal trends in twinning and triplet rates in Sweden (1751–2000). During 1750–1890 the rates are rather similar, but during the period 1900–1970, there is a deficit in the TRR. After 1970, the TRR shows an excess.

The temporal trends in the twinning and triplet trends in Sweden (1751–2000) are presented in **Figure 3**. During 1750–1890 the rates are rather similar, but during the period 1900–1970, there is a deficit in the TRR. After 1970, the TRR shows an excess.

Following [37] we present in **Figure 4** the temporal trends in the twinning and triplet trends in Portugal (1930–2011). One changing point can be found in 1950. After 1950, TRR shows an excess.

Fellman [3] presented the temporal trends in the twinning and triplet trends in the Netherlands (1950–2003). The findings are given in **Figure 5**. An excess among TRR can be observed after 1970. At the end of the twentieth century, there is a marked deficit in the TRR.

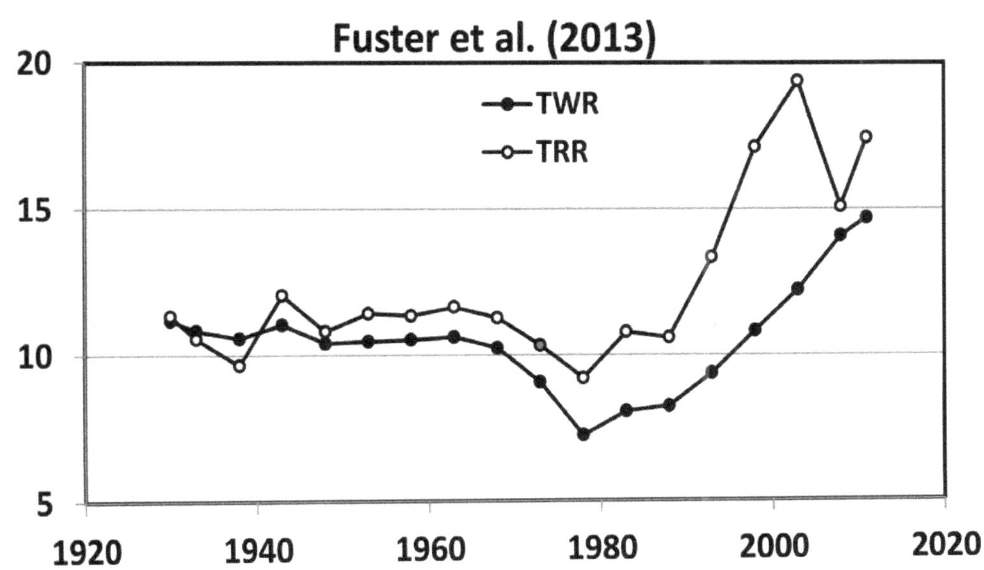

Figure 4. Temporal trends in twinning and triplet trends in Portugal (1930–2011). One changing point can be found at 1950. After 1950, the TRR shows an excess [37].

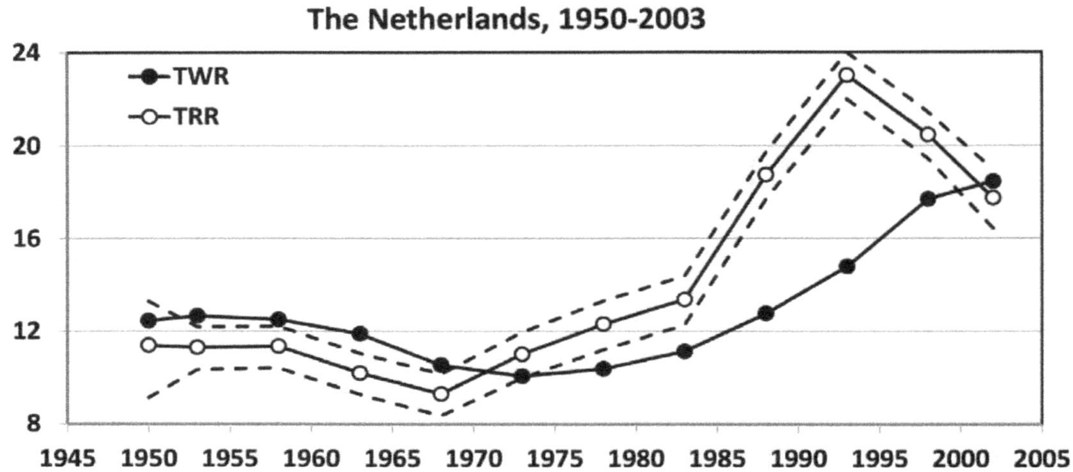

Figure 5. Temporal trends in the twinning and triplet rates in the Netherlands (1950–2003). An excess among TRR can be observed after 1970.

Eriksson and Fellman [33] compared the rates of twin, triplet and quadruplet maternities in England and Wales for the period 1938–2003. In this study, we develop these findings. In **Figure 6**, one observes that before 1970 the graph lines are close to another, but after 1970 the lines rise and diverge. QUR shows the strongest increase and TWR the slightest. Furthermore, **Figure 6** indicates that during the last years, TRR and QUR show a slight decline. Our opinion is that this change is caused by changes in fertilization policies, especially a reduction in the number of fertilized eggs implanted. To clarify the fluctuations, trend lines of sixth degree are included in the figure. Furthermore, **Figure 6** indicates that for data sets after 1970, the TRRs and QURs are markedly too high. It is a remarkable finding that the rates are too high rather

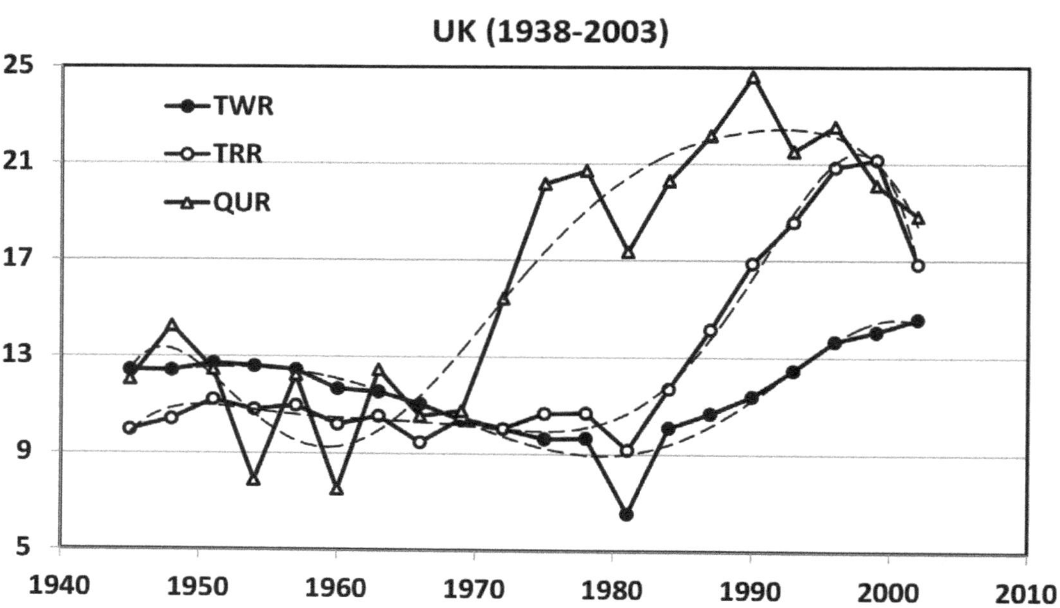

Figure 6. Temporal trends in the twinning, triplet and quadruplet rates in the UK (1938–2003). During 1938–1970 the rates are rather similar, but after 1970 the rates increase. QUR shows the strongest increase and TWR the slightest. In order to clarify the fluctuations, trend lines of sixth degree are included in the figure.

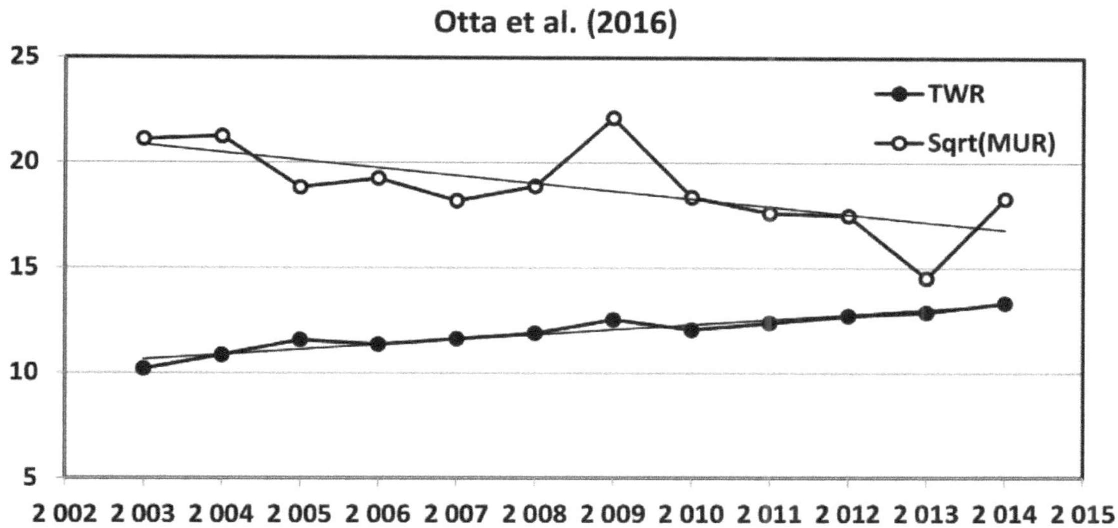

Figure 7. Temporal trends in TWR and the Hellin-transformed rate of multiple maternities (MUR). The figure indicates that the TWR is still increasing, but the transformed MUR is decreasing [38].

than too low, but fertilization policies may result in the extreme sets of multiple maternities. The decreases at the end of the twentieth century are ascribed to changes in the treatment policies discussed above.

Otta et al. [38] analyzed the TWR and the MUR for Brazil data (2003–2014). They discussed the influence of artificial reproduction technologies, particularly the use of fertility-enhancing drugs. They included in their analyses the effect of maternal age. In this study, we look at their data from a different point of view. In **Figure 7**, we present the TWR and the Hellin-transformed rate of multiple maternities (MUR). We assume that the number of multiple maternities is dominated by triplet maternities, and we use the square root transformation. **Figure 7** indicates that the TWR is still increasing, but that the MUR decreases. The excesses coincided with the introduction of subfertility treatments, mainly ovulation inductions. Our opinion is that the difference in the changes between TWR and MUR is caused by changes in fertilization policies, especially a reduction in the number of fertilized eggs implanted. Finally, there is common agreement that discrepancies obtained during the era of fertility treatments are of less interest when Hellin's law is considered because no natural stochastic model is applicable. For the whole period 2003–2014, the TWR = 11.96 per 1000 and MUR = 357.97 per 10^6. Hence, HR = 2.50 indicates a marked excess of multiple maternities.

6. Discussion

A problem that complicates the discussion of Hellin's law is that the law is a mathematical rule concerning theoretical rates, but all checks of the law must be based on empirically obtained rates. In fact, one can only check whether the discrepancies are too large and cannot be explained by random errors. Although the discrepancies are small, Hellin's law cannot be accepted as a theoretical one. In this way, no exact proof to support the law can be obtained [32].

Jenkins ([35], Figure 8) and later Fellman and Eriksson [1] presented the association between the TWRs and the TRRs in the Prussian data [16]. They observed marked fluctuations for the different annual data but a good agreement between the TRR and the TWR for the total data set [32].

Our impression is that the finding already noted by Strassmann [20] was the birth of Hellin's law. Furthermore, Jenkins [35] stressed that Hellin's law is a first approximation. It is generally agreed that the main argument for Hellin's law is that the probabilities of additional ovulations and the fissions of fertilized eggs can be explained by stochastic models. Consequently, in large data sets, the averages could be stable and formulated by a mathematical relation (Hellin's law). A common argument for the discrepancies is that after the conceptions, there is a long process influenced by disturbing factors (intrauterine deaths, spontaneous abortions, etc., of one or more fetuses). Jenkins [35] and Komai and Fukuoka [39], for instance, assumed that differential mortality in utero of twins and triplets could be one such factor. Consequently, the final result often shows only a weak resemblance to the outcome of a simple stochastic process associated with the initial conceptions. Excesses of higher multiple maternities in old birth registers must be considered paradoxical. One explanation can be the results of the comparisons between the changes in the rates of singletons, twins and triplets during the time from conception to confinement discussed above. Another probable explanation is that systematic errors in the registers may cause biases in the data. This explanation is less plausible if the data are collected in different countries, as is the case in data in ([32, 35], **Table 1** and **Figure 1**).

In his study of the rates of multiple maternities for total, "white" and "colored" in US populations (1922–1936), Strandskov [40] evaluated how well his data satisfy Hellin's law. Applying χ^2 tests, he found that in none of the populations tested did the observed plural birth frequencies agree closely with Hellin's law [3].

Based on hospital data, Sarkar [41] studied the TWR in India and on Ceylon (Sri Lanka). His paper is interesting because he defined the TWR as $1 : n$ and the triplet rate as $1 : m^2$, that is, he indirectly used a modified Hellin's law without any reference to Hellin. One finds a deficit of triplet maternities ($m > n$). In addition, one observes that on Ceylon the TWR was low ($1 : 161.1$), yielding a TWR of 6.21 per 1000. On Ceylon, the TRR followed Hellin's law more exactly because it was $1 : 154.4^2$.

Das [42] formulated Hellin's law such that "the frequency of twin confinements bears to that of total confinements a ratio which is equal to the ratio borne by the frequency of the triplet confinements to that of the twin confinements". This modified definition is in congruence with Strassmann's version of the law. He reviewed earlier studies concerning Hellin's law and stressed the discrepancies presented in them [3]. Das concluded that Hellin's law has no sound basis and that exceptions to the rule have been the rule. In a later paper, Das [43] also considered the relation $\text{TRR} = (\text{TWR})^2$. He constructed an advanced model based on the zygosity of both twins and triplets. His mathematical analyses of these models did not support Hellin's law [1].

Fellman and Eriksson [2] compared in **Figure 3** the TWR and the transformed TRR and QUR for Sweden (1751–2000). For the period 1871–1960, there is a deficiency in the TRR. Fellman and Eriksson [32] discuss this deficiency in more detail. There is almost constantly an excess in the QUR for the whole period. After 1970, both the TRR and QUR show excesses, but this is mainly caused by the influence of the artificial reproduction technologies, particularly the use of fertility-enhancing drugs. For references, see [14, 32].

Above the HR is defined as HR = TRR/TWR^2. Agreements between TWR and transformed TRR can show remarkable variations. Eriksson [12] studied the TWR and the TRR in the southwestern part of Finland. On the Åland islands, the TWR was continuously high. For the period 1653–1949, the TWR was 19.21 per 1000, and the TRR was 375 per 10^6. According to Hellin's law, the expected TRR was 369 per 10^6. For the Åland data, HR = 1.02, showing a good agreement with Hellin's law. In the Åboland (Turunmaa in Finnish) archipelago, close to the Åland islands, the TWR was also high. For the period 1655–1949, the TWR was 20.90 per 1000. For the same period, the TRR was 252 per 10^6. According to Hellin's law, the expected TRR was 437 per 10^6, yielding HR = 0.58, and consequently, the Åboland archipelago data showed a marked deficit in TRR with respect to Hellin's law [32].

Lam and Ho [44] noted an increase in the number of multiple maternities in Hong Kong in 1981–1995. They also stressed the marked discrepancy between the observed data and Hellin's law. Zhang et al. [45] have observed similar increases in the rates of multiple maternities among older mothers in the USA in 1995–1997, and they also attributed this finding to the increased use of assisted reproductive technology. Simmons et al. [46] noted a dramatic decrease in the proportion of triplet and higher-order births since 1998 [32].

7. Conclusion

It is generally agreed that the main argument for Hellin's law is that the probabilities of additional ovulations and the fissions of fertilized eggs can be explained by stochastic models. Consequently, in large data sets, the averages could be stable and formulated by a mathematical relation (Hellin's law). A common argument for the discrepancies is that after the conceptions, there is a long process influenced by disturbing factors (intrauterine deaths, spontaneous abortions, etc., of one or more fetuses) [32]. The discussion of Hellin's law is complicated by the fact that the law is a mathematical rule concerning theoretical rates, but all checks have to be based on empirically obtained rates. In fact, one can only check if the discrepancies are so large that they cannot be explained by random errors. If the discrepancies are small, an exact Hellin's law cannot be accepted. In this way, no exact proof to support the law can be obtained [32].

Acknowledgements

This work was supported in part by grants from the Magnus Ehrnrooth Foundation. I am very grateful to the personnel of the National Library of Health Sciences, University of Helsinki

(Terkko), for providing copies of old publications concerning twin studies in the nineteenth century, otherwise difficult to obtain.

Author details

Johan Fellman

Address all correspondence to: fellman@hanken.fi

Hanken School of Economics, Helsinki, Finland

References

[1] Fellman J, Eriksson AW. The history of Hellin's law. Twin Research and Human Genetics. 2009;**12**:183-190

[2] Fellman J, Eriksson AW. Temporal variation in rates of multiple maternities in Sweden (1751-2000). JP Journal of Biostatistics. 2014;**11**(2):143-156

[3] Fellman J. Aspects on the history of twin research: Statistical congresses in the 19th century and Hellin's law. Twin Research and Human Genetics. 2017;**21**(1):57-66

[4] Levi L. Resume of the Statistical Congress, held at Brussels, September 11th, 1853, for the Purpose of Introducing Unity in the Statistical Documents of all Countries. Journal of the Statistical Society of London. 1854;**17**(1):14

[5] Brown S. Report on the Eighth International Statistical Congress, St. Petersburg, August, 1872. Journal of the Statistical Society of London. 1872;**35**:431-457

[6] Westergaard H. Contribution to the history of statistics. London: PS King and Son; 1932

[7] Droesbeke JJ. Personal communication. About the First International Statistical Meeting (Brussels – 1853). 4 pp

[8] Randeraad N. The International Statistical Congress (1853-1876): Knowledge Transfers and their Limits. European History Quarterly. 2011;**41**:50-65

[9] Arosenius E. The History of Organization of Swedish Official Statistics. In: The History of Statistics. Their Development and Progress in Many Countries. The Macmillan Company of New York: The American Statistical Association; 1918. pp. 537-569

[10] Hofsten E. Pehr Wargentin och grundandet av den svenska befolkningsstatistiken [Pehr Wargentin and the foundation of the Swedish population statistics], 11–58. In: Pehr Wargentin den svenska statistikens fader [Pehr Wargentin the father of the Swedish Statistics], Borås; 1983. 180 pp

[11] Berg FT. Om flerfostriga barnsbörder [On multiple maternities, in Swedish]. Hygiea (Stockholm). 1880;**42**:331-342

[12] Eriksson AW. Human twinning in and around the Åland Islands. Commentationes Biologicae. 1973;**64**:1-159

[13] Eriksson AW, Fellman J. Factors influencing the stillbirth rates in singleton and multiple births in Sweden, 1869 to 1967. Twin Research and Human Genetics. 2006;**9**:591-596

[14] Fellman J, Eriksson AW. Stillbirth rates in singleton, twins and triplets in Sweden, 1869 to 2001. Twin Research and Human Genetics. 2006;**9**:260-265

[15] Fellman J, Eriksson AW. Temporal differences in the regional twinning rates in Sweden after 1750. Twin Research. 2003;**6**:183-191

[16] Veit G. Beiträge zur Geburtshülflichen Statistik (Contributions to the obstetric statistics). Monatsschrift für Geburtskunde und Frauenkrankheiten. Bd 6 Heft. 1855;**2**:101-132

[17] Wappäus JE. Algemeine Bevölkerungsstatistik. Vorlesungen (General population statistics. Lectures). Leipzig; 1859. 581 pp

[18] Bertillon M. Des combinaisons de sexe dans les grossesses gémelláres (doubles et triples), de leur cause et de leur caractère ethnique [Sex combination in multiple maternities (twin and triplet), their causes and their ethnic characteristics]. Bulletins de la Société d'Anthropologie de Paris. 1874;**9**:267-290

[19] Neefe M. Zur Statistik der Mehrgeburten (Statistics of multiple maternities). Jahrbücher für Nationalökonomie und Statistik. 1877;**28**:168-194

[20] Strassmann P. Zur Lehre von der mehrfachen Schwangerschaft (On multiple maternities). Thesis, Berlin; 1889

[21] Hellin D. Die Ursache der Multiparität der uniparen Tiere überhaupt und der Zwillingsschwangerschaft beim Menschen insbesondere [The etiology of multiple maternities among unipair animals and especially twinning maternities in man]. München: Seitz & Schauer; 1895

[22] Drejer P. Om tvillinger [About twins]. Kristiania: Tillægshefte til 'Norsk Magazin for Lægevidenskaben'; 1895

[23] Stigler SM. Stigler's law of eponymy. Transactions of the New York Academy of Sciences, Series II. 1980;**39**:147-158

[24] Merton RK. The sociology of science: Theoretical and empirical investigations. In: Storer NW, editor. Priorities of scientific discovery (Chapter 14). Chicago, IL: University of Chicago Press; 1973

[25] Zeleny C. The relative numbers of twins and triplets. Science. 1921;**53**:262-263

[26] Jenkins RL. Twin and triplet birth ratios. A further study of the interrelations of the frequencies of plural births. Journal of Heredity. 1929;**20**:485-494

[27] Jenkins RL, Gwin J. Twin and triplet births ratios. Journal of Heredity. 1940;**31**:243-248

[28] Allen G, Firschein IL. The mathematical relations among plural births. American Journal of Human Genetics. 1957;**9**:181-190

[29] Bulmer MG. The biology of the twinning in man. London: Oxford University Press; 1970

[30] Fellman J, Eriksson AW. Association between the rates of multiple maternities. Twin Research. 2004;**7**:387-397. DOI: 10.1375/twin.7.5.387

[31] Peller S. A new rule for predicting the occurrence of multiple births. American Journal of Physical Anthropology. 1946;**4**:99-105

[32] Fellman J, Eriksson AW. Statistical analyses of Hellin's law. Twin Research and Human Genetics. 2009;**12**:191-200

[33] Eriksson AW, Fellman J. Temporal trends in the rates of multiple maternities in England and Wales. Twin Research and Human Genetics. 2007;**10**:626-632

[34] Fellman JO, Eriksson AW. Biometric analysis of the multiple maternities in Finland, 1881–1990 and in Sweden since 1751. Human Biology. 1993;**65**:463-479

[35] Jenkins RL. The interrelations of the frequencies of plural births. Journal of Heredity. 1927; **8**:387 and 504

[36] Dahlberg G. Twin births and twins from a hereditary point of view. Stockholm: Bokförlags A–B. Tidens Tryckeri; 1926

[37] Fuster V, Santos C, Román-Busto J, Magalhaes M. A study of multiple deliveries in Portugal: Indications of an Iberian Peninsula Pattern. Twin Research and Human Genetics. 2013;**16**(5): 998-1007

[38] Otta E, Fernandes ES, Acquaviva TG, Lucci TK, Kiehl LC, Varella MAC, Segal NL, Valentova JV. Twinning and Multiple Birth Rates According to Maternal Age in the City of São Paulo, Brazil: 2003–2014. Twin Research and Human Genetics. 2016;**19**(6):679-686

[39] Komai T, Fukuoka G. Frequency of multiple births among the Japanese and related people. American Journal of Physical Anthropology. 1936;**21**:433-447

[40] Strandskov HH. Plural birth frequencies in the total, the 'white' and the 'colored' U.S. populations. American Journal of Physical Anthropology. 1945;**3**:49-55

[41] Sarkar SS. The frequency of multiple births in India and Ceylon. Transactions of the Bose Research Institute, XV. 1945:1-9

[42] Das SR. A mathematical analysis of the phenomena of human twins and higher plural births. Part I: Twins. Metron. 1953;**17**:65-88

[43] Das SR. A mathematical analysis of the phenomena of human twins and higher plural births. Part II: Triplets and the application of the analysis in the interpretation of the twin and the triplet data. Metron. 1955;**17**:67-91

[44] Lam H, Ho PC. A comparison of pregnancy outcome between high-order multiple and twin pregnancies: Matched-pair retrospective study. Hong Kong Medical Journal. 1999;**5**: 16-20

[45] Zhang J, Meikle S, Grainger DA, Trumble A. Multifetal pregnancy in older women and perinatal outcomes. Fertility and Sterility. 2002;**78**:562-568

[46] Simmons R, Doyle P, Maconochie N. Dramatic reduction in triplet and higher order births in England and Wales. BJOG: An International Journal of Obstetrics & Gynaecology. 2004; **111**:856-858

5

Judicious Fertility Treatment to Minimise the Risk of Multiple Pregnancy

Fiona Langdon and Roger Hart

Abstract

Pregnancies resulting from fertility treatment are associated with higher rates of multiple pregnancy and have higher rates of pregnancy complications than spontaneously conceived pregnancies. Methods exist to make fertility treatment safer and less likely to result in multiple pregnancy and practitioners should be practicing fertility treatment with the aim to produce a healthy, term, singleton pregnancy. Approaches to minimising the risk of multiple pregnancy include carefully monitoring ovulation induction (OI) cycles to produce mono-follicular ovulation. Identifying patients at risk of excessive response to ovulation induction and treating them with low dose therapies and close monitoring is a critical step in practicing safe OI treatment. Performing single embryo transfer in all but exceptional cases of in-vitro fertilisation (IVF), and never transferring more than two embryos, is the single, most successful way to reduce the multiple pregnancy rate with IVF. An appreciation of the increased risk of mono-chorionic twinning with IVF is also important. This chapter will explore ways to minimise the risk of multiple pregnancy with a variety of fertility treatments.

Keywords: ART, multiple pregnancy, ovulation induction, single embryo transfer

1. Introduction

Assisted Reproductive Technology (ART) has, since its inception, been associated with increased rates of multiple pregnancy as the treating doctors struggled to balance an acceptable live birth rate with the risk of multiple pregnancy. A multiple pregnancy results in increased rates of both maternal and neonatal morbidity compared with a singleton pregnancy. Further, multiple pregnancy is associated with increased rates of prematurity, especially an increased rate of severe prematurity, low birth weight, neonatal death and longer term developmental concerns [1]. Women with a multiple pregnancy are at risk of nearly every complication of pregnancy in comparison to women pregnant with a singleton pregnancy. Pre-eclampsia, gestational diabetes and operative delivery are all associated with significant increased maternal morbidity in multiple pregnancies.

A multiple pregnancy, for patients who have suffered through months or years of infertility and treatment, can often be seen as a "double blessing" and may indeed result in a successful outcome for many patients. For many years rates of multiple pregnancy for women undergoing ART were accepted as a necessary part of treatment. With ongoing development of fertility treatment, employing better processes and therapies, the success rate of ART has improved, and thus the impetus for using methods that also run the risk of high rates of multiple pregnancy are no longer warranted or accepted. Now when determining the success of an ART technique or an ART service provider, the rate of singleton, term, live birth should be seen as the gold standard of measurement and the aim of successful treatment [2]. Strategies to achieve this are now the cornerstone in research, development and guidelines in ART techniques and stricter regulations and protocols are in place to implement safer methods.

This chapter will explore ways in which ART, in particular ovulation induction, super-ovulation and intra-uterine insemination (IUI) and in-vitro fertilisation (IVF), can be delivered to ensure low rates of multiple pregnancy and make ART and the pregnancy that results safer for mother and baby.

2. Ovulation induction

Ovulation induction involves stimulating the ovary with the aim to induce mono-follicular-ovulation in a sub-fertile woman who is anovulatory. A trigger injection, to mimic the mid-cycle luteinising hormone (LH) surge, is given to initiate release of the ovum and timed intercourse is advised.

Multiple pregnancy may occur with ovulation induction secondary to unintended over-stimulation of the ovary and the development of more than one follicle and the release and subsequent fertilisation of more than one oocyte. Rates of multiple pregnancy with ovarian stimulation depend greatly on the treatment protocol used, but for all methods has been approximated at up to 9 times the rate of natural conception in fertile women [3].

A recent 5-year review of multiple pregnancy rates in the United States revealed 22% of the nation's twin pregnancies were due to ovulation induction and 40% of triplet pregnancies were as a result of ovulation induction treatment [4]. The rates of multiple pregnancy secondary to ovulation induction are falling as better techniques and practices are introduced however, not as quickly as is being seen with more invasive ART techniques such as IVF. Stricter controls and more stringent regulations are being enforced in many countries towards IVF treatments in the hope of stalling the multiple pregnancy rate, however this has not been replicated in the field of ovulation induction, as this is often performed outside of large fertility clinics, or without strict tracking protocols. Hence it is believed that ovulation induction accounts for up to 65% of the world's higher order multiple pregnancies [5].

Ovulation induction agents are usually divided into oral and injectable agents with the historical belief being that injectable agents, usually recombinant or urinary derived follicular stimulating hormone (FSH), being associated with higher rates of both multiple pregnancy and ovarian hyper-stimulation syndrome.

2.1. Clomiphene citrate

Clomiphene citrate was until recently the first line fertility treatment for anovulatory women undergoing ovulation induction [6]. Clomiphene is a selective oestrogen receptor modulator that blocks negative feedback of rising oestrogen levels at the level of the hypothalamus thereby resulting in ongoing FSH secretion and follicular development. Clomiphene citrate has historically had rates of multiple pregnancy quoted at 7%, with higher order multiple pregnancies rates occurring in less than 1% of confirmed pregnancies. [7] Newer data however suggests that multiple pregnancy rates with the use of clomiphene may be as high as 9% and higher order multiple pregnancy rates closer to 2%, as often ultrasound monitoring of the stimulated cycles is not performed [8]. Clomiphene, unlike other ovulation induction agents, does not have a higher rate of multiple pregnancy rates with higher dosing. The anti-oestrogenic properties exhibited by clomiphene on both the cervical mucus and endometrial lining with increased dosing have a negative impact on the rate of conception and implantation. Hence, although ovulation rates may increase, successful pregnancy, including multiple pregnancy, are not necessarily increased. Thus, for clomiphene, unlike other ovulation induction agents, simply prescribing lower doses of the agent will do little to reduce multiple pregnancy rates.

2.2. Letrozole

Letrozole is an aromatase inhibitor that is now recommended as a first line ovulation induction agent [6]. It is associated with higher rates of mono-ovulation than clomiphene and thus lower rates of multiple pregnancy, at around 3.5% [9], but with overall similar if not higher live birth rates [10]. It has a shorter half-life than clomiphene and, unlike clomiphene, during treatment endogenous FSH is suppressed by rising oestrogen levels thus reducing the risk of multiple follicles developing. Due to the benefit of increased live birth rates and a reduction in the rates of multiple pregnancy letrozole should be the oral agent for first line use in anovulatory women undergoing ovulation induction. However, letrozole must be used under informed consent as ovulation induction is not an approved indication for the drug.

2.3. Metformin

Metformin has, over the last few years, been increasingly used for the management of women with PCOS, having potential benefits with regard to its metabolic consequences [11] and androgenic side-effects [12]. However, with respect to anovulatory infertility as a sole agent the benefit of increasing the chance of a live birth is not clear, other than perhaps as an adjuvant to clomiphene citrate in overweight women [13], or as an adjuvant to FSH ovulation induction [14].

2.4. Follicular stimulation hormone (FSH)

Injectable agents, usually recombinant FSH, have historically been associated with higher rates of multiple pregnancy. When first described dosing regimes in the realm of 225 IU of FSH were used to induce ovulation in anovulatory women with multiple pregnancy rates of around 25% [15]. As greater experience was gained using FSH and with a clear distinction being made between dosing for the aim of mono-ovulation in ovulation induction, versus ovarian hyper-stimulation for IVF cycles initial dosages fell dramatically. Low dose, step up protocols are now the recommended regime with close monitoring to observe response [16]. Unlike oral agents that are given for a limited number of days in the early follicular phase, FSH can be given for an extended period until follicular development is seen. With this method rates of multiple pregnancy can be as low, or lower, than with oral agents and can be achieved with higher live birth rates. In countries with good health insurance and state funding for fertility treatments out of pocket costs to patients are comparable to oral agents and are thus often used as a first line treatment due to their increased success rates.

In our unit, after exclusion of other potential infertility factors, we aim to induce mono-ovulation with a low dose step up protocol. We start all women on a low dose of gonadotropin, on average 25 IU FSH, and monitor women with oestrogen levels and ultrasound tracking of developing follicles. Dosing is increased if no response is seen after 10 days, with dose increments of 12.5 IU, until a threshold is reached whereby mono-follicular development occurs and the dose is not increased further. If more than 2 follicles of 10 mm are noted the cycle is cancelled, and in patients under 35 years consideration is given to cancelling with two follicles. Review of our data has showed that our rate of multiple pregnancy using this method for ovulation induction is below 4% [17]. This is with a cumulative live birth rate of close to 50% over 3 cycles and a cycle cancellation rate of around 10%. After 3 cycles the live birth rate per cycle falls significantly as the patients with additional reproductive pathology start to make up a greater percentage of remaining patients. If after 3 cycles a successful pregnancy has not occurred we give consideration to switching to IVF treatment. This allows a low rate of multiple pregnancy and a close to 50% rate of successful pregnancy for our patients without exposing them to the increased risk of IVF unless it is warranted.

The hallmark of reducing rates of multiple pregnancy with ovulation induction is to closely monitor follicular development both with hormone levels and ultrasound tracking to ensure only a single dominant follicle, or a maximum of two, will develop and ultimately ovulate. It would be assumed that with close monitoring a clinician could predict when a patient was at risk of releasing more than one oocyte and could act prudently to avoid conception in such cases. Existing guidelines surrounding risk adverse practice in regard to tracking are sparse and not overly cautious. The American College of Obstetricians and Gynaecologists (ACOG) guideline recommends abandoning an ovulation induction cycle if there are more than 3 follicles measuring more than 15 mm [18]. Studies have shown that follicles as small as 7 mm at time of trigger can result in successful ovulation and impact the multiple pregnancy rate, although it is generally believed that follicles of 14 mm in size or greater will have a mature oocyte [19]. Capping the recommended maximum number of follicles before cancellation of the cycle at more than 3 is doing little to reduce the rate of multiple pregnancy and indeed risks, not just a multiple pregnancy but a higher order multiple pregnancy.

More judicious care can be taken to actively avoid multiple pregnancy by ensuring mono-ovulation by very closely monitoring oestrogen levels and follicular development on ultrasound. By cancelling cycles when more than 2 follicles of greater than 10 mm are present has been shown to actively reduce multiple pregnancy rates. Oestrogen levels above 600 pg/mL have been associated with increased rates of multiple pregnancy [20] and higher than 2000 pg/mL with higher order multiple pregnancy. [21] Using both ultrasound follicle tracking and serum oestradiol measurements to carefully track cycles is imperative to minimise multiple pregnancy.

As a general rule, younger women, women with a greater antral follicle count or higher anti-mullerian hormone (AMH) levels are more likely to have a greater response to a lower dose of induction agent and thus should be started at a minimum dose on the first cycle and tracked accordingly.

All couples should be worked up prior to embarking on ovulation induction to confirm tubal patency and adequate semen analysis, and to ensure a more invasive form of ART may not be a better first line therapy. The group of women for who ovulation induction is most widely used is those with anovulation secondary to poly-cystic ovarian syndrome (PCOS.) This is often a group of patients that are of a younger age than the average infertility patient and have a high antral follicle count and in reflection of that, often a high AMH. These women may also benefit from the additional use of metformin during their stimulation to improve outcomes [14]. It is critical that these women are identified as high risk for responding excessively to even small doses of ovulation induction agents and should be started on very low doses of ovulation induction agents and very carefully monitored. Being younger also means the rate of fecundity per ovulation is high and therefore every effort should be made to aim for mono-ovulation.

Options available when development of an excessive number of follicles is observed include cancelling the cycle, aspirating the excess follicles or switching to an egg collection and IVF cycle. None of these options are ideal for a patient hoping to achieve a pregnancy but need to be discussed with the patient before embarking on treatment. Cancellation of the cycle can be devastating to the patient from a financial and emotional cost, however a cancelled cycle due to hyper-stimulation of the ovary gives valuable information to the practitioner for management of the next cycle in regard to dosing and monitoring. Follicular aspiration for either reduction in follicle number, or for transfer to an IVF cycle is difficult if it has not been discussed as an option pre-treatment, and has ethical implications in regard to informed consent for a patient who is now being faced with either cancellation of the cycle or conversion to a more complicated and costly treatment. It is imperative that as part of the consent process for ovulation induction the risk of multiple follicle development is discussed and the options and recommendations when an excessive number of follicles develop are considered.

Having an absolute maximum cut off of 2 follicles, and for high risk couples one follicle, will be a huge step forward in reducing the multiple pregnancy rates with ovulation induction. Such an approach has been associated with multiple pregnancy rates below 5% and no higher order multiple pregnancies [22]. This compares with rates up to 30% if no intervention is made until follicular numbers reach more than three [23]. High risk couples, for whom more than one follicle should be the threshold for cancellation include young women undergoing their first few cycles and who have an expected high fecundity per follicle, but also patients for whom multiple pregnancy would be particularly dangerous. This includes women with an independent risk of pre-term birth and women with underlying medical conditions making them more susceptible to the pregnancy complications of multiple pregnancy.

3. Super ovulation and intra-uterine insemination (IUI)

Super ovulation and IUI involves stimulating the ovary with ovulation induction agents with the aim to produce two follicles, then with ovulation trigger performing IUI to allow the sperm to bypass the cervical environment. It is usually performed in patients with unexplained subfertility or mild male factor subfertility. Consequently, the purpose of the treatment is to increase the chance of a successful pregnancy by increasing the number of oocytes ovulated and the availability of sperm.

Given it is used in women that are already ovulating, prudent use of ovulation induction agents is imperative and careful monitoring of the cycle with ultrasound and oestrogen levels is important, as in ovulation induction, to prevent multiple pregnancy and higher order multiple pregnancy. Unlike ovulation induction, where the aim is to produce a single dominant follicle, super-ovulation is aimed at producing two follicles, with well controlled cycles accepting up to three follicles, but certainly no more. The reason is in this situation there is a potentially as yet unrecognised factor limiting conception, whereas in standard ovulation induction treatment for the anovulatory woman, it is only the absence of ovulation that is limiting conception, hence when that is overcome the woman should conceive. Once four follicles are present there is no increase in the live birth rate, but a significant increase in the multiple pregnancy and higher order multiple pregnancy rate [21].

As the aim is to produce more than one follicle the risk of multiple pregnancy is high, higher than that is seen with IVF or ovulation induction. Overall rates of multiple pregnancy are around 14% in well controlled cycles, involving cancellation when more than three follicles are identified [24]. This is higher than is seen with IVF cycles, even in well controlled ovarian hyperstimulation protocols. Like ovulation induction the discussion regarding switching to an IVF treatment course, or cancellation of the cycle is required to be had with the patient prior to embarking on treatment. Often the decision around opting for IVF, to minimise the risk of a multiple pregnancy, or to adopt the cheaper treatment of super ovulation and IUI, but a greater risk of a multiple, revolve around the costs to the patient. This situation is unfortunate as the cost to the health care system and the family, ultimately, are greater when a multiple pregnancy results.

4. In-vitro fertilisation

In vitro fertilisation resulted in the first live birth in 1978. Since that time the use of IVF technology has changed dramatically and the increased success and its widespread use to treat all manner of subfertility issues has meant currently in Australia 1 in 25 children born are the result of an IVF cycle [25]. Like ovulation induction and super ovulation, IVF is associated with increased rates of unintended multiple pregnancy, in comparison to spontaneous conception, plus there is also a greater risk of an embryo splitting and resulting in monozygotic twinning.

While the key to reducing rates of multiple pregnancy with ovulation induction and superovulation and IUI lies with careful monitoring of the cycle and judicious cancellation of cycles when multiple follicles develop, the cornerstone to reducing multiple pregnancy rates in IVF treatment is to ensure single embryo transfer is the norm.

As IVF technology has developed and successful live birth rates have increased the need to transfer more than one embryo has rapidly declined. There is no significant difference in the live birth rate for women aged under 37 years undergoing a single embryo transfer (sET) compared with a double embryo transfer (dET), only an increase in the multiple pregnancy rate and subsequent increased pregnancy complication rate [26]. For women aged under 37 years the rate of multiple pregnancy with a double embryo transfer is as high as 25% [27], compared with less than 6% for women undergoing single embryo transfer [28].

Although implantation rate is not the gold standard by which to measure success of a fertility treatment, when compared with sET, dET has been reported to be associated with lower implantation rates suggesting a deleterious effect on the intrauterine environment when dET is employed [29]. This observation is further supported by the increased rates of poor pregnancy outcome when dET is performed but only one embryo implants. This scenario is associated with increased rates of growth restriction and preterm delivery compared with singleton pregnancies resulting from a single embryo transfer [30]. A review of the American Society for Assisted Reproductive Technology outcomes between 2004 and 2013, of over 180,000 IVF cycles concluded that although the live birth rate may increase with a dET, this is substantially out-weighed by the risk of multiple gestations [31]. They demonstrated that for patients with favourable prognostic factors; including younger maternal age, transfer of a blastocyst, and additional embryos cryopreserved, the gain in the live birth rate from sET to dET was approximately 10–15%, however, the multiple birth rate increased from approximately 2% to almost 50% for both fresh and frozen embryo transfer cycles.

Single embryo transfer is associated with not just a reduction in multiple pregnancy rates, but also a reduction in overall pregnancy complication rates with little effect on the live birth rate compared with double or higher number embryo transfer rates [32]. Double embryo transfer rates are occasionally recommended or supported when a patient has particular barriers to implantation success and thus have a perceived lower rate of risk to multiple pregnancy with dET. These may include advanced maternal age, poor embryo quality or multiple previous unsuccessful attempts at single embryo transfer.

The barrier to implementing universal single embryo transfer appears to lie in the cost of IVF treatment to the patient. In countries or regions where state funded or supported fertility treatment exists, the rates of single embryo transfer are far higher. The factor most influencing the likelihood a patient will undergo a single embryo transfer over a double or greater number embryo transfer is whether or not they have health insurance, a greater influencing factor than that of maternal age [33]. In Australia where fertility treatment is subsidised by the state and rates of health insurance are high, the rate of single embryo transfer is over 75% and reflected in the multiple pregnancy rate from IVF being below 6% [34]. In comparison, in the United States sET recorded in the same year was less than 25% [35]. This is also a reflection of the strict regulations that exist in Australia governing IVF treatment.

Regulations and policy governing single embryo transfer also exist in many Scandinavian and some European countries, such as Belgium, as well as Australia, with reflective low rates of multiple pregnancy and high rates of cycle success. The transfer of more than two embryos is banned in Australia and double embryo transfer only allowed in the setting of significant advanced maternal age or multiple failed attempts at single embryo transfer [36]. In comparison, other European countries like Greece, Montenegro and Lithuania have few regulations governing IVF protocols and treatment and overall data from Europe show rates of double embryo transfer well over 50% and rates of transfer of three or more embryos as high as 12.5% [37]. The multiple birth rate is reflected in this practice with the multiple birth rate following IVF being 18.7% in Europe compared with 5.6% in Australia and New Zealand [37]. The multiple birth rate following IVF is even higher in the United States at 26.6% [35]. This is despite slightly higher rates of double embryo transfer in Europe, however this is thought to reflect the high rate of fetal reductions that occur in Europe as a management strategy for multiple pregnancy.

Despite implementing a single embryo transfer an IVF cycle may still result in a multiple pregnancy due to monozygotic twinning. Monozygotic twins are at increased risk of significant complications including Twin-Twin Transfusion Syndrome (TTTS) and Twin Anaemia-Polycythaemia Sequence (TAPS), fetal anomalies and perinatal morbidity. The rate of monozygotic twinning is increased in IVF pregnancy by 6 times compared with spontaneously conceived pregnancies [38], occurring at a rate of around 2.5% [39]. The reason for this is likely multifactorial. Culture media, embryo quality, use of gonadotropins and manipulation of the zona pellucida are all thought to play a role in the increased rates of monozygotic twinning following IVF [40].

In natural conception the rate of monozygotic twinning increases with age, likely a reflection of egg quality, however the inverse has been seen in pregnancies conceived with IVF. Women under 35 are twice as likely to have a monochorionic twin pregnancy following IVF treatment compared with women aged over 35 [41]. The mechanism for this may include the zona pellucida experiencing increased thickening with advancing maternal age, resulting in the embryo of an older patient being more robust to the manipulation exerted on it during IVF or Intracytoplasmic Sperm Injection (ICSI), or during embryo biopsy. This is an important observation and further supports the argument for single embryo transfer for younger patients with a good chance of implantation per embryo transfer. If a patient is at increased risk of monozygotic twinning, and has a double embryo transfer the risk of a higher order multiple pregnancy, with the added complication of a monozygotic twin pair develops.

The stress that a developing blastocyst and embryo undergoes during an IVF cycle may rationalise the increased rates of monozygotic twinning. Monozygotic twin pregnancies are more likely in day 5 blastocyst transfer than day 2 or 3 cleavage stage transfer, perhaps reflective of the strain that may be put on the embryo the day of transfer. Monozygotic twinning occurs due to the embryo splitting anywhere from Day 4 through to Day 8. Transfer in the middle of this time period involves subtle changes to the pH, temperature and nutrient environment that could explain the increased rate during blastocyst transfer. The actual mechanics of the transfer may also play a role in making the embryo more likely to split. Blastocyst transfer is associated with nearly a three times increased chance of embryo splitting and resultant monozygotic twinning compared with cleavage stage transfer [42]. This finding has not lead to a change in practice due to the significantly greater live birth rate seen overall with blastocyst transfer due to the ability to select an embryo that has survived until day 5 of development and also result in transfer at a similar time to when the blastocyst would be reaching the uterine cavity in a natural conception [43].

The increased rate of monozygotic twinning for blastocyst transfer is not replicated, or at least not as pronounced, when the transfer is a result of a frozen cycle, rather than a fresh transfer [41]. An explanation for this is the freezing/thawing cycle may harden the zona pellucida making the blastocyst more robust against the process of embryo transfer and reduce the chance of splitting. A regime of 'freeze all' may be worthwhile to further reduce rates of multiple pregnancy from monozygotic twinning with blastocyst transfer.

Micro-manipulation techniques of the egg and embryo such as ICSI and pre-implantation genetic diagnosis have long been thought to play a role in increased rates of monozygotic twinning through weakening of the zona pellucida making it prone to splitting. Like blastocyst transfer, if this effect exists, it is likely associated with fresh transfers rather than frozen transfers. Because of this it is recommended that conventional IVF be used over ICSI unless significant male factor fertility issues exist.

Embryo quality has an association with the chance of monozygotic twinning. Poorer embryo quality has been shown to increase the rate of monozygotic twinning [44]. An appreciation of this is important when considering double embryo transfer due to poorer embryo quality. An awareness that the resultant pregnancy may develop into a higher order pregnancy, such as a dichorionic-triamniotic triplet pregnancy is crucial.

Not all multiple pregnancies that develop after single embryo transfers are monozygotic. A review of twin pregnancies following single embryo transfer found 18% of twin pregnancies were dizygotic [45]. The explanation for this was likely concurrent spontaneous conception with a frozen transfer or ovulation of uncollected eggs and subsequent fertilisation with fresh transfers. This hypothesis is supported by the fact that unexplained subfertility, with an underlying chance of conception, and obesity, that increases chance of uncollected oocytes due to limitations of ultrasound, was the main risk factors for dizygotic twinning in this scenario. The importance of abstaining from unprotected sexual intercourse at time of transfer is imperative when counselling couples on how to reduce the risk of multiple pregnancy.

5. Conclusion

The rate of multiple pregnancy associated with ART has fallen steadily with the implementations of better practices. As pregnancy success rates have increased the belief that more follicles or more embryos equates to better outcomes has been disproven. Close monitoring of ovulation stimulation protocols, and a practice of single embryo transfer for IVF has resulted in far lower multiple pregnancy rates and safer practices for women. An awareness of the risk of multiple pregnancy with ART and the ways in which this can be avoided is paramount to the future direction of ART, both for research and regulatory bodies.

Author details

Fiona Langdon[1,2,3] and Roger Hart[2,3]*

*Address all correspondence to: roger.hart@uwa.edu.au

1 King Edward Memorial Hospital, Subiaco, WA, Australia

2 Fertility Specialists of Western Australia, Bethesda Hospital, Claremont, WA, Australia

3 Division of Obstetrics and Gynaecology, University of Western Australia, Perth, WA, Australia

References

[1] Kogan MD et al. Trends in twin birth outcomes and prenatal care utilization in the United States, 1981-1997. Journal of the American Medical Association. 2000;**284**:335-341

[2] Min JK et al. What is the most relevant standard of success in assisted reproduction? The singleton, term gestation, live birth rate per cycle initiated: The BEST endpoint for assisted reproduction. Human Reproduction. 2004;**19**:3-7

[3] Zhu JL et al. Infertility, infertility treatment and twinning: The Danish national birth cohort. Human Reproduction. 2007;**22**:1086-1090

[4] Dickey RP. The relative contribution of assisted reproductive technologies and ovulation induction to multiple births in the United States 5 years after the Society for Assisted Reproductive Technology/American Society for Reproductive Medicine recommendation to limit the number of embryos transferred. Fertility and Sterility. 2007;**88**: 1554-1561

[5] Chaabane S et al. Association between ovarian stimulators with or without intrauterine insemination, and assisted reproductive technologies on multiple births. American Journal of Obstetrics and Gynecology. 2015;**213**:511

[6] Balen AH. The management of anovulatory infertility in women with polycystic ovary syndrome: An analysis of the evidence to support the development of global WHO guideline. Human Reproduction Update. 2016;**22**:687-708

[7] Schenker JG et al. Multiple pregnancies following ovulation induction. Fertility and Sterility. 1981;**35**:105-123

[8] Dickey RP et al. Effect of diagnosis, age, sperm quality, and number of preovulatory follicles on the outcome of multiple cycles of clomiphene citrate-intrauterine insemination. Fertility and Sterility. 2002;**78**:1088-1095

[9] Legro RS et al. Letrozole versus clomiphene for infertility in the polycystic ovary syndrome. NEJM. 2014;**371**:119-129

[10] Fisher SA et al. A randomized double-blind comparison of the effects of clomiphene citrate and the aromatase inhibitor letrazole on ovulatory function. Fertility and Sterility. 2002;**78**:280-285

[11] Misson ML et al. Metformin in women with PCOS. Endocrine. 2015;**48**:428-433

[12] Costello M et al. Insulin-sensitising drugs versus the combined oral contraceptive pill for hirsutism, acne and risk of diabetes, cardiovascular disease, and endometrial cancer in polycystic ovary syndrome. Cochrane Database of Systematic Reviews. 2007;**24**(1):CD005552

[13] Misson ML et al. Status of clomiphene citrate and metformin for infertility in PCOS. Trends in Endocrinology and Metabolism. 2012;**23**:533-543

[14] Bordewijk EM et al. Metformin during ovulation induction with gonadotrophins followed by timed intercourse or intrauterine insemination for subfertility associated with polycystic ovary syndrome. Cochrane Database of Systematic Reviews. 2018 Jul 1; **24**(4):468-483. DOI: 10.1093/humupd/dmy006. PMID:29538675

[15] Dodson WC et al. Superovulation with intrauterine insemination in the treatment of infertility: A possible alternative to gamete intrafallopian transfer and invitro fertilization. Fertility and Sterility. 1987;**48**:441-445

[16] Homburg R et al. Clomiphene citrate or low dose FSH for the first-line treatment of infertile women with anovulation associated with polycystic ovary syndrome: A prospective randomized multinational study. Human Reproduction. 2012;**27**:468-473

[17] Langdon FH et al. The management of anovulatoy infertility for women with PCOS. In: Darwish AM, editor. Testes and Ovaries - Discrepancies and Similarities. Rijeka, Croatia: InTechOpen; 2018. pp. 61-75. ISBN:978-953-51-5409-9

[18] ACOG. Practice Bulletin. Clinical Management Guidelines for Obstetricians-Gynaecologists Nmber 34. Management of Infertility Caused by Ovulatory Dysfunction. American College of Obstetricians and Gynecologists; 2002

[19] Gleicher N et al. Reducing the risk of high-order multiple pregnancy after ovarian induction with gonadotrophins. NEJM. 2000;**343**:2-7

[20] Tur R et al. Risk factors for high-order multiple implantation after ovarian induction with gonadotrophins: Evidence from a large series of 1878 consecutive pregnancies in a single center. Human Reproduction. 2001;**16**:2124-2129

[21] Dickey RP et al. Risk factors for high-order multiple pregnancy and multiple birth after controlled ovarian hyperstimulation: Results of 4,062 intrauterine insemination cycles. Fertility and Sterility. 2005;**83**:671

[22] Dickey RP. Strategies to reduce multiple pregnancies due to ovulation stimulation. Fertility and Sterility. 2009;**91**:1-14

[23] Fauser BCJM, Devroey P, Macklon NS. Multiple birth resulting from ovarian stimulation for infertility treatment. Lancet. 2005;**365**:1807-1816

[24] Nandi A et al. Intrauterine insemination with gonadotropin stimulation or in vitro fertilization for the treatment of unexplained subfertility: A randomized controlled trial. Fertility and Sterility. 2017;**107**:1329-1335

[25] Hart R, Norman RJ. The longer-term health outcomes for children born as a result of IVF treatment. Part I-general health outcomes. Human Reproduction Update. 2013;**19**:232-243

[26] Kissin DM et al. Number of embryos transferred after in vitro fertilization and good perinatal outcome. Obstetrics and Gynecology. 2014;**123**:239-247

[27] Sunderam S et al. Assisted reproductive technology surveillance—United States, 2012. MMWR Surveillance Summaries. 2015;**64**:1-29

[28] Bensdorp AJ et al. Prevention of multiple pregnancies in couples with unexplained or mild male subfertility: Randomised controlled trial of in vitro fertilisation with single embryo transfer or in vitro fertilisation in modified natural cycle compared with intrauterine insemination with controlled ovarian hyperstimulation. BMJ. 2015;**350**:1-14

[29] Styer AK et al. Single-blastocyst transfer decreases twin gestation without affecting pregnancy outcome. Fertility and Sterility. 2008;**89**:1702-1708

[30] Brown LB et al. Effect of embryo transfer number on singleton and twin implantation pregnancy outcomes after assisted reproductive technology. The Journal of Reproductive Medicine. 2010;**55**:387-394

[31] Merereau J et al. Patient and cycle characteristics predicting high pregnancy rates with single-embryo transfer: An analysis of the Society for Assisted Reproductive Technology outcomes between 2004 and 2013. Fertility and Sterility. 2017;**108**:750-756

[32] Takeshima K et al. Impact of single embryo transfer policy on perinatal outcomes in fresh and frozen cycles-analysis of the Japanese Assisted Reproduction Technology registry between 2007 and 2012. Fertility and Sterility. 2016;**105**:337-346

[33] Styer AK et al. Factors associated with the use of elective single embryo transfer and pregnancy outcomes in the United States, 2004-2012. Fertility and Sterility. 2016;**106**:80-89

[34] Fitzgerald O, Harris K, Paul RC, Chambers GM. Assisted reproductive technology in Australia and New Zealand 2015. Sydney: National Perinatal Epidemiology and Statistics Unit, the University of New South Wales Sydney; 2017

[35] CDC, Centres for Disease Control and Prevention. Reproductive Health. Assisted Reproductive Technology. National Summary and Fertility Clinic Reports. 2013

[36] Code of Practice for Assisted Reproductive Technology Units. Fertility Society of Australia, Reproductive Technology Accreditation Committee. 2014

[37] Calhaz-Jorge C et al. Assisted reproductive technology in Europe, 2013: Results generated from European registers by ESHRE. Human Reproduction. 2017;**32**:1957-1973

[38] Aston KI et al. Monozygotic twinning associated with assisted reproductive technologies: A review. Reproduction. 2008;**136**:377-386

[39] Sobek A et al. High incidence of monozygotic twinning in infertility treatment. Biomedical Papers of the Medical Faculty of the University Palacky, Olomouc, Czech Republic. 2016;**160**:358-362

[40] Hviid KVR et al. Determinants of monozygotic twinning in ART: A systematic review and a meta-analysis. Human Reproduction Update. 2017 Nov 6;**12**(11):e0186813. DOI: 10.1371/journal.pone.0186813. eCollection 2017. PMID:29107981

[41] Song B et al. Prevalence and risk factors of monochorionic diamniotic twinning after assisted reproduction: A six year experience base on a large cohort of pregnancies. PLoS One. 2017 Jan 24;**1**:CD009090. DOI: 10.1002/14651858.CD009090.pub2. Review. PMID: 28118681

[42] Chang HJ et al. Impact of blastocyst transfer on offspring sex ratio and the monozygotic twinning rate: A systematic review and meta-analysis. Fertility and Sterility. 2009;**91**:2381

[43] Papanikolaou EG et al. Live birth rates after transfer of equal number of blastocysts or cleavage-stage embryos in IVF. A systematic review and meta-analysis. Human Reproduction. 2008;**23**:91

[44] Franasiak JM et al. Blastocyst transfer is not associated with increased rates of monozygotic twins when controlling for embryo cohort quality. Fertility and Sterility. 2015;**103**:95-100

[45] Vega M et al. Not all twins are monozygotic after elective single embryo transfer: Analysis of 32,600 elective single embryo transfer cycles as reported to the Society for Assisted Reproductive Technology. Fertility and Sterility. 2018;**109**:118-122

6

Complications in Monochorionic Pregnancies

Bruno Rodrigues Toneto

Abstract

Monochorionic (MC) pregnancies have higher rates of fetal morbidity and mortality when compared to dichorionic (DC) ones. Therefore, the early diagnostic of chorionicity is of great importance. Monochorionic pregnancies have specific complications such as twin to twin transfusion syndrome (TTTS), selective fetal growth restriction (sFGR), twin anemia polycythemia sequence (TAPS), and twin reversed arterial perfusion sequence (TRAPS). MC pregnancies have several unique and serious complications that contribute to a perinatal mortality rate of 11%. The pathophysiology of most of these complications is related to the placental angio-architecture, and it results from an unbalanced perfusion between the fetuses. The screening of TTTS starts in 16 weeks with a sonographic follow-up every 2 weeks. In the last decade, there was an improvement in the treatment of TTTS. With the advent of the fetoscopic laser photocoagulation (FLPC), there was a drastic increase in the survival rate of the fetuses with TTTS when compared with serial amnioreduction. Besides that, in TRAPS, fetoscopic procedures such as cord occlusion improve the outcome of the normal fetus. We will also discuss sFGR and its classification and management. The aim of this chapter is to review the most important complications in MC pregnancies.

Keywords: monochorionic, twin to twin transfusion syndrome, TTTS, twin anemia polycythemia sequence, TAPS, selective fetal growth restriction, multiple pregnancy

1. Introduction

Multiple pregnancies are the result of one of the three possibilities: a fertilization of two or more oocytes from different spermatozoids, a single fertilization followed by a splitting of the zygote, or a combination of both [1]. These pregnancies have an increased risk of several complications for both mother and fetuses, such as diabetes mellitus, hypertensive disorders associated with pregnancy, preeclampsia, anemia, hyperemesis, hemorrhage, and cesarean delivery [2–5] in the maternal side and higher risk of fetal anomalies, fetal demise, neonatal death [6], and preterm birth in the fetal side [7].

It is known that monochorionic (MC) pregnancies have higher rates of fetal morbidity and mortality when compared to dichorionic (DC) ones [1, 8, 9]. Besides that, the MC pregnancies have specific complications such as the twin to twin transfusion syndrome (TTTS), the selective fetal growth restriction (sFGR), the twin anemia polycythemia sequence (TAPS), and the twin reversed arterial perfusion sequence (TRAPS). Most of these complications can be managed and treated in order to decrease the fetal morbimortality.

2. Importance of multiple pregnancy

In the last years, the rate of multiple pregnancies has raised all over the globe. In the USA, it rose from 18.9in 1980 to 33.4 twins per 1000 births in 2016. The twin birth rates were higher in black women, followed by non-Hispanic white women. The triplet and high-order multiple birth rate has decreased about 48% in the last 8 years, from 193.5 in 1998 to 101.4 twins per 100.000 births in 2016 [7]. This decrease in high-order multiple pregnancies illustrates the reproductive medicine societies' strategies for reducing the risk of high-order pregnancies, like single-embryo transfer and multifetal pregnancy reduction [10–12].

In England, there is also an increase in multiple births. From 1998 to 2016, the multiple maternity rate rose from 14.4 to 15.9 twins per 1000 births. Since 1993, women aged 45 and over have consistently recorded the highest multiple maternity rate. These changes in the multiple pregnancy rates are due to the increase in ART. It is estimated that in vitro fertilization (IVF) conceptions are 11 times more likely to result in a multiple birth than natural conceptions. In 2014, 16% of IVF pregnancies resulted in multiple birth, with nearly 19,000 IVF babies born in the UK in 2014 [13].

This trend was largely attributed to an elevated amount of dizygotic pregnancies, without significant variations in monozygotic births over the past few decades. The dizygotic twinning rate is affected by many factors such as race, previous multiple pregnancy, maternal age and parity, lifestyle, season, use of fertility drugs and treatments, genetics, and others [14–16].

The high number of multiple births impacts directly in rate of preterm birth and low birthweight. Data from 2016 show that among twin pregnancies, 59.9% are born before complete 37 weeks of gestation, while in singletons, only 8% are preterm births. In singleton births, 6.4% were born with weight less than 2500 g. This percentage is 55.4 in twins and more than 95% in triplets [7].

3. Complications

The MC pregnancies have several unique and serious complications that contribute to a perinatal mortality rate of 11% [17, 18]. The pathophysiology of most of these complications is related to the placental angio-architecture [19]. Placental anastomoses are described since the 1600s.

The term "third circulation" that represents an "area of transfusion" and the potential harmful effect of vascular connections between the fetuses was first described by Schatz in 1896 [20]. In 1965, Naeye [21] identified the effect of chronic nutritional deprivation on the size of organs in one twin while appreciating that transfusion to the other increased the hemoglobin concentration and hematocrit, with subsequent cardiomyopathy and hypertension. Since then, several authors have proposed diagnosis criteria and different kinds of treatments of the MC pregnancy problems. In this session, the main complications of the MC gestations will be discussed.

3.1. Twin to twin transfusion syndrome

One of the first suggestions of this disease in history lies in a Dutch painting from 1617 named the Early-Deceased Children of Jacob de Graeff and Aeltge Boelens that illustrates two children. One of them is pale and the other plethoric (**Figure 1**). Twin to twin transfusion syndrome is one of the main complications that occurs in about 10–15% of the MC pregnancies with an overall incidence of 3 in 10,000 pregnancies [22, 23].

If left untreated, TTTS mortality rates are about 70–100%. Perinatal mortality is the result of either miscarriage or very preterm delivery as a consequence of severe polyhydramnios and uterine distention or fetal demise due to severe cardiovascular disturbances [24, 25].

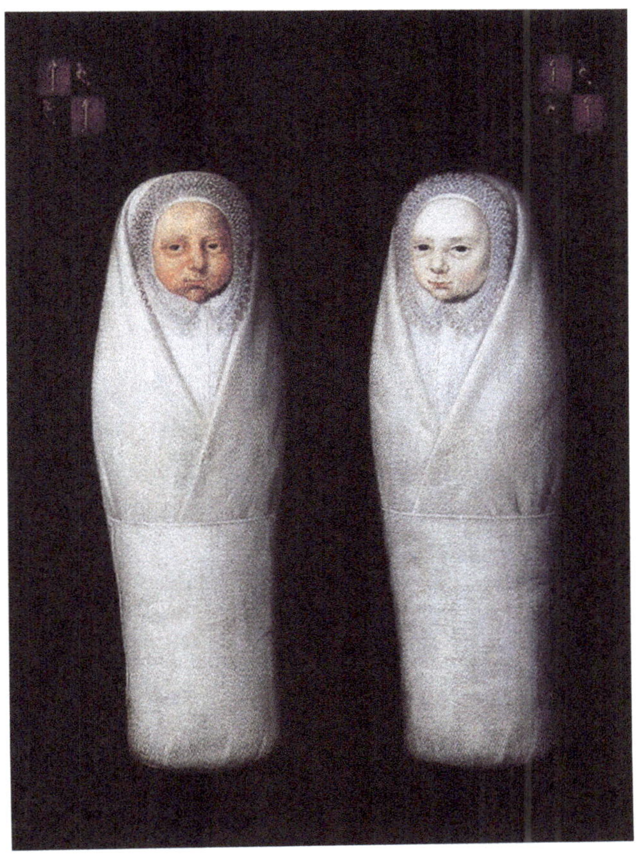

Figure 1. The Dutch painting the Early-Deceased Children of Jacob de Graeff and Aeltge Boelens shows two male twins: one pale and the other plethoric.

3.1.1. Pathophysiology

The pathophysiology underlies in the placental angio-architecture which is characterized by individual placental territory size, cord insertion location, and the quantity, size, and direction of intertwin anastomoses which are the most important factors in the pathogenesis because when unbalanced, they may cause hemodynamic changes that end in TTTS [26].

All MC placentas have intertwin anastomoses that are formed in the first trimester. They are important because they allow transfer of volume, red blood cells, vasoactive substances, and hormones. There are three type of intertwin anastomoses, and their flow may be unidirectional or bidirectional. Arteriovenous (AV) anastomoses are unidirectional but they exist in both directions (from donor to recipient or from recipient to donor). AV anastomoses end in a shared cotyledon where the arterial villous circulation of one twin links to the venous villous return of the other at the level of the intervillous space. Artery-to-artery (AA) and vein-to-vein (VV) are more superficial and bidirectional anastomoses (**Figure 2**). The flow direction depends on the types of connection, vessel calibers, and the pulse pressure. TTTS results from an unbalanced chronic perfusion from donor to recipient twin across placental anastomoses. This blood transfer is more likely in those placentas with more AV anastomoses and a lack of superficial balancing AA or VV anastomoses or when these bidirectional anastomoses are unusually small [26, 28].

3.1.2. Clinical manifestations of TTTS

The principal clinical feature in TTTS is hypervolemia in the recipient and hypovolemia in the donor twin that may progress to cardiovascular impairment, hydrops, and fetal death. In the

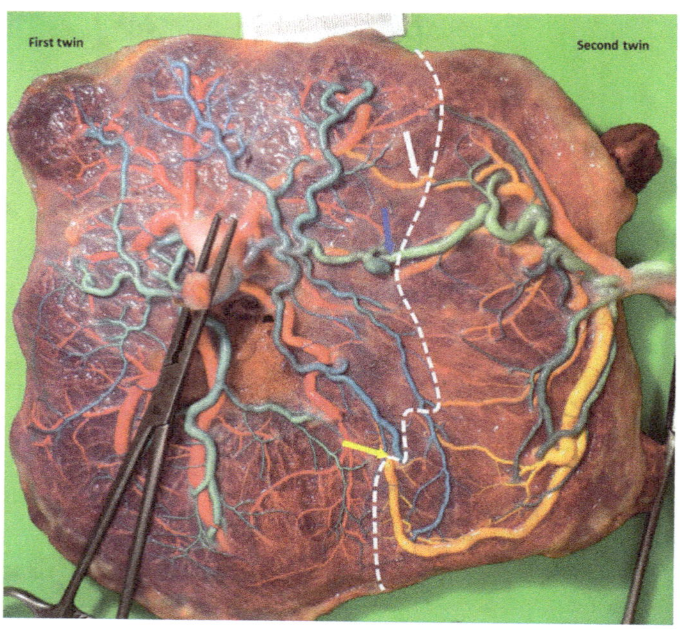

Figure 2. Monochorionic placenta of not complicated twin pregnancy. The blue, white, and yellow arrows represent AA, VV, and AV anastomoses, respectively. Adapted from twin research and human genetics, Zhao et al. [27].

first trimester, diagnosis is difficult, since the amniotic fluid is usually normal in both fetuses. Some sonographic markers such as discordance in nuchal translucency thickness (NT) and abnormalities in ductus venosus (DV) may be early signs of TTTS, but they have a low predictive value [29–31]. The sonographic manifestations usually may be noted as early as 16 weeks of gestation, but they can appear in the third trimester as well. TTTS manifestations are rare after 28 weeks of gestation.

In the second trimester, the oligohydramnios in the donor twin, as well as the polyhydramnios in the recipient twin, can easily be noted by ultrasound examination. The donor becomes hypovolemic; therefore, renal perfusion decreases. This hypoperfusion activates the renin-angiotensin system (RAS), producing vasoconstriction, oliguria, and oligohydramnios. As the disease progresses, the fetus becomes anuric and gets "stuck" against the uterine walls (**Figure 3**). The circulation becomes hyperdynamic with an increased vascular resistance in the fetus and in the placenta, leading to fetal growth restriction (FGR), cerebral redistribution, and abnormal arterial Doppler assessment. The recipient twin becomes hypervolemic and, by myocardial stretching, releases atrial natriuretic peptide (ANP) and brain natriuretic peptide (BNP), which are also biomarkers associated with heart failure. Elevated levels of these biomarkers and troponin are found in the amniotic fluid of the recipient, suggesting the presence of myocardial damage [26, 32, 33]. Despite the hypervolemia, vascular resistance in the recipient twin is increased. This hypertension is attributed to vasoactive mediators such as endothelin and also a paradoxically high level of renin. The source of endothelin and renin is probably partly from the placenta and partly from the donor via the vascular communications [34, 35]. These changes in fetal hemodynamics may cause a progressive cardiomyopathy that increases the heart size, reduces the myocardial compliance, and causes atrioventricular valvar regurgitation and abnormal venous Doppler findings. Several studies show that in early Quintero stages or even before the diagnostic of TTTS, the cardiac function in the recipient twin may be impaired [36–38]. A recent study noted that in the recipient twin, left ventricular filling pressures are elevated and systolic function is decreased before abnormalities in the

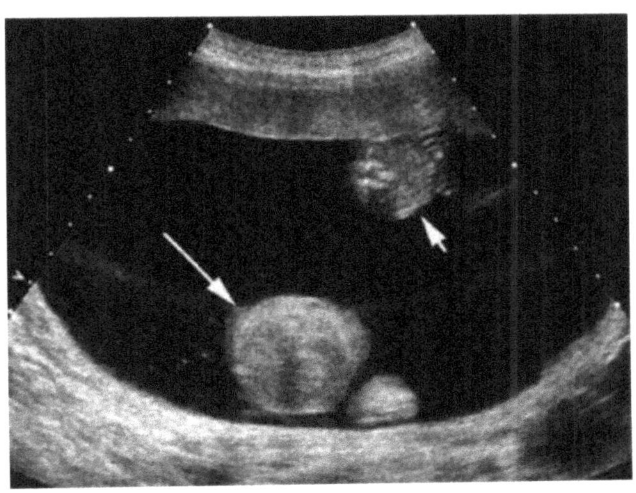

Figure 3. Two fetal abdomens. The smaller one (short arrow) is stuck in the anterior uterine wall and has no amniotic fluid. The bigger fetus (long arrow) has polyhydramnios. Adapted from: https://radiologykey.com/complications-of-multiple-gestations/.

right heart become apparent. They also described an improvement after fetoscopic laser photocoagulation (FLPC) in these fetuses [38].

In the third trimester, fetal discordance in amniotic fluid and growth may occur, increasing uterine distension and causing shortened cervical length and preterm birth. Also, the mirror syndrome, a rare condition that presents itself as a sudden maternal edema, loss of renal and cardiac function, hypertension, and fetal hydrops, may appear in women with TTTS [26, 39, 40].

There is another rare form of TTTS described as "acute peripartum TTTS" which is defined as the intertwin hemoglobin difference at birth >8 g/dl. Since it is a rare condition (2.5% of all the MC pregnancies), there are a few studies and the pathogenesis remains unclear. Some studies says that in theory, acute fetal blood loss from the donor twin into the circulation of the recipient twin may occur as a result of variations in blood pressure due to uterine contractions or fetal positions [41].

3.1.3. *Diagnostic criteria and staging*

In the past, TTTS was diagnosed at the time of birth based on neonatal criteria that included a growth discordance of 15–20% associated with discordant cord or neonatal hemoglobin concentrations of ≥5 g/dl [42]. In 1992, another study showed that these criteria are present in other conditions such as uteroplacental insufficiency, infection, and malformations and therefore should not be used as diagnostic criteria for TTTS [43].

The screening for TTTS should begin with an early ultrasound in order to confirm the chorionicity. The first trimester scan should be performed to look for morphology abnormalities and discordance in the NT measurement, abnormalities in the DV, and even crown-rump length discordances [44]. Unlike dichorionic pregnancies, where ultrasound can be performed every 4 weeks until the end of the second trimester, monochorionic pregnancies should be examined by ultrasound every 2 weeks beginning in the 16th week. An analysis of fetal growth, amniotic fluid deepest vertical pocket (DVP), umbilical artery pulsatility index (UA-PI), medium cerebral artery pulsatility index (MCA-PI), and peak systolic velocity (MCA-PSV) should be obtained [45, 46]. Besides that, a fetal echocardiography should be performed, since cardiac abnormalities are the most common defect in MC pregnancies. The fetal growth and the MCA-PSV are important parameters in the differential diagnosis of sFGR and TAPS, respectively. The early diagnosis is extremely important, since it allows timely treatment with FLPC.

In 1999, Quintero et al. standardized the diagnostic criteria and classification system of TTTS (**Table 1**) [47]. The diagnosis is made when a discordance in the DVP of the twins is visualized. The DVP of the donor twin should be <2 cm; meanwhile the DVP of the recipient, before 20 weeks, should be >8 cm, and after 20 weeks, it should be >10 cm in the European criteria and > 8 cm in the US criteria. The fetal bladders should also be evaluated since there might be a discordance in the size of the fetal bladders (larger in the recipient and smaller in the donor). It is worth reminding that weight discordance is not a diagnostic criterion for TTTS, but it also can be noted in the ultrasound examination.

Stage	Sonographic findings
I	DVP > 8 cm in the recipient* and < 2 cm in the donor twin
II	Absent bladder filling in the donor
III	Critically abnormal Doppler studies of either fetus**
IV	Hydrops of either fetus
V	Intrauterine fetal demise of either fetus

*Before 20 weeks the universal cutoff is 8 cm, and between 21 and 26 weeks, the cutoff is 8 cm in the USA and 10 cm in Europe.

**Absent-reverse diastolic flow in the umbilical artery and/or absent/reverse flow in the ductus venosus or pulsatile flow in the umbilical vein.

Table 1. TTTS staging system. Adapted from Journal of Perinatology, Quintero et al. [44].

There are some critics about it because this staging system is not progressive (e.g., stage I can go to stage IV without passing through stages II and III) [45], and it does not correlate well with survival chance in twins treated with FLPC [48]. Nevertheless, these criteria are the most used to classify TTTS.

3.1.4. Management of TTTS

The natural history of TTTS shows high rates of fetal morbidity and mortality. The perinatal death in some series of cases is about 70–100%, depending on the stage of disease [26]. In stage I, it is known that nearly 70% of the pregnancies remain stable or regress, but in 5% of cases of stages I or II, there is fetal death of one or both twins without warning. Besides that, only 30% of pregnancies managed expectantly have double survivors. In the other stages, mortality increases and treatment is necessary [49]. There are several ways to manage TTTS, which include FLPC, amnioreduction, selective reduction, and pregnancy termination.

The FLPC is the preferred option because its outcomes are better when compared to serial amnioreduction [50, 51]. For stage I, there is no consensus regarding the use of FLPC, so the cases should be individualized [52]. For stages II to IV, FLPC of placental anastomoses is the primary treatment between 16 and 26 weeks of gestation. In 2004, Senat et al. have shown that the mortality rate of fetuses treated with FLPC when compared with serial amnioreduction is significantly lower (RR 0.71; 95% CI 0.55; 0.92). This study also showed a decreased risk of intraventricular hemorrhage and neurological impairment in the laser group. Probably it is because there is a higher rate of prematurity in the amnioreduction group [51]. The procedure consists in inserting a fetoscope in the amniotic sac of the recipient, locating the donor twin and the intertwin membrane, coagulating (with Nd:YAG or diode laser) the intertwin anastomoses along the placental vascular equator, and, after that, removing amniotic fluid from the recipient sac [26, 51].

The quality of fetoscopy images in the early 1990s, when the first FLPC for TTTS was performed, was not good; therefore, the vascular anastomoses were not so easy to identify. The so-called nonselective technique for vessel coagulation was proposed [53]. This technique consisted in coagulating all of the vessels that crossed the intertwin membrane. It did not attempt to differentiate anastomotic from non-anastomotic vessels but rather to catch as many anastomoses as possible (**Figure 4**). With the development of new techniques and advance in fetoscopy technology, another approach was proposed: the selective fetoscopic laser photocoagulation (SFLP) [54, 55]. In this method, the vascular equator is visualized and only intertwin anastomoses are coagulated. This technique differs from the "nonselective" FLPC because the equator does not always coincide with the membrane; therefore, not all the vessels that cross the intertwin membrane should be coagulated; thus, theoretically, more placental tissue will be available for the donor twin after the procedure (**Figure 4**). In 2000, Quintero et al. compared the SFLP with the "nonselective" FLPC and found that the selective method yielded superior results, with survival of at least 1 infant in 83% of patients against 61% in the "nonselective" group [56]. The order of anastomoses coagulation was also studied. Some authors claim that the sequential method, which is a technique where the AV (donor to recipient) are coagulated before the VA, improves the survival rate of both fetuses [57–59] and the survival rate of at least on fetus [58–60]. A recent meta-analysis showed that there may be an improved double neonatal survival as well as a decreased donor and recipient fetal demise with the use of the sequential technique, although all the studies are small and underpowered to confirm the hypothesis [61]. Although the SFLP improved neonatal outcomes, there is about 18% of surgical failure, defined as postoperative symptomatic patent anastomoses (**Figure 5**) [62–65], which could result in several complications such as recurrent TTTS (7–9%) [61, 65], TAPS (13–16%) [66, 67], and fetal death. This is a very delicate situation, because

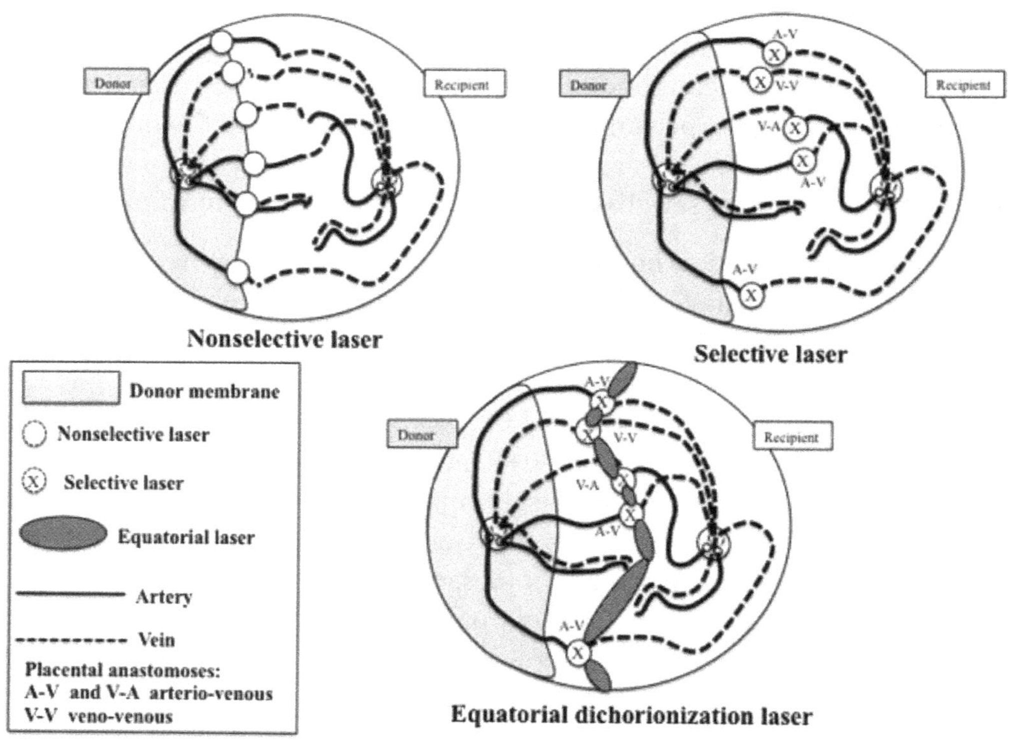

Figure 4. Types of fetoscopic laser techniques in the treatment of TTTS. The nonselective method coagulates all vessels crossing the intertwin membrane. SFLP occlude anastomoses where they occur, sparing placental tissue of the donor. The equatorial laser dichorionization or Solomon technique separates the fetal circulations by coagulating the vascular equator. Adapted from Am J Perinatol. Benoit et al. [26].

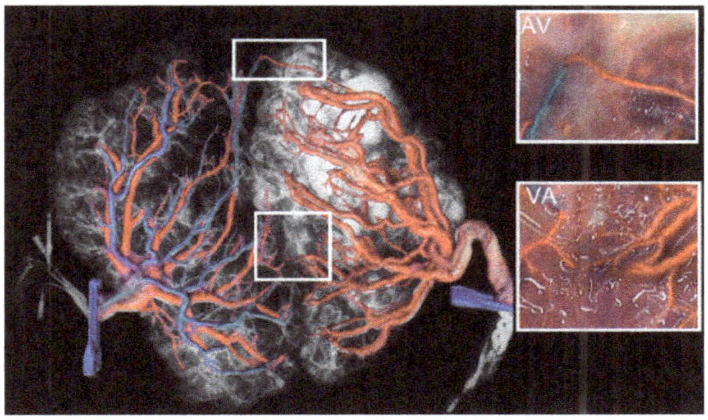

Figure 5. Digitally modified image of placenta with recurrent TTTS with missed AV and VA anastomoses. Adapted from Am J Obstet Gynecol. Lewi et al. [62].

repeating the procedure is more difficult for several reasons such as the size of the uterus and the fetuses. Furthermore, it is associated with an overall perinatal survival rate of 50% [67].

Recently, a new fetoscopic technique in which superficial coagulation of microvasculature on the chorionic plate between ablated anastomotic sites following SFLP was described [68] (**Figure 4**). Some authors compared the SFLP with this new technique in cohort studies and showed a trend toward the latter group [69, 70]. A subsequent randomized trial by Slaghekke et al. compared this new approach called the Solomon technique *versus* the SFLP and found no difference in the overall survival rates. However, a decrease in recurrent TTTS and TAPS after the procedure was observed in the Solomon group (4 vs. 21%) [66].

The main early complications of laser photocoagulation are unintentional septostomy in 8–12%, premature rupture of membranes (PROM) in about 1–9%, and amnion dehiscence (membrane separation) in 5–10% of cases.

The time of delivery in cases of laser photocoagulation varies between 31 and 34 weeks and most of them (60–80%) are not elective. The most common indication is the onset of labor followed by nonreassuring fetal testing and PROM. The mode of delivery is usually by cesarean section, in 57–70% of cases [26, 51, 60, 69, 70].

Unfortunately, in low-income countries, the laser therapy is not widely known and there are no teaching facilities. One Brazilian study showed the initial experience of a single center and found a single twin and both twins' survival rate 1 month after birth is 87.5 and 45.8%, respectively. These reported data are in line with those obtained in major centers worldwide, considering the learning curves and infrastructures [71]. In order to extend the range of the laser therapy to all the MC pregnancies, more teaching centers should be opened, and telemedicine should be used to aid low-income places to achieve the excellence in fetoscopy techniques.

3.1.5. *Perinatal outcomes after treatment*

The perinatal outcomes after the use of SFLP or Solomon technique are very satisfactory. Baschat et al. [70] found that the double survival rates at 6 months of age were 68% in the Solomon group and 50% in the SFLP. Ruano et al. [69] showed an overall neonatal survival rate from 61.8% in the SFLP group to 86.5% when Solomon technique was used. This difference could be due to the increased experience with fetoscopic laser in general and not to the use of the Solomon technique. In the only randomized trial, the single twin and both twins' survival rates after 1 month in the SFLP were 87% and 60%, while in the Solomon group these rate were 85% and 64%, respectively [66].

The neurologic outcomes in the neonatal period following laser procedures, such as intraventricular hemorrhage, periventricular leukomalacia, cerebral white matter cysts, ventricular dilatation, and cerebral atrophy, range from 8 to 18% [51, 72, 73]. The long-term neurodevelopmental outcomes vary between 3 and 12% for cerebral palsy and 4 and 18% for neurodevelopmental impairment [73]. In one study, the neurodevelopmental scores in preterm-born children treated with laser therapy for TTTS were similar in preterm-born DC children, suggesting that prematurity has the main role in the neurologic impairment in fetus treated with laser photocoagulation [74]. Other authors have suggested risk factors for poorer neurodevelopmental outcomes [75, 76]. Lopriore et al. analyzed 212 pregnancies treated with fetoscopic laser surgery and found that advanced gestational age at laser surgery, low gestational age at birth, low birthweight, and high Quintero stage are risk factors of poor neurological development at 2 years of age [76].

Several studies report a rapid cardiac function recovery in the recipient and in the donor twin [36, 38, 77–80]. The coagulation of vascular anastomoses stops the volume exchange, as well as the vasoactive mediators, allowing cardiac output, cardiac size, valvular regurgitation, and ventricular inflow to normalize in the recipient twin in about half of the cases [38, 77]. The donor twin shows an increase in left ventricular filling pressure and cardiac output, which can temporarily cause a relative volume overload. It can worsen the cardiac function and cause ductus venosus alterations and even hydrops; however, these changes tend to disappear by 2 to 4 weeks after the laser procedure [79, 81, 82].

There are other types of treatment, such as septostomy. This procedure increases the risk of severe complications like cord entanglement and disruption of the membrane. This procedure has generally been abandoned [64, 83]. The selective reduction is another therapeutic option that tries to improve the outcome of the surviving twin whenever there is an imminent risk of spontaneous intrauterine death of one fetus. It can be performed either by ultrasound-guided vascular embolization or cord clamping through fetoscopy. A maximum of 50% survival is reached and most services have not supported this technique [68].

The fetoscopic laser coagulation is the gold standard treatment in stage II to stage IV TTTS affected pregnancies; the SFLP and Solomon technique are the best options for lowering the mortality and morbidity in theses fetuses. For Quintero stage I, there is not enough data that favors laser surgery, and more powered studies should be done comparing it to other kinds of treatment; therefore, the treatment for this stage has to be individualized.

3.2. Selective intrauterine growth restriction

Selective intrauterine growth restriction happens in 10–25% of MC gestations and it considerably increases perinatal morbidity and mortality [84–86]. The diagnostic criteria for sFGR differ among clinicians; therefore, it is hard to compare the findings of existing studies, to combine their results, or to establish robust evidence-based management. The pathophysiology in sFGR in MC and DC twins seems to be different. While DC sFGR have conventionally been managed as FGR in a singleton pregnancy, MC twin pregnancies sFGR is thought to result mainly from an unequal placental share. In most cases the origin is in the placental territory discrepancy (**Figure 6**). Vascular anastomoses between both fetuses intrinsically justify IUGR, and one twin receives better oxygenated blood [87].

3.2.1. Diagnostic criteria and staging

Since many authors have proposed different diagnostic criteria, in 2017, the International Society of Ultrasound in Obstetrics and Gynecology (ISUOG) published a guideline for the sFGR diagnostic. It is defined as a condition in which one fetus has estimated fetal weight (EFW) < 10th centile and the intertwin EFW discordance is >25%. EFW discordance is calculated by the following formula: (weight of larger twin – weight of smaller twin) × 100)/weight of larger twin [45]. This weight discordance was proposed by an expert consensus, mainly based on data that show that an 18% EFW discordance reflects poorer outcomes both in DC and MC pregnancies [88]. Curiously, the charts used to monitor the fetal growth should be the same as those used in singleton pregnancies [45, 89], although specific multiple pregnancy charts are available [90]. However, there is a reduction in fetal growth in twin compared with singleton pregnancy, particularly in the third trimester. The key question for clinicians is whether this difference in growth represents adaptation or restriction [91]. Once the diagnosis is made, a detailed anomaly scan and screening for viral infections (cytomegalovirus, rubella, and toxoplasmosis) should be made. Amniocentesis may also be required to exclude chromosomal abnormalities as a cause of FGR [45, 92].

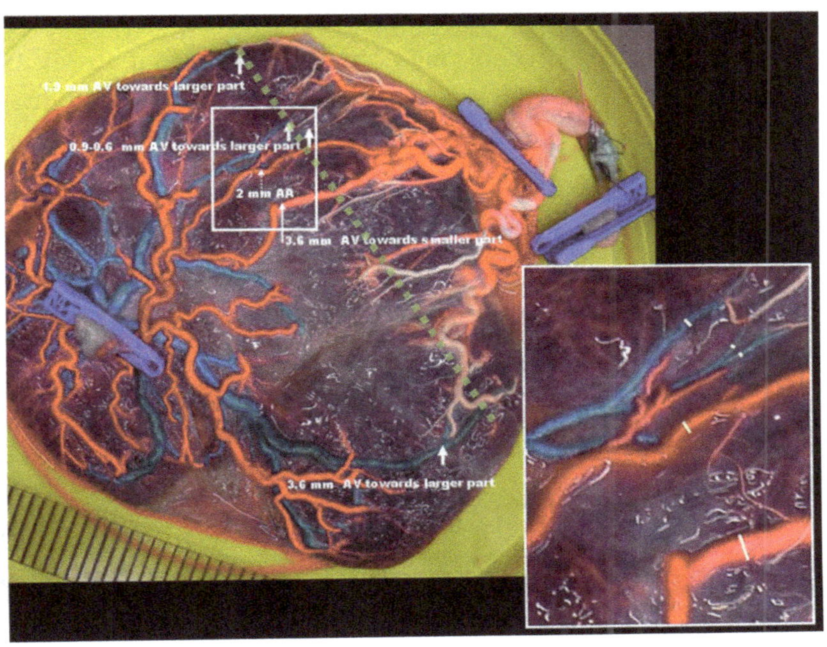

Figure 6. Macroscopic photograph demonstrates the measurement of the vascular anastomoses. There is a 2-mm arterioarterial anastomosis (dashed arrow) and 5 AV anastomoses (arrows). A macroscopic placental surface discordance is also visible (green dashed line: Vascular equator). Adapted from Am J Obstet Gynecol. Lewi et al. [86].

In order to follow up the sFGR pregnancies, as well as in singleton pregnancies, umbilical artery Doppler waveforms and UA-PI are accessed. In pregnancies complicated with sFGR, there are particularities in the umbilical artery Doppler probably because of the variability in the intertwin vascular anastomoses resistance [93, 94]. Three patterns are observed in the umbilical artery Doppler: positive end-diastolic flow, absent or reversed end-diastolic flow (AREDF), and intermittent absent or reversed end-diastolic flow (iAREDF) [95]. The latter pattern though is to result from the presence of transmitted waveforms from the larger into the smaller twin's cord due to the existence of placental large AA anastomoses (**Figure 6**) [93–95]. Based on these three Doppler types, Gratacós et al. proposed a three-stage classification system of the sFGR fetuses. In stage I, the umbilical artery in the smaller twin has a positive end-diastolic flow; in stage II, there is an AREDF; and stage III is characterized by iAREDF (**Figure 7**) [95].

The stage I prognosis is better, with an overall intrauterine mortality rate of 3–4% and a 97% rate of intact survival-free from neurological complications according to two recent meta-analyses. The neonatal morbidity, defined as abnormal brain imaging, respiratory distress syndrome (RDS), admission to the neonatal intensive care unit (NICU), or retinopathy of prematurity (ROP), was reported in about 9% of newborns. The neurologic outcome in this stage seems to be better when compared to the others as well as the gestational age at delivery [84, 93–95, 97]. Stage II sFGR has a poorer prognostic. It is reported that these fetuses tend to have a high risk of hypoxic deterioration and consequently overall, single, and double intrauterine death rates of 16.6%, 8.2%, and 10.4% of cases managed expectantly [97] and a 21% perinatal mortality [84]. The double survival rate in this stage is about 25% [98]. The iAREDF pattern has an intrauterine mortality rate similar to stage II. The overall, single, and double intrauterine death occurred in 13.2%, 7.2%, and 5.5% of cases managed expectantly although this stage is more unpredictable than the others [86, 93, 95, 97, 98]. Some ultrasound markers can be used as adverse predictors such as ductus venosus Z score [98], velamentous cord insertion (**Figure 8**) [99, 100], and weight discordance. A recent meta-analysis found that, in MC twin pregnancies, excluding cases affected by twin to twin transfusion syndrome, twins with birthweight discordance ≥25% were at higher risk of intrauterine death (OR 3.2, 95%CI, 1.5–6.7) and neonatal

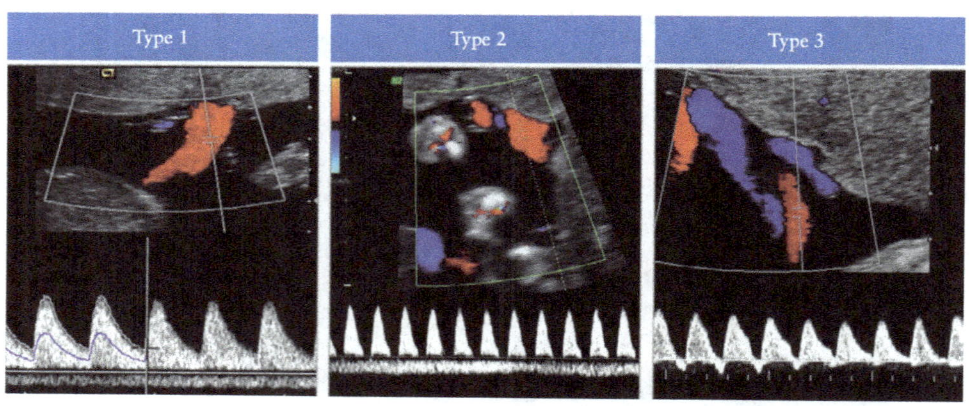

Figure 7. Classification of selective fetal growth restriction in monochorionic twin pregnancy. In type I, the umbilical artery Doppler waveform has positive end-diastolic flow, while in type II there is absent or reversed end-diastolic flow (AREDF). In type III there is a cyclical/intermittent pattern of AREDF. Extracted from ISUOG. https://www.isuog.org/uploads/assets/uploaded/b4ce0129-a7e8-40a9-8543c4243fb7638f.pdf [45].

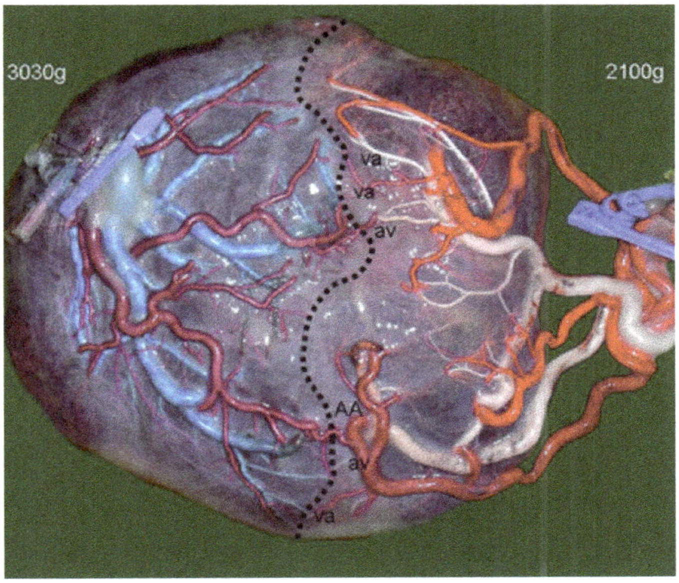

Figure 8. Monochorionic placenta with velamentous cord insertion in the smaller twin side. AV and VA anastomoses are seen and on big AA anastomoses. Adapted from Am J Obstet Gynecol. Lewi et al. [96].

death (OR 4.66, 95% CI, 1.8–12.4) compared with controls [101]. Gratacós et al. [93] found a 15% unexpected intrauterine death rate in the smaller twin on stage III sFGR compared with 2.6% and 0 in stages I and II, respectively. On the other hand, other authors show a better prognosis. Rustico et al. [102] showed a 0% rate in double fetal death at stage III as well as better rates in overall survival and lower neonatal death in the smaller twin (8% and 62%, respectively).

3.2.2. *Management of sFGR*

When sFGR presents with an umbilical artery positive end-diastolic flow, the prognosis is good, and therefore it is a consensus that the expectant management based on a weekly fetal growth and UA-PI evaluation should be done to look for progression to more severe stages which can occur in up to 25% of cases. For stages II and III, several studies compared SFLP with cord occlusion or expectant management, but there are not powered studies to support a gold standard treatment. In a retrospective study with 142 stage II sFGR fetuses treated with SFLP, there was survival rate of the smaller, larger, and both twins of 38.7, 67.6, and 34.5%, respectively. The survival rate of at least one twin was 71.8% [103]. When compared to expectant management, SFLP for stage III sFGR showed a higher overall intrauterine death (14.5 vs. 36%, respectively) as well as a higher death rate in the smaller twin which is 19% for the expectant group and 66% for the SFLP group [104]. Other prospective trial with ten pregnant women with sFGR stages II or III and oligohydramnios treated with SFLP showed that only three newborns of the restricted group survived and all of the newborns in the larger twin group were well and alive at 28 days of age [105].

Cord occlusion of the smaller twin is an option for early diagnosed sFGR, when the spontaneous death of the restricted fetus is most likely to happen, but it is the most difficult decision for the parents to make since they give up the life of one child to protect the other. Chalouhi et al.

[106] found a 90% survival rate in the larger twin after cord occlusion and a 4.5% neurologic complication rate which is much lower than the 26% rate when a spontaneous intrauterine death occurs [107].

The sFGR treatment is not yet defined. Several factors should be evaluated together with parents such as weight discordance, time of diagnosis (early vs. late), hemodynamic state of the restricted fetus at the time of diagnosis, and the will to protect the larger twin since the adverse outcomes are very low after a cord occlusion [94]. If FLPC or expectant management is elected, parent counseling should be made regarding complications and outcomes to both fetus.

3.3. Twin anemia polycythemia sequence

The placental angio-architecture is responsible for most of the complications in MC pregnancies. The intertwin vascular anastomoses have a key role in the pathogenesis of TTTS and sFGR. In 2007, a new MC pregnancy complication was described by Lopriore et al. [108] that involves a discordance in postnatal hemoglobin and hematocrit levels, a difference in neonate reticulocyte levels, and small AV anastomoses in the placenta after colored dye injection (**Figure 9**). This condition was named twin anemia polycythemia sequence. TAPS happens when blood from one twin is slowly transfused to the other by small AV anastomoses at a 5–15 ml/ 24 h rate [108]. Unlike TTTS, there is a less acute and well-compensated intertwin transfusion process leading to a discordance in hemoglobin levels without hemodynamic or amniotic fluid alterations [110]. The reticulocyte levels are also increased in the donor newborn and decreased in the recipient, which differ from other acute diseases, such as acute peripartum TTTS [41]. Another characteristic of TAPS is that after colored dye injection in MC placentas after TAPS, AA anastomoses are observed in about 11% and all of them are small (<1 mm). In comparison, the incidence of AA anastomoses in uncomplicated MC pregnancies and TTTS pregnancies is 80 and 25%, respectively [111, 112], which suggests that AA anastomoses protect against TAPS and TTTS. The maternal side of the TAPS placenta also shows an important color difference. The donor side is more white than the recipient side that shows a plethoric aspect like the respective twin (**Figure 10**) [113].

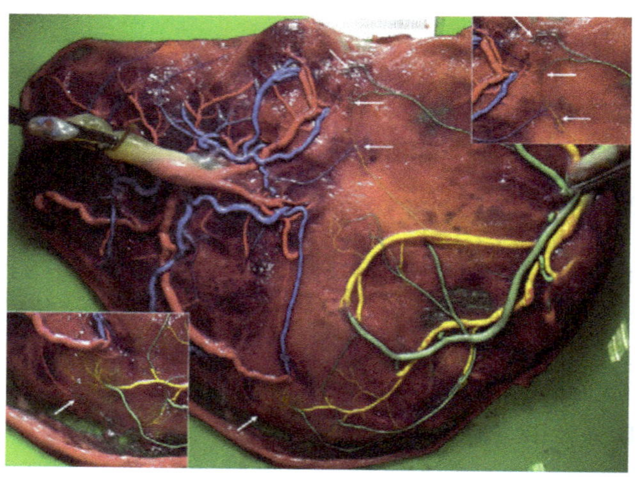

Figure 9. TAPS placenta after colored dye injection (blue or green for arteries and pink or yellow for veins). The white arrows indicate the small AV and VA anastomoses. Adapted from placenta. de Villiers et al. [109].

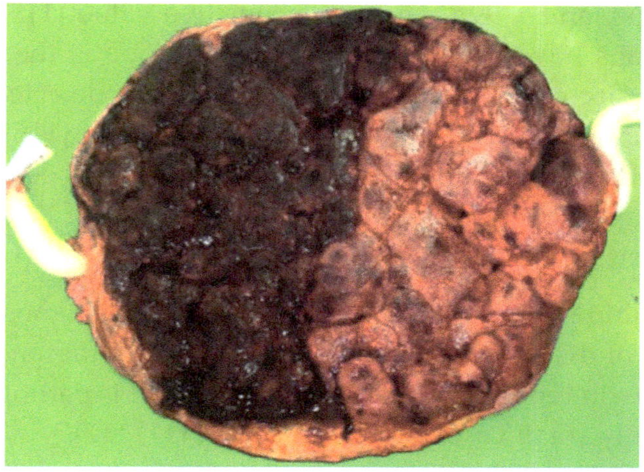

Figure 10. Maternal side of the TAPS placenta showing the difference in color between the plethoric share of the recipient (left side of the placenta) and the anemic share of the donor (right side of the placenta). Adapted from twin research and human genetics. Tollenaar et al. [113].

TAPS may occur spontaneously or post-laser surgery. The prevalence of spontaneous TAPS is about 1.6–5% [18, 68, 114], while post-laser TAPS occurs in 3–16% [66], depending on the technique used. The possible pathophysiology for the latter is the inability to identify all AV anastomoses, therefore leaving some small AV anastomoses without coagulation. The Solomon trial showed a significant decrease in post-laser TAPS in the placental dichorionization group, supporting this hypothesis [66].

3.3.1. *Diagnostic criteria and classification*

TAPS can be diagnosed either antenatally or postnatally. Antenatal diagnosis (**Table 2**) is based in MCA-PSV measurement in both fetuses showing an increased velocity in the anemic and a decreased velocity in the polycythemic twin. The most used criteria of TAPS diagnosis are an MCA-PSV > 1.5 MoM for the donor twin and <1.0 MoM for the recipient twin [111, 115]. Slaghekke et al. analyzed 43 twin pregnancies complicated by TAPS and found that a MCA-PSV > 1.5 MoM correlated with anemia (hemoglobin levels >5 SD below the mean) with a 94% sensitivity, a 74% specificity, a 76% positive predictive value, and a 94% negative predictive value. In the same study, MCA-PSV ≤ 1.0 MoM correlated with polycythemia (hemoglobin levels >5 SD above the mean) with a 97% sensitivity, a 96% specificity, a 93%

Antenatal criteria	Postnatal criteria
Donor MCA-PSV ≥ 1.5 MoM	Intertwin hemoglobin difference > 8 g/dl
AND	**AND 1 of the following**
Recipient MCA-PSV ≤ 1.0 MoM	Reticulocyte count ratio > 1.7
	Placenta with only small (diameter < 1 mm) vascular anastomoses

Table 2. Antenatal and postnatal diagnostic criteria for TAPS. Adapted from ultrasound Obstet Gynecol. Slaghekke et al. [111].

positive predictive value, and a 99% negative predictive value [115]. In some TAPS cases, other ultrasound findings have been reported. The first one is the difference in placental thickness, and echodensity on ultrasound examination was detected [110]. Another ultrasound finding described in TAPS is the so-called starry sky liver [116] which is characterized by clearly identified portal venules and diminished parenchymal echogenicity. More studies are needed to further investigate the validity and significance of these antenatal ultrasound findings for the diagnosis of TAPS.

The postnatal criteria (**Table 2**) can be used when TAPS is not diagnosed by MCA Doppler. It is based on the finding of discordant hemoglobin levels (Hb difference > 8.0 g/dl) associated with an increased intertwin reticulocyte count ratio > 1.7 that is pathognomonic for TAPS and placental evidence of only small vascular anastomoses [111, 117].

The classification for TAPS was proposed by Slaghekke et al. in 2010 [111] based on the difference in hemoglobin levels postnatally (**Table 3**).

3.3.2. Management of TAPS

There is no optimal treatment for TAPS. Options include expectant management and early delivery; intrauterine transfusion (IUT) in the donor, with or without partial exchange transfusion (PET) in the recipient; selective feticide; and fetoscopic laser surgery.

Expectant management is made with closing ultrasound monitoring with serial MCA-PVS evaluation and an early delivery when necessary. It leads to a 75 to 83% survival rate [111, 118].

Another kind of treatment is IUT that can be performed intravascularly or intraperitoneal. It seems the latter may be superior to intravascular intrauterine transfusions because it is technically easier and can be performed as early as 15 weeks [119]. Although this method is commonly used, it is a palliative option, since it temporarily meliorates the donor anemia. Furthermore, the raise in blood viscosity in the recipient twin can lead to embolic complications [67]. These complications can be managed by partial exchange transfusion (PET) that decreases the viscosity of the blood of the polycythemic recipient. The perinatal survival rate in some studies is generally good, reaching 85–100% [111, 118].

Antenatal stage	Doppler ultrasound
Stage I	MCA-PSV donor >1.5 MoM and MCA-PSV recipient <1.0 MoM, without other signs of fetal compromise
Stage II	MCA-PSV donor >1.7 MoM and MCA-PSV recipient <0.8 MoM, without other signs of fetal compromise
Stage III	As stage I or II, with cardiac compromise of donor, defined as critically abnormal flow*
Stage IV	Hydrops of donor
Stage V	Intrauterine demise of one or both fetuses preceded by TAPS

*Critically abnormal Doppler is defined as absent or reversed end-diastolic flow in umbilical artery, pulsatile flow in the umbilical vein, and increased pulsatility index or reversed flow in ductus venosus.

Table 3. Antenatal TAPS classification. Adapted from Ultrasound Obstet Gynecol. Slaghekke et al. [111].

The only causal treatment for both spontaneous and post-laser TAPS is laser surgery. It is technically more difficult because of the absence of polyhydramnios and a stuck twin, which makes the visualization of the vascular equator more challenging as well as the size of anastomoses, which is difficult to visualize during fetoscopy [111]. The results in small studies are satisfactory, with a survival rate of 94–100% [111, 118, 120, 121] and an apparent improvement in perinatal outcome by prolonging pregnancy and reducing respiratory distress syndrome [117].

The TAPS management should be made after evaluation of different factors, including TAPS stage, gestational age, and the clinician experience in the different types of treatments. In early stages, TAPS can be managed expectantly. If gestational age is below 26–28 weeks, laser treatment should be considered [113]. When laser treatment is not possible, IUT should be considered. When repeated IUT is expected or in case of severe polycythemia in the recipient, PET of the recipient can be done.

3.4. Twin reversed arterial perfusion sequence

Twin reversed arterial perfusion sequence resulting in an acardiac twin is a rare condition and occurs in 1:35,000 births or 1% of all monozygotic twins [122]. It consists in one health twin (the "pump" twin) and one acardiac mass which is perfused by the other fetus' heart. This acardiac twin most often has an underdeveloped head and upper body and impressive edema also mostly of the upper body. In some cases, there might be fetal movements. In rare cases, a rudimentary pulsating cardiac structure may be seen. It is though that the VV and AA bidirectional anastomoses are responsible for the perfusion of the acardiac fetus. One study analyzed the TRAPS placenta and found big AA anastomoses as well as veins in direct continuity with each other. They also noted that umbilical cords were attached, with insertion adjacent to each other [123]. The blood from the pump twin flows through the umbilical artery to the umbilical artery of the acardiac twin and then it flows back to the recipient twin through the umbilical vein. The returning blood bypasses the placenta and returns to the pump twin via VV anastomoses, without passing through the placenta. This condition may cause a hyperdynamic circulation and progressive high output cardiac failure in the pump twin causing fetal death in about half of cases if not treated [122, 124, 125].

The diagnostic is made by turning on the color Doppler and showing the inverse direction of blood flow in the aorta of the acardiac twin [92] (**Figure 11**). TRAPS is usually diagnosed in the 11–13 weeks scan or even in the early endovaginal ultrasound [126–128]. Given the fact that 50% of pump twin dies if expectant management is made and that in 33% of the TRAPS pregnancies diagnosed at the first trimester the healthy twin dies before 18 weeks [123, 129], several intrauterine interventions have been tested in order to improve the perinatal outcomes. The overall survival of the treatment methods is similar among several studies and varies between 71 and 86% [130–134]. The methods used to manage TRAPS are cord ligation; monopolar, bipolar, or laser cord coagulation; and fetoscopic laser coagulation of placental anastomoses. However, intrafetal techniques such as intrafetal laser ablation and intrafetal radiofrequency ablation (RFA) are preferred because, when compared to cord occlusion

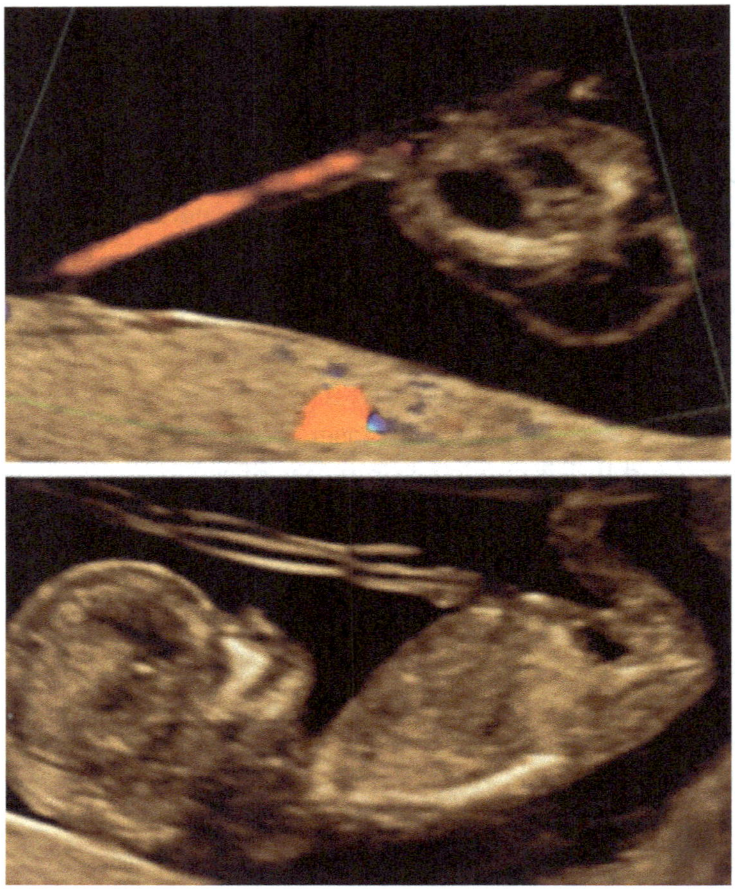

Figure 11. Upper image: Acardiac twin with retrograde flow in the umbilical cord. Lower image: Normal recipient twin. Adapted from ultrasound Obstet Gynecol. Pagani et al. [124].

techniques, they are associated with a lower technical failure rate (13 vs. 35%), lower rate of preterm birth or rupture of membranes before 32 weeks (23 vs. 58%), and higher rate of clinical success (77 vs. 50%) [135].

There are some doubts about the optimal time to do the treatment. Performing any procedure before the obliteration of the coelomic cavity increases the risk of talipes and miscarriage [136]; therefore, most of the authors perform the intervention between 13 and 16 weeks [124]. In one study in which the median gestational age at intervention (intrafetal laser ablation) was 13.2 weeks, there was a 41% mortality rate in the first 72 h after the procedure; therefore, surgery before 13 weeks of gestation should be avoided [136]. Some studies showed that expectant management could be offered in special cases. Jelin et al. [125] found a 100% survival when the acardiac twin had less than 50% of the pump twin's weight. Other studies suggested that discordance between crown-rump length of the pump twin and upper pole-rump length of the TRAP twin could be potential predictors of pregnancy outcome [137].

The optimal approach should be an early diagnosis and a proper parental counseling and an intrafetal intervention, by laser or RFA in 13–16 weeks. The expectant management could be considered if the TRAP twin is smaller (about half the size) than the pump twin.

4. Conclusion

Monochorionic pregnancies are at a great risk of complications such as preterm birth, fetal and neonatal death, and neurological injury. The early sonographic screening is extremely important to diagnose some of the most important complications which can lead to death of one or both siblings. It should begin in the first trimester, where the confirmation of chorionicity should be done and the search for potential predictors of adverse outcomes such as NT discordance should be accessed. Some complications such as TRAPS can be diagnosed and managed in this period. Beginning in the 16th week, a biweekly detailed ultrasound examination is extremely important since it can detect early stages of TTTS, sFGR, and TAPS. Most of these complications can be treated in the mid-trimester improving the survival rate of one or both fetuses.

The fetoscopic approach is the main method to manage MC twin complications and should be available in specialized fetal medicine centers with trained staff to perform the laser surgery. Several laser techniques have been tested in the last years and the improvement in the outcomes is clear. Although the results are satisfactory, the complication rates, such as PROM and unintentional septostomy, are still relatively high as well as the both twins' survival rate.

Future directions in the management of TTTS are likely to involve refinements in the prediction of the disease, clarification of the optimum frequency of surveillance, technique of laser therapy, prediction of adverse outcome after treatment, and development of other vascular ablative techniques.

Although the treatment efficacy is rapidly improving in big centers, in most parts of the world, there is a lack of specialized centers and trained personnel. In order to achieve an optimal management in MC pregnancy complications, it is important to improve the early screening and diagnosis and the referral system, mainly in low-income countries.

Author details

Bruno Rodrigues Toneto

Address all correspondence to: brunotoneto@yahoo.com.br

Federal University of São Paulo, São Paulo, Brazil

References

[1] Gary Cunningham F. Multifetal pregnancy. In: Williams Obstetrics. 24th ed. McGraw-Hill Education; 2014. pp. 891-924

[2] Schwartz DB, Daoud Y, Zazula P, Goyert G, Bronsteen R, Wright D. Gestational diabetes mellitus: Metabolic and blood glucose parameters in singleton versus twin pregnancies. American Journal of Obstetrics and Gynecology. 1999;**181**(4):912-914

[3] Bailit JL. Hyperemesis gravidarum: Epidemiologic findings from a large cohort. American Journal of Obstetrics and Gynecology. 2005;**193**(3 Pt 1):811-814. DOI: 10.1016/j.ajog.2005.02.132

[4] Conde-Agudelo A, Belizán JM, Lindmark G. Maternal morbidity and mortality associated with multiple gestations. Obstetrics and Gynecology. 2000;**95**(6 Pt 1):899-904

[5] Sibai BM, Hauth J, Caritis S, Lindheimer MD, MacPherson C, Klebanoff M. Hypertensive disorders in twin versus singleton gestations. National Institute of Child Health and Human Development network of maternal-Fetal medicine units. American Journal of Obstetrics and Gynecology. 2000;**182**(4):938-942

[6] Scher AI, Petterson B, Blair E, Ellenberg JH, Grether JK, Haan E. The risk of mortality or cerebral palsy in twins: A collaborative population-based study. Pediatric Research. 2002;**52**:671-681. DOI: 10.1203/00006450-200211000-00011

[7] Martin JA, Hamilton BE, Osterman MJ, Driscoll AK, Drake P. Births: Final data for 2016. National Vital Statistics Reports. 2018;**67**(1):1-55

[8] McPherson JA, Odibo AO, Shanks AL, Roehl KA, Macones GA, Cahill AG. Impact of chorionicity on risk and timing of intrauterine fetal demise in twin pregnancies. American Journal of Obstetrics and Gynecology. 2012;**207**(3):190.e1-6. DOI: 10.1016/j.ajog.2012.07.031

[9] Lee YM, Wylie BJ, Simpson LL, D'Alton ME. Twin Chorionicity and the risk of stillbirth. Obstetrics and Gynecology. 2008;**111**(2, Part 1):301-308. DOI: 10.1097/AOG.0b013e318160d65d

[10] Committee on ethics. Committee opinion No. 719. Obstetrics & Gynecology. 2017;**130**(3):e158-e163. Available from: http://www.ncbi.nlm.nih.gov/pubmed/28832490 [Accessed: 2018-10-06]

[11] Blondel B, Kaminski M. Trends in the occurrence, determinants, and consequences of multiple births. Seminars in Perinatology. 2002;**26**(4):239-249

[12] Haines N. Birth characteristics in England and Wales - Office for National Statistics [Internet]. 2017. Available from: https://www.ons.gov.uk/peoplepopulationandcommunity/birthsdeathsandmarriages/livebirths/bulletins/birthcharacteristicsinenglandandwales/2016 [Accessed: 2018-10-06]

[13] Kulkarni AD, Kissin DM, Adashi EY. Fertility treatments and multiple births in the United States. The New England Journal of Medicine. 2014;**370**(11):1069-1071. DOI: 10.1056/NEJMc1400242

[14] Bortolus R, Parazzini F, Chatenoud L, Benzi G, Bianchi MM, Marini A. The epidemiology of multiple births. Human Reproduction Update;**5**(2):179-187

[15] Multiple gestation pregnancy. The ESHRE Capri workshop group. Human Reproduction. 2000;**15**(8):1856-1864

[16] Gan J-P, Wu Z-H, Tu Z-M, Zheng J. The comparison of twinning rates between urban and rural areas in China. Twin Research and Human Genetics. 2007;**10**(4):633-637. DOI: 10.1375/twin.10.4.633

[17] Hack KE, Derks JB, Elias SG, et al. Increased perinatal mortality and morbidity in monochorionic versus dichorionic twin pregnancies: Clinical implications of a large Dutch cohort study. BJOG. 2008;**115**:58-67. DOI: 10.1111/j.1471-0528.2007.01556.x

[18] Lewi L, Jani J, Blickstein I, et al. The outcome of monochorionic diamniotic twin gestations in the era of invasive fetal therapy: A prospective cohort study. American Journal of Obstetrics and Gynecology. 2008;**199**:514-518. DOI: 10.1016/j.ajog.2008.03.050

[19] Denbow ML, Cox P, Taylor M. Placental angioarchitecture in monochorionic twin pregnancies: Relationship to fetal growth, fetofetal transfusion syndrome, and pregnancy outcome. American Journal of Obstetrics and Gynecology. 2000;**182**:417-426

[20] Glennon CL, Shemer SA, Palma-Dias R, Umstad MP. The history of treatment of twin-to-twin transfusion syndrome. Twin Research and Human Genetics. 2016;**19**(3):168-174. DOI: 10.1017/thg.2016.27

[21] Naeye RL. Organ abnormalities in a human parabiotic syndrome. The American Journal of Pathology. 1965;**46**(5):829-842

[22] Danskin FH, Neilson JP. Twin-to-twin transfusion syndrome: What are appropriate diagnostic criteria? American Journal of Obstetrics and Gynecology. 1989;**161**:365-369

[23] Blickstein I. Monochorionicity in perspective. Ultrasound in Obstetrics & Gynecology. 2006;**27**(3):235-238. DOI: 10.1002/uog.2730

[24] WAPM Consensus Group on Twin-to-Twin Transfusion, Baschat A, Chmait RH, Deprest J, Gratacós E, Hecher K. Twin-to-twin transfusion syndrome (TTTS). Journal of Perinatal Medicine. 2011;**39**(2):107-112. DOI: 10.1515/JPM.2010.147

[25] Berghella V, Kaufmann M. Natural history of twin-twin transfusion syndrome. The Journal of Reproductive Medicine. 2001;**46**(5):480-484

[26] Benoit RM, Baschat AA. Twin-to-twin transfusion syndrome: Prenatal diagnosis and treatment. American Journal of Perinatology. 2014;**31**(7):583-594. DOI: 10.1055/s-0034-1372428

[27] Zhao D, Lipa M, Wielgos M, Cohen D, Middeldorp JM, Oepkes D, et al. Comparison between monochorionic and dichorionic placentas with special attention to vascular anastomoses and placental share. Twin Research and Human Genetics. 2016;**19**(3): 191-196. DOI: 10.1055/s-0029-1215430

[28] De Paepe ME, Shapiro S, Greco D, Luks VL, Abellar RG, Luks CH, et al. Placental markers of twin-to-twin transfusion syndrome in diamniotic-monochorionic twins: A morphometric analysis of deep artery-to-vein anastomoses. Placenta. 2010;**31**(4):269-276. DOI: 10.1016/j.placenta.2009.12.024

[29] Matias A, Montenegro N, Loureiro T, Cunha M, Duarte S, Freitas D, et al. Screening for twin-twin transfusion syndrome at 11-14 weeks of pregnancy: The key role of ductus venosus blood flow assessment. Ultrasound in Obstetrics & Gynecology. 2010;**35**(2): 142-148. DOI: 10.1002/uog.7533

[30] Memmo A, Dias T, Mahsud-Dornan S, Papageorghiou AT, Bhide A, Thilaganathan B. Prediction of selective fetal growth restriction and twin-to-twin transfusion syndrome in monochorionic twins. BJOG. 2012;**119**:417-421

[31] Maiz N, Staboulidou I, Leal AM, Minekawa R, Nicolaides KH. Ductus venosus Doppler at 11 to 13 weeks of gestation in the prediction of outcome in twin pregnancies. Obstetrics and Gynecology. 2009;**113**:860-865

[32] Van Mieghem T, Doné E, Gucciardo L, Klaritsch P, Allegaert K, Van Bree R, et al. Amniotic fluid markers of fetal cardiac dysfunction in twin-to-twin transfusion syndrome. American Journal of Obstetrics and Gynecology. 2010;**202**(1):48.e1-48.e7. DOI: 10.1002/uog.7533

[33] Habli M, Cnota J, Michelfelder E, Salisbury S, Schnell B, Polzin W, et al. The relationship between amniotic fluid levels of brain-type natriuretic peptide and recipient cardiomyopathy in twin–twin transfusion syndrome. American Journal of Obstetrics and Gynecology. 2010;**203**(4):404.e1-404.e7. DOI: 10.1016/j.ajog.2010.06.070

[34] Mahieu-Caputo D, Meulemans A, Martinovic J, Gubler M-C, Delezoide A-L, Muller F, et al. Paradoxic activation of the renin-angiotensin system in twin-twin transfusion syndrome: An explanation for cardiovascular disturbances in the recipient. Pediatric Research. 2005;**58**(4):685-688. DOI: 10.1203/01.PDR.0000180558.03164.E8

[35] Galea P, Barigye O, Wee L, Jain V, Sullivan M, Fisk NM. The placenta contributes to activation of the renin angiotensin system in twin–twin transfusion syndrome. Placenta. 2008;**29**(8):734-742. DOI: 10.1016/j.placenta.2008.04.010

[36] Manning N, Archer N. Cardiac manifestations of twin-to-twin transfusion syndrome. Twin Research and Human Genetics. 2016;**19**(3):246-254. DOI: 10.1017/thg.2016.20

[37] Habli M, Michelfelder E, Cnota J, Wall D, Polzin W, Lewis D, et al. Prevalence and progression of recipient-twin cardiomyopathy in early-stage twin-twin transfusion syndrome. Ultrasound in Obstetrics & Gynecology. 2012;**39**(1):63-68. DOI: 10.1016/j.ajog.2018.05.008

[38] Wohlmuth C, Boudreaux D, Moise KJ, Johnson A, Papanna R, Bebbington M, et al. Cardiac pathophysiology in twin-twin transfusion syndrome: New insights into its evolution. Ultrasound in Obstetrics & Gynecology. 2018;**51**(3):341-348. DOI: 10.1002/uog.17480

[39] Braun T, Brauer M, Fuchs I, et al. Mirror syndrome: A systematic review of fetal associated conditions, maternal presentation and perinatal outcome. Fetal Diagnosis and Therapy. 2010;**27**(4):191-203. DOI: 10.1159/000305096

[40] Ortiz LFL, Elito Júnior J, Araujo Júnior E, Peixoto AB, Sass N, Moron AF. Mirror syndrome in Monochorionic twin pregnancy with Acardiac Fetus. Case Reports in Obstetrics and Gynecology. 2018;**2018**:1302041. DOI: 10.1155/2018/1302041

[41] Lopriore E, Holtkamp N, Sueters M, Middeldorp JM, Walther FJ, Oepkes D. Acute peripartum twin-twin transfusion syndrome: Incidence, risk factors, placental characteristics and neonatal outcome. The Journal of Obstetrics and Gynaecology Research. 2014;**40**(1):18-24. DOI: 10.1111/jog.1211

[42] Rausen AR, Seki M, Strauss L. Twin transfusion syndrome. A review of 19 cases studied at one institution. The Journal of Pediatrics. 1965;**66**:613-628

[43] Wenstrom KD, Tessen JA, Zlatnik FJ, Sipes SL. Frequency, distribution, and theoretical mechanisms of hematologic and weight discordance in monochorionic twins. Obstetrics and Gynecology. 1992;**80**(2):257-261

[44] Mackie FL, Hall MJ, Morris RK, Kilby MD. Early prognostic factors of outcomes in monochorionic twin pregnancy: Systematic review and meta-analysis. American Journal of Obstetrics and Gynecology. 2018;**219**(5):436-446. DOI: 10.1016/j.ajog.2018.05.00

[45] ISUOG Practice Guidelines: Role of Ultrasound in Twin Pregnancy. 2015 [Internet]; Available from: https://www.isuog.org/uploads/assets/uploaded/b4ce0129-a7e8-40a9-8543c4243fb7638f.pdf [Accessed: 2018-10-07]

[46] Sueters M, Middeldorp JM, Lopriore E, Oepkes D, Kanhai HHH, Vandenbussche FPHA. Timely diagnosis of twin-to-twin transfusion syndrome in monochorionic twin pregnancies by biweekly sonography combined with patient instruction to report onset of symptoms. Ultrasound in Obstetrics & Gynecology. 2006;**28**(5):659-664. DOI: 10.1002/uog.15821

[47] Quintero RA, Morales WJ, Allen MH, Bornick PW, Johnson PK, Kruger M. Staging of twin-twin transfusion syndrome. Journal of Perinatology. 1999;**19**(8 Pt 1):550-555

[48] Rossi A, D'Addario V. The efficacy of Quintero staging system to assess severity of twin–twin transfusion syndrome treated with laser therapy: A systematic review with meta-analysis. American Journal of Perinatology. 2009;**26**(07):537-544. DOI: 10.1055/s-0029-1215430

[49] O'Donoghue K, Cartwright E, Galea P, Fisk NM. Stage I twin-twin transfusion syndrome: Rates of progression and regression in relation to outcome. Ultrasound in Obstetrics & Gynecology. 2007;**30**(7):958-964. DOI: 10.1016/j.ajog.2018.05.008

[50] Hecher K, Diehl W, Zikulnig L, Vetter M, Hackelöer BJ. Endoscopic laser coagulation of placental anastomoses in 200 pregnancies with severe mid-trimester twin-to-twin transfusion syndrome. European Journal of Obstetrics, Gynecology, and Reproductive Biology. 2000;**92**(1):135-139

[51] Senat M-V, Deprest J, Boulvain M, Paupe A, Winer N, Ville Y. Endoscopic laser surgery versus serial Amnioreduction for severe twin-to-twin transfusion syndrome. The New England Journal of Medicine. 2004;**351**(2):136-144. DOI: 10.1016/j.ajog.2018.05.008

[52] Khalil A, Cooper E, Townsend R, Thilaganathan B. Evolution of stage 1 twin-to-twin transfusion syndrome (TTTS): Systematic review and meta-analysis. Twin Research and Human Genetics. 2016;**19**(3):207-216. DOI: 10.1016/j.ajog.2018.05.008

[53] De Lia JE, Cruikshank DP, Keye WR. Fetoscopic neodymium: YAG laser occlusion of placental vessels in severe twin-twin transfusion syndrome. Obstetrics and Gynecology. 1990;**75**(6):1046-1053

[54] Quintero RA, Morales WJ, Mendoza G, Allen M, Kalter CS, Giannina G, et al. Selective photocoagulation of placental vessels in twin-twin transfusion syndrome: Evolution of a surgical technique. Obstetrical & Gynecological Survey. 1998;**53**(12 Suppl):S97-S103

[55] Thilaganathan B, Gloeb DJ, Sairam S, Tekay A. Sono-endoscopic delineation of the placental vascular equator prior to selective fetoscopic laser ablation in twin-to-twin transfusion syndrome. Ultrasound in Obstetrics & Gynecology. 2000;**16**(3):226-229. DOI: 10.1046/j.1469-0705.2000.00272.x

[56] Quintero RA, Comas C, Bornick PW, Allen MH, Kruger M. Selective versus non-selective laser photocoagulation of placental vessels in twin-to-twin transfusion syndrome. Ultrasound in Obstetrics & Gynecology. 2000;**16**(3):230-236. DOI: 10.1046/j.1469-0705.2000.00265.x

[57] Chmait RH, Khan A, Benirschke K, Miller D, Korst LM, Goodwin TM. Perinatal survival following preferential sequential selective laser surgery for twin-twin transfusion syndrome. The Journal of Maternal-Fetal & Neonatal Medicine. 2010;**23**(1):10-16. DOI: 10.3109/14767050903128618

[58] Nakata M, Murakoshi T, Sago H, Ishii K, Takahashi Y, Hayashi S, et al. Modified sequential laser photocoagulation of placental communicating vessels for twin-twin transfusion syndrome to prevent fetal demise of the donor twin. The Journal of Obstetrics and Gynaecology Research. 2009;**35**(4):640-647. DOI: 10.1111/j.1447-0756.2009.01034.x

[59] Quintero RA, Ishii K, Chmait RH, Bornick PW, Allen MH, Kontopoulos EV. Sequential selective laser photocoagulation of communicating vessels in twin–twin transfusion syndrome. Journal of Maternal-Fetal and Neonatal Medicine. 2007;**20**(10):763-768. DOI: 10.1080/14767050701591827

[60] Murata S, Takano M, Kagawa Y, Sumie M, Nakata M. The experience of modified sequential selective laser photocoagulation of communicating vessels technique for twin-twin transfusion syndrome. Journal of Maternal-Fetal and Neonatal Medicine. 2018;**31**(9):1137-1141. DOI: 10.1080/14767058.2017.1311309

[61] Akkermans J, Peeters SH, Klumper FJ, Middeldorp JM, Lopriore E, Oepkes D. Is the sequential laser technique for twin-to-twin transfusion syndrome truly superior to the standard selective technique? A meta-analysis. Fetal Diagnosis and Therapy. 2014; **37**(4):251-258. DOI: 10.1159/000365212

[62] Stirnemann JJ, Nasr B, Quarello E, Ortqvist L, Nassar M, Bernard J-P, et al. A definition of selectivity in laser coagulation of chorionic plate anastomoses in twin-to-twin

transfusion syndrome and its relationship to perinatal outcome. American Journal of Obstetrics and Gynecology. 2008;**198**(1):62.e1-62.e6. DOI: 10.1016/j.ajog.2007.06.009

[63] Chalouhi GE, Essaoui M, Stirnemann J, Quibel T, Deloison B, Salomon L, et al. Laser therapy for twin-to-twin transfusion syndrome (TTTS). Prenatal Diagnosis. 2011;**31**(7): 637-646. DOI: 10.1002/pd.2803

[64] Chalouhi GE, Stirnemann JJ, Salomon LJ, Essaoui M, Quibel T, Ville Y. Specific complications of monochorionic twin pregnancies: Twin-twin transfusion syndrome and twin reversed arterial perfusion sequence. Seminars in Fetal & Neonatal Medicine. 2010;**15**(6):349-356. DOI: 10.1016/j.siny.2010.09.003

[65] Lewi L, Jani J, Cannie M, Robyr R, Ville Y, Hecher K, et al. Intertwin anastomoses in monochorionic placentas after fetoscopic laser coagulation for twin-to-twin transfusion syndrome: Is there more than meets the eye? American Journal of Obstetrics and Gynecology. 2006;**194**(3):790-795. DOI: 10.1016/j.ajog.2013.05.034

[66] Slaghekke F, Lopriore E, Lewi L, Middeldorp JM, Van Zwet EW, Weingertner AS, et al. Fetoscopic laser coagulation of the vascular equator versus selective coagulation for twin-to-twin transfusion syndrome: An open-label randomised controlled trial. Lancet. 2014;**383**(9935):2144-2151. DOI: 10.1016/j.ajog.2007.06.009

[67] Robyr R, Lewi L, Salomon LJ, Yamamoto M, Bernard J-P, Deprest J, et al. Prevalence and management of late fetal complications following successful selective laser coagulation of chorionic plate anastomoses in twin-to-twin transfusion syndrome. American Journal of Obstetrics and Gynecology. 2006;**194**(3):796-803. DOI: 10.1016/j.ajog.2005.08.069

[68] Lopriore E, Slaghekke F, Middeldorp JM, Klumper FJ, Oepkes D, Vandenbussche FP. Residual anastomoses in twin-to-twin transfusion syndrome treated with selective fetoscopic laser surgery: Localization, size, and consequences. American Journal of Obstetrics and Gynecology. 2009;**201**(1):66.e1-4. DOI: 10.1016/j.ajog.2009.01.010

[69] Ruano R, Rodo C, Peiro JL, Shamshirsaz AA, Haeri S, Nomura ML, et al. Fetoscopic laser ablation of placental anastomoses in twin-twin transfusion syndrome using 'Solomon technique'. Ultrasound in Obstetrics & Gynecology. 2013;(4):42. n/a-n/a. DOI: 10.1002/uog.12492

[70] Baschat AA, Barber J, Pedersen N, Turan OM, Harman CR. Outcome after fetoscopic selective laser ablation of placental anastomoses vs equatorial laser dichorionization for the treatment of twin-to-twin transfusion syndrome. American Journal of Obstetrics and Gynecology. 2013;**209**(3):234.e1-8. DOI: 10.1016/j.ajog.2013.05.034

[71] Barbosa MM, Martins Santana EF, Milani VHJF, Elito Júnior J, Araujo Júnior E, Moron AF, et al. Fetoscopic laser photocoagulation for twin-to-twin transfusion syndrome treatment: Initial experience in tertiary reference Center in Brazil. Obstetrics & Gynecology Science. 2018;**61**(4):461-467

[72] Van Klink JMM, Koopman HM, Rijken M, Middeldorp JM, Oepkes D, Lopriore E. Long-term neurodevelopmental outcome in survivors of twin-to-twin transfusion syndrome. Twin Research and Human Genetics. 2016;**19**(3):255-261. DOI: 10.1017/thg.2016.26

[73] Lopriore E, van Wezel-Meijler G, Middeldorp JM, Sueters M, Vandenbussche FP, Walther FJ. Incidence, origin, and character of cerebral injury in twin-to-twin transfusion syndrome treated with fetoscopic laser surgery. American Journal of Obstetrics and Gynecology. 2006;**194**(5):1215-1220. DOI: 10.1016/j.ajog.2005.12.003

[74] Lenclen R, Ciarlo G, Paupe A, Bussieres L, Ville Y. Neurodevelopmental outcome at 2 years in children born preterm treated by amnioreduction or fetoscopic laser surgery for twin-to-twin transfusion syndrome: Comparison with dichorionic twins. American Journal of Obstetrics and Gynecology. 2009;**201**(3):291.e1-291.e5. DOI: 10.1016/j.ajog.2009.05.036

[75] Salomon LJ, Rtqvist L, Aegerter P, Bussieres L, Staracci S, Stirnemann JJ, et al. Long-term developmental follow-up of infants who participated in a randomized clinical trial of amniocentesis vs laser photocoagulation for the treatment of twin-to-twin transfusion syndrome. American Journal of Obstetrics and Gynecology. 2010;**203**(5):444.e1-444.e7. DOI: 10.1016/j.ajog.2010.08.054

[76] Lopriore E, Ortibus E, Acosta-Rojas R, Le Cessie S, Middeldorp JM, Oepkes D, et al. Risk factors for neurodevelopment impairment in twin-twin transfusion syndrome treated with fetoscopic laser surgery. Obstetrics and Gynecology. 2009;**113**(2 Pt 1):361-366. DOI: 10.1097/AOG.0b013e318195873e

[77] Van Mieghem T, Lewi L, Gucciardo L, Dekoninck P, Van Schoubroeck D, Devlieger R, et al. The fetal heart in twin-to-twin transfusion syndrome. International Journal of Pediatrics. 2010;**2010**:8 pages. DOI: 10.1016/j.ajog.2010.08.054

[78] Baschat AA, Gungor S, Glosemeyer P, Huber A, Hecher K. Changes in umbilical venous volume flow after fetoscopic laser occlusion of placental vascular anastomoses in twin-to-twin transfusion syndrome. American Journal of Obstetrics and Gynecology. 2010;**203**(5):479.e1-6. DOI: 10.1016/j.ajog.2009.11.013

[79] Van Mieghem T, Klaritsch P, Doné E, Gucciardo L, Lewi P, Verhaeghe J, et al. Assessment of fetal cardiac function before and after therapy for twin-to-twin transfusion syndrome. American Journal of Obstetrics and Gynecology. 2009;**200**(4):400.e1-400.e7. DOI: 10.1016/j.ajog.2009.01.051

[80] Van Mieghem T, Martin AM, Weber R, Barrea C, Windrim R, Hornberger LK, et al. Fetal cardiac function in recipient twins undergoing fetoscopic laser ablation of placental anastomoses for stage IV twin-twin transfusion syndrome. Ultrasound in Obstetrics & Gynecology. 2013;**42**(1):64-69. DOI: 10.1002/uog.12454

[81] Gratacós E, Van Schoubroeck D, Carreras E, Devlieger R, Roma E, Cabero L, et al. Transient hydropic signs in the donor fetus after fetoscopic laser coagulation in severe twin-twin transfusion syndrome: Incidence and clinical relevance. Ultrasound in Obstetrics & Gynecology. 2002;**19**(5):449-453. DOI: 10.1046/j.1469-0705.2002.00642.x

[82] Gray PH, Ward C, Chan F-Y. Cardiac outcomes of hydrops as a result of twin-twin transfusion syndrome treated with laser surgery. Journal of Paediatrics and Child Health. 2009;**45**(1-2):48-52. DOI: 10.1046/j.1469-0705.2002.00642.x

[83] Saade GR, Belfort MA, Berry DL, Bui T-H, Montgomery LD, Johnson A, et al. Amniotic septostomy for the treatment of twin oligohydramnios-polyhydramnios sequence. Fetal Diagnosis and Therapy. 1998;**13**(2):86-93. DOI: 10.1046/j.1469-0705.2002.00642.x

[84] Buca D, Pagani G, Rizzo G, Familiari A, Flacco ME, Manzoli L, et al. Outcome of monochorionic twin pregnancy with selective intrauterine growth restriction according to umbilical artery Doppler flow pattern of smaller twin: Systematic review and meta-analysis. Ultrasound in Obstetrics & Gynecology. 2017;**50**(5):559-568. DOI: 10.1046/j.1469-0705.2002.00642.x

[85] Lewi L, Van Schoubroeck D, Gratacós E, Witters I, Timmerman D, Deprest J. Monochorionic diamniotic twins: Complications and management options. Current Opinion in Obstetrics & Gynecology. 2003;**15**(2):177-194. DOI: 10.1046/j.1469-0705.2002.00642.x

[86] Gratacós E, Carreras E, Becker J, Lewi L, Enríquez G, Perapoch J, et al. Prevalence of neurological damage in monochorionic twins with selective intrauterine growth restriction and intermittent absent or reversed end-diastolic umbilical artery flow. Ultrasound in Obstetrics & Gynecology. 2004;**24**(2):159-163. DOI: 10.1046/j.1469-0705.2002.00642.x

[87] Lewi L, Cannie M, Blickstein I, Jani J, Huber A, Hecher K, et al. Placental sharing, birthweight discordance, and vascular anastomoses in monochorionic diamniotic twin placentas. American Journal of Obstetrics and Gynecology. 2007;**197**(6):587.e1-587.e8. DOI: 10.1046/j.1469-0705.2002.00642.x

[88] Breathnach FM, McAuliffe FM, Geary M, Daly S, Higgins JR, Dornan J, et al. Definition of intertwin birth weight discordance. Obstetrics and Gynecology. 2011;**118**(1):94-103. DOI: 10.1046/j.1469-0705.2002.00642.x

[89] Khalil A, Beune I, Hecher K, Wynia K, Ganzevoort W, Reed K, et al. Consensus definition and essential reporting parameters of selective fetal growth restriction in twin pregnancy: A Delphi procedure. Ultrasound in Obstetrics & Gynecology. 2018. DOI: 10.1002/uog.19013

[90] Araujo Júnior E, Ruano R, Javadian P, Martins WP, Elito J Jr, Pires CR, et al. Reference charts for fetal biometric parameters in twin pregnancies according to chorionicity. Prenatal Diagnosis. 2014;**34**(4):382-388

[91] Stirrup OT, Khalil A, D'Antonio F, Thilaganathan B. Fetal growth reference ranges in twin pregnancy: Analysis of the Southwest Thames obstetric research collaborative (STORK) multiple pregnancy cohort. Ultrasound in Obstetrics & Gynecology. 2015;**45**(3):301-307. DOI: 10.1002/uog.14640

[92] Sueters M, Oepkes D. Diagnosis of twin-to-twin transfusion syndrome, selective fetal growth restriction, twin anemia-polycythaemia sequence, and twin reversed arterial perfusion sequence. Best practice and research. Best Practice & Research. Clinical Obstetrics & Gynaecology. 2014;**28**:215-226

[93] Gratacós E, Lewi L, Muñoz B, Acosta-Rojas R, Hernandez-Andrade E, Martinez JM, et al. A classification system for selective intrauterine growth restriction in monochorionic pregnancies according to umbilical artery Doppler flow in the smaller twin. Ultrasound in Obstetrics & Gynecology. 2007;**30**(1):28-34

[94] Wee LY, Taylor MJ, Vanderheyden T, Talbert D, Fisk NM. Transmitted arterio-arterial anastomosis waveforms causing cyclically intermittent absent/reversed end-diastolic umbilical artery flow in monochorionic twins. Placenta. 2003;**24**(7):772-778

[95] Gratacos E, Lewi L, Carreras E, Becker J, Higueras T, Deprest J, et al. Incidence and characteristics of umbilical artery intermittent absent and/or reversed end-diastolic flow in complicated and uncomplicated monochorionic twin pregnancies. Ultrasound in Obstetrics & Gynecology. 2004;**23**:456-460. DOI: 10.1002/uog.1013

[96] Lewi L, Gucciardo L, Huber A, Jani J, Van Mieghem T, Doné E, et al. Clinical outcome and placental characteristics of monochorionic diamniotic twin pairs with early- and late-onset discordant growth. American Journal of Obstetrics and Gynecology. 2008;**199**(5): 1-7. DOI: 10.1002/uog.18966

[97] Townsend R, D'Antonio F, Sileo FG, Kumbay H, Thilaganathan B, Khalil A. Perinatal outcome of monochorionic twin pregnancies complicated by selective fetal growth restriction according to management: A systematic review and meta-analysis. Ultrasound in Obstetrics & Gynecology. 2018. DOI: 10.1002/uog.20114

[98] Monaghan C, Kalafat E, Binder J, Thilaganathan B, Khalil A. Prediction of adverse pregnancy outcome in monochorionic- diamniotic twin pregnancies complicated by selective fetal growth restriction. Ultrasound in Obstetrics & Gynecology. 2018. DOI: 10.1002/uog.19078

[99] Couck I, Mourad Tawfic N, Deprest J, De Catte L, Devlieger R, Lewi L. Does site of cord insertion increase risk of adverse outcome, twin-to-twin transfusion syndrome and discordant growth in monochorionic twin pregnancy? Ultrasound in Obstetrics & Gynecology. 2018;**52**(3):385-389. DOI: 10.1002/uo.18926

[100] Kalafat E, Thilaganathan B, Papageorghiou A, Bhide A, Khalil A. Significance of placental cord insertion site in twin pregnancy. Ultrasound in Obstetrics & Gynecology. 2018;**52**(3):378-384. DOI: 10.1002/uog.18914

[101] D'Antonio F, Odibo AO, Prefumo F, Khalil A, Buca D, Flacco ME, et al. Weight discordance and perinatal mortality in twin pregnancy: Systematic review and meta-analysis. Ultrasound in Obstetrics & Gynecology. 2018;**52**(1):11-23. DOI: 10.1002/uog.18966

[102] Rustico MA, Consonni D, Lanna M, Faiola S, Schena V, Scelsa B, et al. Selective intrauterine growth restriction in monochorionic twins: Changing patterns in umbilical artery Doppler flow and outcomes. Ultrasound in Obstetrics & Gynecology. 2017;**49**(3):387-393. DOI: 10.1002/uog.15933

[103] Peeva G, Bower S, Orosz L, Chaveeva P, Akolekar R, Nicolaides KH. Endoscopic placental laser coagulation in monochorionic diamniotic twins with type II selective fetal growth restriction. Fetal Diagnosis and Therapy. 2015;**38**(2):86-93. DOI: 10.1002/uog.15933

[104] Gratacós E, Antolin E, Lewi L, Martínez JM, Hernandez-Andrade E, Acosta-Rojas R, et al. Monochorionic twins with selective intrauterine growth restriction and intermittent

absent or reversed end-diastolic flow (type III): Feasibility and perinatal outcome of fetoscopic placental laser coagulation. Ultrasound in Obstetrics & Gynecology. 2008;**31**(6): 669-675. DOI: 10.1002/uog.15933

[105] Ishii K, Nakata M, Wada S, Murakoshi T, Sago H. Feasibility and preliminary outcomes of fetoscopic laser photocoagulation for monochorionic twin gestation with selective intrauterine growth restriction accompanied by severe oligohydramnios. The Journal of Obstetrics and Gynaecology Research. 2015;**41**(11):1732-1737. DOI: 10.1002/uog.15933

[106] Chalouhi GE, Marangoni MA, Quibel T, Deloison B, Benzina N, Essaoui M, et al. Active management of selective intrauterine growth restriction with abnormal Doppler in monochorionic diamniotic twin pregnancies diagnosed in the second trimester of pregnancy. Prenatal Diagnosis. 2013;**33**(2):109-115. DOI: 10.1002/uog.15933

[107] Hillman SC, Morris RK, Kilby MD. Co-twin prognosis after single fetal death: A systematic review and meta-analysis. Obstetrics and Gynecology. 2011;**118**(4):928-940. DOI: 10.1002/uog.15933

[108] Lopriore E, van den Wijngaard JPHM, Middeldorp JM, Oepkes D, Walther FJ, van Gemert MJ, et al. Assessment of feto-fetal transfusion flow through placental arterio-venous anastomoses in a unique case of twin-to-twin transfusion syndrome. Placenta. 2007;**28**(2-3):209-211. DOI: 10.1016/j.placenta.2006.03.006

[109] De Villiers SF, Slaghekke F, Middeldorp JM, Walther FJ, Oepkes D, Lopriore E. Placental characteristics in monochorionic twins with spontaneous versus post-laser twin anemia-polycythemia sequence. Placenta. 2013;**34**(5):456-459. DOI: 10.1016/j.placenta.2013.02.005

[110] Lopriore E, Deprest J, Slaghekke F, Oepkes D, Middeldorp JM, Vandenbussche FPHA, et al. Placental characteristics in monochorionic twins with and without twin anemia–Polycythemia sequence. Obstetrics and Gynecology. 2008;**112**(4):753-758. DOI: 10.1097/AOG.0b013e318187e1ff

[111] Slaghekke F, Kist WJ, Oepkes D, Pasman SA, Middeldorp JM, Klumper FJ, et al. Twin anemia-polycythemia sequence: Diagnostic criteria, classification, perinatal management and outcome. Fetal Diagnosis and Therapy. 2010;**27**(4):181-190. DOI: 10.1159/000304512

[112] Zhao DP, de Villiers SF, Slaghekke F, Walther FJ, Middeldorp JM, Oepkes D, et al. Prevalence, size, number and localization of vascular anastomoses in monochorionic placentas. Placenta. 2013;**34**(7):589-593. DOI: 10.1159/000304512

[113] Tollenaar LSA, Slaghekke F, Middeldorp JM, Klumper FJ, Haak MC, Oepkes D, et al. Twin anemia polycythemia sequence: Current views on pathogenesis, diagnostic criteria, perinatal management, and outcome. Twin Research and Human Genetics. 2016;**19**(3):222-233. DOI: 10.1017/thg.2016.18

[114] Yokouchi T, Murakoshi T, Mishima T, Yano H, Ohashi M, Suzuki T, et al. Incidence of spontaneous twin anemia-polycythemia sequence in monochorionic-diamniotic twin

pregnancies: Single-center prospective study. The Journal of Obstetrics and Gynaecology Research. 2015;**41**(6):857-860. DOI: 110.1111/jog.12641

[115] Slaghekke F, Pasman S, Veujoz M, Middeldorp JM, Lewi L, Devlieger R, et al. Middle cerebral artery peak systolic velocity to predict fetal hemoglobin levels in twin anemia-polycythemia sequence. Ultrasound in Obstetrics & Gynecology. 2015;**46**(4):432-436. DOI: 10.1002/uog.14925

[116] Soundararajan LP, Howe DT. Starry sky liver in twin anemia-polycythemia sequence. Ultrasound in Obstetrics & Gynecology. 2014;**43**(5):597-599. DOI: 10.1002/uog.13276

[117] Lopriore E, Slaghekke F, Oepkes D, Middeldorp JM, Vandenbussche FPHA, Walther FJ. Hematological characteristics in neonates with twin anemia-polycythemia sequence (TAPS). Prenatal Diagnosis. 2010;**30**(3):251-255. DOI: 10.1002/pd.2453

[118] Slaghekke F, Favre R, Peeters SHP, Middeldorp JM, Weingertner AS, van Zwet EW, et al. Laser surgery as a management option for twin anemia-polycythemia sequence. Ultrasound in Obstetrics & Gynecology. 2014;**44**(3):304-310. DOI: 10.1002/uog.6334

[119] Herway C, Johnson A, Moise K, Moise KJ. Fetal intraperitoneal transfusion for iatrogenic twin anemia-polycythemia sequence after laser therapy. Ultrasound in Obstetrics & Gynecology. 2009;**33**(5):592-594. DOI: 10.1002/uog.6334

[120] Groussolles M, Sartor A, Connan L, Vayssire C. Evolution of middle cerebral artery peak systolic velocity after a successful laser procedure for iatrogenic twin anemia-polycythemia sequence. Ultrasound in Obstetrics & Gynecology. 2012;**39**(3):354-356. DOI: 10.1002/uog.6334

[121] Ishii K, Hayashi S, Mabuchi A, Taguchi T, Yamamoto R, Murata M, et al. Therapy by laser equatorial placental dichorionization for early-onset spontaneous twin anemia-polycythemia sequence. Fetal Diagnosis and Therapy. 2013;**35**(1):65-68. DOI: 10.1002/uog.6334

[122] Moore TR, Gale S, Benirschke K. Perinatal outcome of forty-nine pregnancies complicated by acardiac twinning. American Journal of Obstetrics and Gynecology. 1990; **163**:907-912

[123] Steffensen TS, Gilbert-Barness E, Spellacy W, Quintero RA. Placental pathology in trap sequence: Clinical and pathogenetic implications. Fetal and Pediatric Pathology. 2008;**27**(1):13-29. DOI: 10.1002/uog.6334

[124] Pagani G, D'Antonio F, Khalil A, Papageorghiou A, Bhide A, Thilaganathan B. Intrafetal laser treatment for twin reversed arterial perfusion sequence: Cohort study and meta-analysis. Ultrasound in Obstetrics & Gynecology. 2013;**42**(1):6-14. DOI: 10.1002/uog.12495

[125] Jelin E, Hirose S, Rand L, Curran P, Feldstein V, Guevara-Gallardo S, et al. Perinatal outcome of conservative management versus fetal intervention for twin reversed arterial perfusion sequence with a small acardiac twin. Fetal Diagnosis and Therapy. 2010;**27**(3):138-141. DOI: 10.1159/000295176

[126] Zucchini S, Borghesani F, Soffriti G, Chirico C, Vultaggio E, Di Donato P. Transvaginal ultrasound diagnosis of twin reversed arterial perfusion syndrome at 9 weeks' gestation. Ultrasound in Obstetrics & Gynecology. 1993;**3**(3):209-211. DOI: 10.1046/j.1469-0705.1993.03030209.x

[127] Schwärzler P, Ville Y, Moscosco G, Tennstedt C, Bollmann R, Chaoui R. Diagnosis of twin reversed arterial perfusion sequence in the first trimester by transvaginal color Doppler ultrasound. Ultrasound in Obstetrics & Gynecology. 1999;**13**(2):143-146. DOI: 10.1046/j.1469-0705.1999.13020143.x

[128] Coulam CB, Wright G. First trimester diagnosis of acardiac twins. Early Pregnancy. 2000; **4**(4):261-270

[129] Lewi L, Valencia C, Gonzalez E, Deprest J, Nicolaides KH. The outcome of twin reversed arterial perfusion sequence diagnosed in the first trimester. American Journal of Obstetrics and Gynecology. 2010;**203**(3):213.e1-213.e4. DOI: 10.1002/uog.12495

[130] Lee H, Wagner AJ, Sy E, Ball R, Feldstein VA, Goldstein RB, et al. Efficacy of radiofrequency ablation for twin-reversed arterial perfusion sequence. American Journal of Obstetrics and Gynecology. 2007;**196**(5):1-4. DOI: 10.1016/j.ajog.2006.11.039

[131] Hecher K, Lewi L, Gratacos E, Huber A, Ville Y, Deprest J. Twin reversed arterial perfusion: Fetoscopic laser coagulation of placental anastomoses or the umbilical cord. Ultrasound in Obstetrics & Gynecology. 2006;**28**(5):688-691. DOI: 10.1002/uog.3816

[132] Sugibayashi R, Ozawa K, Sumie M, Wada S, Ito Y, Sago H. Forty cases of twin reversed arterial perfusion sequence treated with radio frequency ablation using the multistep coagulation method: A single-center experience. Prenatal Diagnosis. 2016;**36**(5):437-443. DOI: 10.1002/pd.4800

[133] Cabassa P, Fichera A, Prefumo F, Taddei F, Gandolfi S, Maroldi R, et al. The use of radiofrequency in the treatment of twin reversed arterial perfusion sequence: A case series and review of the literature. European Journal of Obstetrics, Gynecology, and Reproductive Biology. 2013;**166**(2):127-132. DOI: 10.1016/j.ejogrb.2012.10.009

[134] Lee H, Bebbington M, Crombleholme TM. The north American fetal therapy network registry data on outcomes of radiofrequency ablation for twin-reversed arterial perfusion sequence. Fetal Diagnosis and Therapy. 2013;**33**(4):224-229. DOI: 10.1159/000343223

[135] Tan TYT, Sepulveda W. Acardiac twin: A systematic review of minimally invasive treatment modalities. Ultrasound in Obstetrics & Gynecology. 2003;**22**(4):409-419

[136] Nicolaides K, Brizot Mde L, Patel F, Snijders R. Comparison of chorionic villus sampling and amniocentesis for fetal karyotyping at 10-13 weeks' gestation. Lancet. 1994; **344**(8920):435-439

[137] Roethlisberger M, Strizek B, Gottschalk I, Mallmann MR, Geipel A, Gembruch U, et al. First-trimester intervention in twin reversed arterial perfusion sequence: Does size matter? Ultrasound in Obstetrics & Gynecology. 2017;**50**(1):40-44

7

Preterm Birth in Twins

Marcelo Santucci Franca,
Tatiana E. N. K. Hamamoto and
Antônio Fernandes Moron

Abstract

Multiple pregnancy differs from singleton pregnancy in several aspects, including increased risk of preeclampsia, fetal malformation, maternal morbidity, and mortality. However, certainly, prematurity is a fundamental concern when twin gestation is approached, due to the frequency of this disease and also to the severity of preterm birth, which unfortunately can also occur near to the fetal viability limit. Labor in twin pregnancy generally occurs before singleton pregnancy. Nevertheless, another factor can contribute to raise even more preterm birth rates in this already high-risk gestation: the short cervix. Although only 1–2% of twin pregnancy present short cervix at transvaginal ultrasound, this association increases the chance of unfavorable outcome for the newborn, frequently causing death of one or both twins. So, many strategies were proposed to minimize this catastrophic situation: follow-up of cervical length to prevent preterm birth, pessary use, progesterone, tocolysis to postpone birth in 48 hours to 7 days in order to use corticosteroids in fetal pulmonary maturation, and magnesium sulfate use to neuroprotection.

Keywords: twin pregnancy, multiple pregnancy, preterm birth, cervical pessary, progesterone, tocolysis, corticosteroids, magnesium sulfate, neuroprotection

1. Introduction

Preterm birth is defined as delivery before 37 weeks of gestation, starting with fetal viability, which is around 23–25 weeks. It is known that prematurity is a great villain among pregnancy diseases due to its extremely high cost. Currently, the technological resources necessary to offer life support to preterm babies in neonatal ICUs cause expenditures of around 2500–5000

American dollars per day of hospitalization. Some preterm babies close to the limit of viability (23–25 weeks) can be hospitalized 100 days, that is, a single preterm baby can cause costs of 250,000–500,000 American dollars to the health system; considering that 10% of deliveries are preterm, we can comprehend that we are dealing with excessively high Figures [1].

Preterm birth may cause a great impact in the life of the affected. Severe complications can be mentioned: death, cerebral palsy, intraventricular hemorrhage (IVH), sepsis, retinopathy of prematurity, behavioral deficits (attention deficit hyperactivity disorder—ADHD) or learning deficits, respiratory distress syndrome (RDS), increase need for mechanical ventilation/CPAP, pulmonary dysplasia, and necrotizing enterocolitis [2].

Twin pregnancy is responsible for 2% of all pregnancies, but 15% of extreme preterm birth (≤32 weeks) occurs in twins. Therefore, measures for preterm delivery prevention are of vital importance in health systems management worldwide [3].

Twin pregnancy for itself is a condition associated with prematurity due to uterine over distension, and usually twins are born before the 37th week of pregnancy. The average time of twin pregnancy in a group not selected by the cervix was 35.83 ± 8.7 weeks, and in 50% of the newborns, delivery was prior to 37 weeks [4].

However, twin pregnancy does not occur frequently in the population in general; it accounts for approximately 1–2% of the deliveries. With the couples decision to postpone pregnancy, which has happened in the last 20 years, giving priority to women's presence in the labor market, the necessity of recurring to assisted reproduction techniques has increased, and the twin pregnancy rates, in their turn, have been increasing [5].

It is important to notice that the association of risk factors may be of extreme importance in multiple pregnancy: smoking, infections, vaginal discharge and association with Mullerian malformations, cervix amputation surgeries, the presence of the previous preterm delivery, or identification of short cervix may be catastrophic if associated with twin pregnancy [6]. Hence, in twin pregnancy anamnesis and physical examination have a more important role in detecting risk patients, and more rigorous observation of the uterine cervix may be considered in cases of duplicated risk factors.

In essence, if during prenatal examinations in the period between the 18th and 24th weeks the presence of short cervix is identified, the patient will receive the indication of the use of vaginal progesterone [7], and cervical pessary will be indicated that besides presenting a low index of collateral effects, promotes an important benefit in extending twin pregnancy and, mainly, significantly improving the condition of delivery of the newborn to the cares of the neonatal ICU in situations of preterm birth. The group of preterm birth treated only with progesterone is generally more severe than preterm birth in association with pessary and progesterone; in our present series of cases, we obtained a mean gain of 34 days in singleton pregnancy, and in twins probably similar gain is obtained, as our data will show below.

We can attempt to modify its incidence prior to the occurrence of any modification to the maternal organism. This prevention is called primary prevention. It is known that smoking is an important cause of preterm birth. So, tobacco should be avoided even before pregnancy, although stopping smoking in due time is also a recommended practice [8].

Another example of primary prevention is the preeclampsia, which causes placental insufficiency and frequently culminates in preterm delivery (spontaneous or iatrogenic). Today, we know that the acetylsalicylic acid (ASA) can modify placentation if started in the 12th week of pregnancy and dramatically reduces the incidence of premature preeclampsia, thus reducing prematurity caused by this process [9].

It is known that the previous spontaneous preterm birth (SPB) is one of the main risk factors for a second spontaneous preterm delivery, and any interventions which are developed or studied with the intention of interfering in this event, modifying its natural course and increasing the final gestation time, will be characterized as primary prevention.

Furthermore, we can prevent prematurity after the beginning of the first signs of maternal modification; however, still prior to preterm birth labor being installed, it is called secondary prevention.

In twin gestation, one of the first signs of maternal modification, which may culminate in preterm delivery, is premature cervical shortening. Therefore, interference in the process of cervix modification can be considered secondary prevention of prematurity. Currently, some aspects in cervix evaluation may increase its risk in case of being detected in concomitance with short cervix (≤25 mm) [10], as the presence of funneling and the presence of intra-amniotic sludge [11].

Thus, interventions which interfere in these aspects of cervix modification, are characterized as secondary prevention. It may be stated that the example of progesterone, which modifies the endocervical glandular echo (EGE) and the speed of cervix diminishing; the cervical pessary, which modifies the uterocervical angle (UCA), may reduce funneling and sustain the uterus upon the perineal striated muscles; cervical cerclage in cases of isthmus-cervical incompetence to maintain uterine cervix closed; or, furthermore, the use of antibiotics in the treatment of intra-amniotic "sludge," which may interfere in cervix inflammation and modify its shortening.

The tertiary prevention of preterm birth consists of interventions when labor has already started and tocolysis, i.e. inhibition of premature labor by drugs, is a good example of it, and normally is preconized between 23-24 and 34 weeks of gestation.

So far, there is no evidence that tocolysis is able to indefinitely extend gestation; however, the therapy is efficient to delay delivery between 48 hours and 7 days, time enough for carrying out and for the effectiveness of corticosteroid application. These drugs, in their term, have the function of effectively acting in fetal pulmonary maturation, reducing the perinatal respiratory complications and also intestinal ones (necrotizing enterocolitis), and of the central nervous system, as, for instance, intraventricular hemorrhage.

Some recent studies reveal that the use of corticoid in gestations with high risk of preterm delivery is of great importance; however, its repetition in multiple doses is not advisable. Its usage is to be restricted to no more than two courses, and the second one is to be carried out only if the fetus effectively and irrevocably is going to be born prematurely.

Repetitive corticoid cycles are banned as evidence in tests with animals and studies in human beings have revealed that neuronal migration and neuronal apoptosis are modified in fetuses exposed to high doses of this drug. Recent studies have revealed that even perinatal mortality increases (RR 1.12) in pregnant women using this medication, single cycle, for protection against complications caused by prematurity [12].

Also is considered another form of tertiary prevention of preterm birth the use of magnesium sulfate for fetal neuroprotection during labor or previous to delivery, in gestations below 32th week, administered between 12 and 24 hours prior to delivery.

2. Prevention of preterm birth

According to the WHO, preterm birth is today the main cause of death in the first 5 years of life in the world. Thus, prevention of prematurity is of extreme importance to minimize the morbidity/mortality perinatal and the high costs involved with this disease.

Primary prevention begins with a good detection index of the problem. The previous preterm birth is undoubtedly a significant predictor of prematurity, and this is also valid for twin pregnancies [6]. The more premature the previous delivery was, the higher the risk of recurrence. In addition, other factors can contribute to increase preterm birth rates in multiple pregnancies, as race, schooling, smoking, and short cervix.

Some studies showed higher prematurity rates in black, younger, and low-schooling level pregnant women [13]. Smoking and primiparity seem to be related to shorter gestational age at birth too in twin pregnancy [8].

In secondary prevention of preterm birth, cervix evaluation is an important strategy, once uterine overdistension in multiple pregnancy can perhaps contribute to higher rates of short cervix and, therefore, higher rates of prematurity. So, many efforts were made to improve the prediction and prevention of preterm birth in twin pregnancy, in order to enhance the newborn prognosis, and cervix evaluation is one of them [14].

Transvaginal ultrasound for uterine cervix evaluation is currently the main tracking method for this severe disease [15], and second trimester ultrasound, between 18 and 24 weeks, is considered the best period to make the cervical transvaginal ultrasound.

A retrospective cohort study in twin pregnancy concludes that cervical shortening between 18 and 25 weeks of gestation was a good predictor of SPB [16].

In twins, the association of preterm birth frequently caused by uterine overdistension is largely aggravated by the presence of short cervix, and this association is more evidenced because of high indexes of preterm birth incompatible with extrauterine life.

It is true that a small performance improvement in this association of problems may completely change the prognostics of the newborn. Therefore, the recommendation of carrying out transvaginal ultrasound of the uterine cervix is of vital importance for diminishing preterm delivery in twin gestation.

In twin pregnancy, with the previous spontaneous preterm birth or late miscarriage but with atypical history of cervical insufficiency, strict follow-up of the uterine cervix is necessary from the 16th week of gestation, with transvaginal sonographic evaluation weekly, until the 24th week. If short cervical length (≤25 mm) is detected, a mechanical treatment (cerclage or cervical pessary) should be performed until 48 hours after diagnosis [7].

In the uterine cervix analysis, the evaluation of the cervical length ≤25 mm is considered the main predictor of preterm birth risk [10]. Also, other factors can be considered as preterm birth predictors, for instance, the presence of funneling signal [17], the presence of intra-amniotic sludge [11], the absence of endocervical glandular echo (EGE) [18], and the presence of uterocervical angle >105° [19], as well as progressive diminishing of the cervix of more than 2 mm/week [15], must be considered also in twin pregnancy (Video https://mts.intechopen.com/download/index/process/279/authkey/236271ca370424655923c0bb7a7179a0).

2.1. Fetal fibronectin (fFN)

The fFN test consists of detection of this cervicovaginal glycoprotein, collected between 24 and 34 weeks and 6 days. In normal conditions, fFN should not be present at high concentrations (cutoff is 50 ng/mL) after 20 weeks, and the objective of this test is to predict spontaneous preterm birth within 7:10 days [20]. False-positive results can occur in the sample contaminated with blood and within 24 hours after intercourse or cervical examination (as transvaginal ultrasound or vaginal examination), and it should not be performed in cases of premature rupture of membranes and cervical dilatation ≤3 cm

The American College of Obstetricians and Gynecologists (ACOG) [7] does not recommend its use in asymptomatic women with multiple pregnancy as routine, and some reviews have failed finding enough evidence to support fFN screening [21], once perinatal outcome was not affected by this intervention, although lower incidence of preterm birth before 37 weeks was reached.

However, in symptomatic women, this test can be useful to decide the best moment to administer antenatal corticosteroids in order to promote fetal pulmonary maturation. Published studies in multiple gestation that evaluated fFN test and cervical changes presented high sensitivity and high negative predictive value in predicting preterm birth [22, 23]. Probably, the association of these factors can enhance the approach of twin pregnancies and should be seriously considered in prevention of prematurity.

2.2. Progesterone

The use of progesterone is the main prophylaxis for preterm birth in singleton pregnancies; however, in twin pregnancies its performance does not seem to be that good. Currently, the most recent study with the highest series of cases—a meta-analysis of individual data—concludes that the utilization of progesterone for twin pregnancies presents favorable evidence when used in twins with short cervix (≤25 mm) as it presents a high number of cases by case studies and different clinical tests participated in this meta-analysis. However, a more detailed case-by-case study shows that 70% of the sample was taken from one clinical study only [24] favorable to utilization and another five studies with lower casuistry (30% of the sample) evidence that the medication does not present benefits in twin pregnancy [25].

A randomized clinical trial published in 2015 [4] with casuistry of about 200 twin pregnancies, not selected by cervix, compared the use of progesterone and expectant management in twin pregnancies and did not find differences between the groups. In another multicenter trial (STOPPIT), 500 twin pregnancies, not selected by cervix also, were randomized, and their perinatal outcomes were statistically not different for none of the evaluated perinatal outcomes [26].

Therefore, according to this author's opinion, we can affirm up to the present moment that isolated progesterone is not efficient in the prevention of preterm birth in not selected twin pregnancies; however, in association with short cervix, it can be considered.

2.3. Cerclage

Prophylactic cervical cerclage in multiple pregnancies is controversial, since the systematic review of randomized trials was not convincing in proving its efficacy in reducing perinatal death and neonatal morbidity. Even ultrasound-indicated cerclage (i.e., in short cervix) does not seem to show benefit in twin gestations. However, care must be taken in this analysis, once there are few trials and the number of patients included was not so impressive [27]. On the other hand, one author suggested improvement in perinatal outcome when cervical cerclage is indicated in asymptomatic twin pregnant women that present cervical dilatation (physical examination-indicated cerclage) at 16–24 weeks [28].

ACOG does not recommend cerclage in the incidental short cervix [7], but there is some evidence of benefit of this procedure when short cervix occurs in suspicious but not typical history of cervical insufficiency. The diagnosis can be performed by weekly transvaginal ultrasound since the 16th week. So, cerclage could be performed after shortening of the cervix in these cases, except in exposed membranes, chorioamnionitis, sepsis, and when there is no cervical length measurable [16].

2.4. Cervical pessary

Therefore, the Federal University of São Paulo (UNIFESP) has opted for treating the selected cases of preterm birth risk by short cervix, associated to the above-stated risk factors or previous preterm delivery. The standard treatment would be naturally micronized progesterone in the dosage of 200 mg/day, vaginally, or the combination of this therapy associated to cervical pessary AM-Ingamed. As of 2014, all the cases have been treated with pessary plus progesterone in the Department of Screening of Preterm Delivery of the UNIFESP.

This conduct was based on the studies of ProTwin and PECEP-Twins, which identified that twins with short cervix could benefit from the usage of the cervical pessary [29, 30].

Since January 2014 we have obtained 30 cases of dichorionic twin gestations with short cervix (≤25 mm). The gestational age of diagnosis varied between 18 and 27 weeks and 6 days (mean age of 24 weeks and 3 days ± 2.8 weeks). The mean cervical length of these gestations at the time of the pessary placement was 14.9 ± 6.8 mm, which reveals an extremely high risk.

In our series of cases, the mean gestational age of delivery was 34.59 ± 2.72 weeks, and in a group of 32 cases of dichorionic twin gestation, not selected by cervix, the mean delivery time was 35.83 ± 8.7 weeks. It shall be pointed out that between the time of delivery of the group with cervical pessary and the group not selected by cervix there was a small difference of 1.24 weeks—despite a big difference among the groups regarding the risk due to the cervix—with statistically no significant difference between the groups (P = 0.11). The mean interval of permanence with cervical pessary was 10.18 ± 3.6 weeks.

The result was 79% of the preterm deliveries below 37 weeks, 42% of premature newborns below 34 weeks, 17% below 32 weeks, and 4% below 28 weeks; in comparison, the study published by Fox et al. (2016) with similar case studies (cervix 11.9 ± 4.5 mm with 25.9 ± 2.1 weeks) obtained 44.4% of prematurity below 34 weeks and 28.6% below 32 weeks in patients treated with vaginal progesterone, only [31]. In the group of twins not selected by cervix, preterm birth below 37 weeks is obtained in 50% of the cases, preterm birth below 34 weeks in 19%, below 32 weeks in 9%, and no preterm delivery was registered below 28 weeks, as shown in **Table 1**.

It is important to notice that before 32 weeks (very high risk for adverse neonatal outcome) the group treated by pessary plus progesterone had a better performance if compared to the group treated only by progesterone, regarding cervical length in this group which was 3.0 mm lower.

A recent randomized clinical trial from Egypt (El-refaie's study), compared to the use of progesterone *versus* expectant management in twin pregnancies with short cervix. The number of SPB was considerably lower in progesterone group below 34 and 32 weeks, respectively, 53% (expectant) *versus* 35% (progesterone) and 30% (expectant) *versus* 12% (progesterone group); the mean cervical length was very similar between groups, close to 22 mm [32].

These data from El-refaie's trial are similar to data of twin pregnancy from UNIFESP. In this study pessary plus progesterone group (mean cervical length 14.3 ± 7.1 mm) presents a better performance when compared to El-refaie controls (with short cervix) and also to progesterone group (with short cervix) below 37, 34, 32, and 28 weeks. It is importantly emphasized that UNIFESP controls are not selected by cervix and its performance is better because this group presents lower risk when compared with all other groups. Another important issue is

Author	Treatment	Cervical length (mm)	Mean gestational age of delivery (weeks)	37weeks	34weeks Birth	32weeks Before	28weeks
UNIFESP short cervix	Pessary plus Progesterone	14.9± 6.8	34.59±2.72	79%	42%	17%	4%
Fox, N short cervix	Progesterone	11.9± 4.5	33.3 ± 3.9	Data not available	44.4%	28.6%	Data not available
UNIFESP not select by cervix	No treatment	Data not available	35.83± 8.7	50%	19%	9%	0

Table 1. Comparison of cervical length, mean gestational age of delivery, and percentage of deliveries according to the gestational age between different groups of treatment: pessary plus progesterone in short cervix twin pregnancy, only progesterone in short cervix twin pregnancy, no selected by cervix, and no treated twin pregnancy.

regarding the mean of cervical length which is lower in UNIFESP pessary plus progesterone group than El-refaie's groups, which cause higher risk to SPB to pessary group; so but the performance is better for pessary, despite high risk mentioned (**Figure 1**).

Considering the birthweight of twins not selected by cervix (n = 32), the mean weight of the biggest twin was 2.492 ± 643 g, and of the smallest twin, it was 2.195 ± 665 g; in comparison, in the twin group with short cervix treated by pessary plus progesterone (n = 24), the weight of the biggest one was 2.148 ± 434 g (p = 0.028), and of the smallest twin, it was 2.037 ± 425 g (p = 0.327), presenting a statistically significant difference between the groups for the biggest newborn, but no statistic difference for the smallest one. This result allows the conclusion that for the most vulnerable newborn (smallest one), the use of the cervical pessary was sufficient to modify the statistic difference expected, by cervical length difference, and in accordance with the difference registered between taller twins.

Furthermore, the use of the cervical pessary did not influence the weight difference between the fetuses. For the group not selected by cervix, the mean difference was 12 ± 6%; for the group of twins with short cervix, the difference was 11 ± 2% (p = 0.375).

This small difference demonstrates clear similarity between treated high-risk cases and cases of habitual twin pregnancy without involvement or diagnosis of complication factors in the prenatal routine (**Table 2**).

This study is according to a prospective, multicenter, randomized clinical trial conducted in Spain (PECEP-Twin). The primary outcome was SPB before 34 weeks of gestation. Neonatal morbidity and mortality were also evaluated. Cervical length was measured in 2287 women.

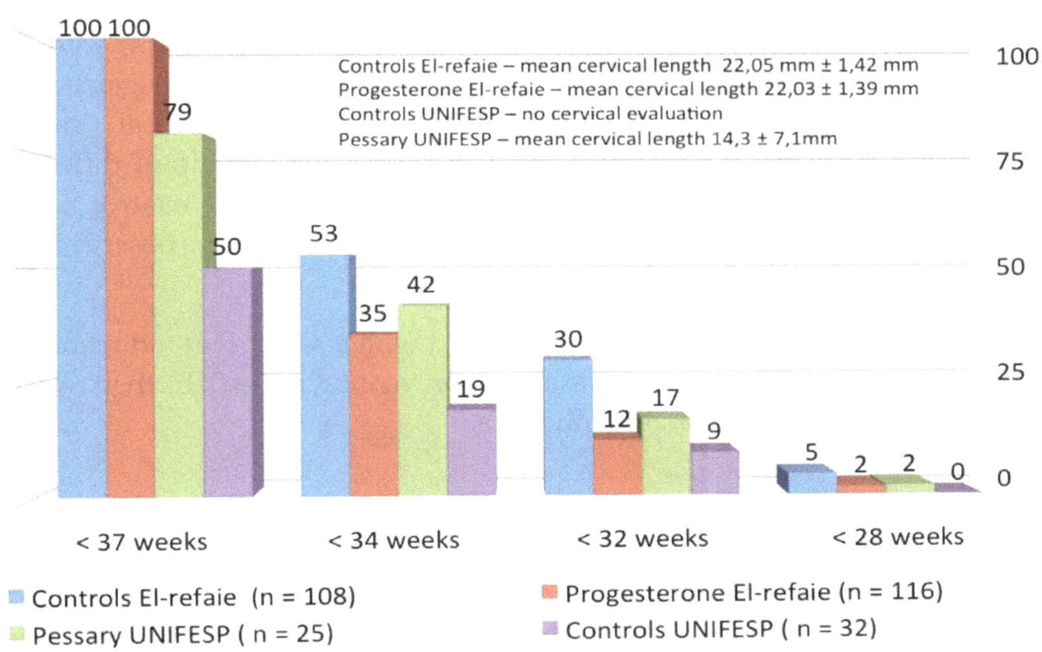

Figure 1. Comparison of percentage of SPB per gestational age between twin pregnancy from El-refaie's trial with short cervix (expectant and progesterone group) and UNIFESP twin pregnancy treated by pessary plus progesterone for short cervix and UNIFESP controls without selection by cervix.

	Not selected by cervix	Short cervix	P
Biggest twin	2.492 ± 643g	2.195 ± 665g	0.028 *
Smallest twin	**2.148 ± 434g**	**2.037 ± 425g**	**NS**
Discordance of weight between twins	12 ± 6%	11 ± 2%	NS

Table 2. Comparison of birthweight and discordance of weight between groups with short cervix/treated by pessary plus progesterone twin pregnancy ***versus*** not selected/not treated twin pregnancy.

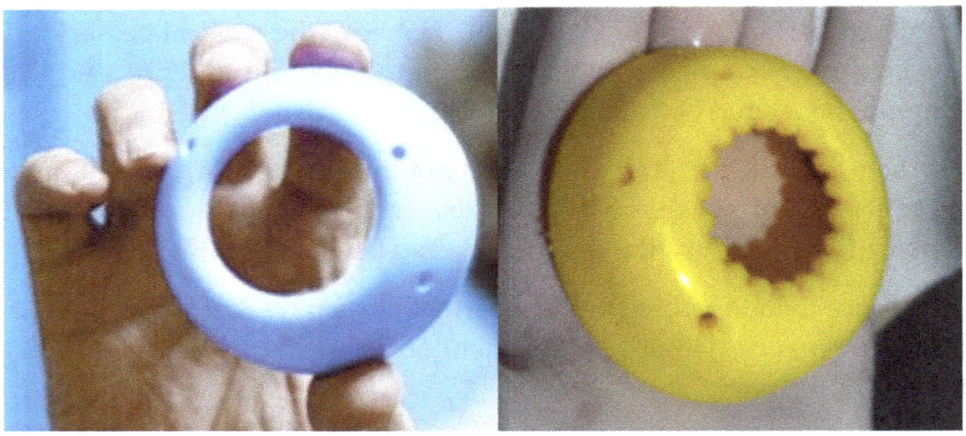

Figure 2. Comparison between the Arabin cervical pessary (blue) and the AM-Ingamed cervical pessary (yellow): They are similar regarding design, size, and texture. The dimensions (largest lower diameter × smallest upper diameter x height) of the most frequently used Arabin pessary are 70 × 32 × 25 mm, and of the Ingamed cervical pessary the dimensions are 70 × 30 × 25 mm.

Pregnant women (n = 137) with a sonographic cervical length (≤25 mm) were randomly selected to receive an Arabin cervical pessary (**Figure 2**) or expectant management (1:1 ratio). SPB < 34 weeks of pregnancy was significantly less frequent in the pessary group than in the expectant group (16.2% *vs.* 39.4%); relative risk, 0.41. No significant differences were observed in composite neonatal morbidity outcome (5.9% *vs.* 9.1%); relative risk, 0.64. No serious adverse effects associated with the use of a cervical pessary were observed or neonatal mortality (none) between the groups.

So, the insertion of a cervical pessary was associated with a significant reduction in the SPB rate. They propose the use of a cervical pessary for preventing preterm birth in twin pregnancies with short cervix [30], corroborating our data.

3. Tocolysis in multiple gestation

When an acute preterm labor is detected, it is possible to use tocolytic drugs to reduce uterine activity, and this is considered part of tertiary prevention. However, the diagnosis of preterm labor is not always simple, being generally defined as painful and regular contractions leading to cervical changes after the 20th week and before the 37th week of pregnancy.

The main goal of tocolysis is not to prevent preterm delivery, once the effectiveness for it is not proven [33]. However, tocolytic drugs can postpone delivery in 48 hours to 7 days, which is essential to manage antenatal corticosteroids to accelerate fetal pulmonary maturation and to transfer the patients to a tertiary care center when necessary [34, 35].

Tocolytic drugs should be administered when there is a clear benefit to the newborn, once the majority of these drugs has side effects to the mother and, sometimes, also to the fetus. So, it can be used from viability (23–24 weeks of pregnancy) until the 34th week, as most guideline recommendations propose. In special cases, they can also be used before viability, for example, in patients after an intra-abdominal surgery, when the cause of preterm labor is self-limited [34, 36, 37].

Contraindications for tocolytics include lethal fetal anomaly, preterm premature rupture of membranes, chorioamnionitis, severe preeclampsia and eclampsia, maternal hemorrhage with hemodynamic instability, suspected placental abruption, intrauterine fetal demise, and compromised fetal status [34].

Nowadays, the main drugs used in tocolysis are beta-agonists (as terbutaline), calcium channel blockers (as nifedipine), cyclooxygenase inhibitors (as indomethacin), and oxytocin receptor antagonist (as atosiban), as exposed in **Table 3**.

The ACOG recommends as first-line treatment in acute preterm labor in multiple pregnancy calcium channel blockers and cyclooxygenase inhibitors due to fewer side effects of these drugs [7]. In UNIFESP, the preference is for calcium channel blockers and oxytocin receptor antagonists.

3.1. Calcium channel blockers

The main drug of this class used in preterm birth inhibition is nifedipine, and many dosing regimens were proposed. Among tocolytics, nifedipine was the only drug that seems to statistically reduce neonatal morbidity and to increase gestational age at birth [38, 39].

In addition to being inexpensive, nifedipine is also administered orally and has less adverse maternal effects when compared to beta-agonists. When present, hypotension, flush, and headaches usually are not severe [37, 39].

The recommendation in UNIFESP is an initial dose of 10 mg orally every 20 minutes (maximum of 30 mg in 1 hour) until inhibition is reached, followed by 20 mg orally every 8 hours for up to 48 hours [40].

3.2. Oxytocin receptor antagonists

Atosiban is an oxytocin receptor antagonist and presents minimum side effects to both mother and fetus in inhibition of preterm labor. This is a positive aspect, since it leads to a better acceptance and compliance to treatment [39].

Meanwhile, this medication has a high cost and is administered intravenously. In the United States, atosiban is not available, because the US Food and Drug Administration (FDA) refused

Drug Class	Recommended Regimen Dose	Characteristics and observations
Calcium Channels Blockers (Nifedipine)	Starting dose: 10mg orally every 20 minutes (maximum 30mg in one hour) until inhibition Maintenance dose: 20mg orally every 8 hours for up to 48h	Few maternal side effects (hypotension, flush, headaches)
Oxytocin receptor antagonists (Atosiban)	bolus of 6.75mg followed by a 300mcg/min infusion for 3 hours, and then 100mcg/min for up to 45 hours	Any contraindication, few side effects. Safety and efficacy questioned before 28 weeks of pregnancy (not available in the USA)
Beta-Agonists (Terbutaline)	Starting dose: 2.5-5.0mcg/min intravenously every 20-30min until inhibition (maximum: 25mcg/min) – maintain this dose for 12 hours After, decrease 2.5-5mcg/min every 20-30min and the minimum dose is maintained for more 12 hours	Many maternal side effects (tachycardia, tremor, palpitations, dyspnea, hyperglycemia, pulmonary edema). We suggest avoid its use in multiple pregnancy when possible
Cyclooxygenase inhibitors (Indomethacin)	Starting dose: 100mg per rectum Maintenance dose: 25mg orally every 6 hours for up to 48h	Should be used before 32 weeks of gestation and for no more than 48 hours, once it is related to premature constriction of the ductus arteriosus of the fetus and can be a cause of oligohydramnios

Table 3. Principal drugs used nowadays in tocolysis, with recommended regimen dose and important characteristics of them.

to approve it as a tocolytic due to the results of one trial, which questioned safety of this drug in pregnancies before 28 weeks. Perhaps, these findings can be explained by the concentration of oxytocin receptors that increases as more advanced the pregnancy is [41].

In UNIFESP, as in Europe, this tocolytic class is considered an interesting choice, and its administration begins with a bolus of 6.75 mg followed by a 300 mcg/min infusion for 3 hours and then 100 mcg/min for up to 45 hours [40].

3.3. Beta-agonists

The beta2-agonists cause relaxation of the myometrium, and the most studied drugs of this tocolytic class were terbutaline and ritodrine, which is no more commercialized in the United States.

Although efficient in postpone preterm labor, terbutaline is also known by many side effects to the mother (as tachycardia, tremor, palpitations, dyspnea, hyperglycemia and pulmonary edema) and to the fetus (tachycardia and neonatal hypoglycemia) [41, 42]. So, if possible, in multiple pregnancy, beta-agonists should be avoided to inhibit preterm labor.

In UNIFESP, when necessary, for example, in the absence of calcium channel blockers and atosiban, terbutaline is used by continuous intravenous infusion. The starting dose is 2.5–5 mcg/min, increasing 2.5–5 mcg/min every 20–30 minutes until inhibition has been reached (maximum dose is 25 mcg/min), and maintain this dose for 12 hours. Then, the infusion can be decreased 2.5–5 mcg/min every 20–30 minutes, and the minimum dose of terbutaline is maintained for more 12 hours [40].

3.4. Cyclooxygenase inhibitors

Indomethacin is considered a first-line drug for acute preterm labor in multiple pregnancy by the ACOG [7], once it is known its efficacy in postpone delivery by at least 48 hours after initiated the treatment.

However, it is important to be aware of adverse effects related to indomethacin. During treatment period, the mother is at higher risk of gastritis, esophageal reflux, and platelet dysfunction. And, the major risk is the premature constriction of the ductus arteriosus of the fetus and oligohydramnios due to reduction of fetal renal blood flow [43, 44].

If necessary, indomethacin can be administered for a maximum period of 48 hours and should be avoided after 32 weeks of gestation; when these complications are more common, it is important to notice that before 32 weeks the risk decreases, but is not zero [37, 41].

Loading dose recommended is 100 mg per rectum and then 25 mg orally every 6 hours up to 48 hours [40].

3.5. Prophylactic tocolysis

There is no evidence of benefit in using prophylactic and long-term tocolytic drugs to avoid preterm birth in multifetal pregnancy. Besides, the prolonged use of these medications leads to increase maternal side effects, including death [7].

4. Corticosteroids

Antenatal glucocorticoid treatment with corticosteroids is routinely used in women at risk of preterm delivery under 34 weeks of gestation [45]. Corticosteroids promote fetal lung development between the 24th and 34th week of gestation [46] and reduce mortality of the preterm infant after delivery [47]. An important consequence of lung immaturity in preterm birth is the respiratory distress syndrome (RDS), and it is the great responsibility for the early neonatal mortality and the high cost of neonatal intensive care [47]. Preterm babies present higher risk of neurological impairment [48], which is the reason why the strategies for reduction of the risk of neonatal RDS and IVH in preterm delivery have received considerable attention [49].

A single course of corticosteroids reduces the risk of RDS from 40 to 21% in babies born before 32 weeks of gestation [46]. In recent publication (2017) of Cochrane Reviews, it was observed that treatment with antenatal corticosteroids was associated with an overall average reduction in IVH of 45%, average reduction in RDS of 34%, moderate to severe RDS was reduced to 41% compared with no exposure to antenatal corticosteroids, with less need for neonatal respiratory support, with a reduction in the need for mechanical ventilation/CPAP, fewer infants receiving corticosteroids needed surfactant, and was associated with a reduction in the incidence of necrotizing enterocolitis, as shown in **Table 4** [2].

However, an experimental study in Wistar rats in UNIFESP [50] evidenced that the groups presented different numbers of apoptotic neurons in the hippocampus, more precisely on the region named cornu ammonis 1 (CA1) and dentate gyrus (DG) after a single course of corticosteroids. The number of apoptotic neurons in the DG region was increased after corticosteroid use (by directly receptor activation), which caused, probably, the decrease in cell death in the CA1, as a compensatory reaction.

The increased apoptosis in DG and reduced cell death in the CA1 region can indicate the existence of an indirect compensatory pattern (statistically significant difference). A new balance was obtained in different areas of the hippocampus. There is no evidence in literature that the decrease in the number of apoptotic cells in CA1 is due to direct action of betamethasone, but the results suggest that this minor mortality is a compensation of a previous lesion in DG [50]. It is possible that inconclusive data referred to neurodevelopmental latency after corticosteroids (RR 0.64) described in Cochrane Review (**Table 4**), can be justified by abnormal neuronal apoptosis in the hippocampus.

Another important finding was described in a multicenter, cluster-randomized trial, within six countries (Argentina, Zambia, India, Kenya, Pakistan, and Guatemala) to standard care or an multifaceted intervention with teaching pregnant women how and when to use corticosteroids, including facilitation of the antenatal corticosteroid use with distribution of a kit with drug, material, and knowledge for application. The primary outcome was 28-day neonatal mortality among infants less than the 5th percentile for birthweight.

Fifty control clusters with 50,743 livebirths (2258 less than 5th percentile for birthweight [4%]) and 51 intervention clusters with 47,394 livebirths (2520 less than 5th percentile [5%]) completed follow-up. About 45% (1052/2327) of women in intervention clusters who delivered less-than-5th-percentile infants received antenatal corticosteroids compared with 10% (215/2062) in control clusters ($p < 0{\cdot}0001$).

Correlation with corticosteroids	Absolut value	RR	95% CI	N participants	Number of studies
Reduction perinatal death	28%	0,72	0.58 - 0.89	6729	15
Reduction neonatal death	31%	0.69	0.59 - 0.81	7188	22
Reduction IVH	45%	0.55	0.40 - 0.76	6093	16
Reduction in RDS	34%	0.66	0.56 - 0.77	7764	28
Reduction severe/mod RDS	41%	0.59	0.38 - 0.91	1686	6
Reduction mechanical ventilation / CPAP	32%	0.68	0.56 - 0.84	1368	9
Reduction necessity of surfactant	32%	0.68	0.51- 0.90	3556	5
Reduction of necrotizing enterocolitis	50%	0.50	0.32 - 0.78	4702	10
Death in childhood after exposure to corticoids	32%	0.68	0.36 - 1.27	1010	4
Neurodevelopmental delay	46%	0.64	0.14 - 2.98	82	1
Increasing tolerance of glucose in group of corticosteroids		2.71	1.14 - 6.46	123	1
Systemic infection in the first 48 hours after birth	40%	0.60	0.41 - 0.88	1753	8
AG had an lower than 7 Apgar score of 5 min.	19%	0.81	0.67 - 0.98	2419	10
Reduction developmental delay in childhood	51%	0.49	0.24 - 1.00	518	2
Increase of cerebral palsy	40%	0.60	0.34 - 1.03	904	5

Table 4. Correlation between complications of SPB and use of corticosteroids (Cochrane Review, 2017 [2]).

Among the less-than-5th-percentile infants, 28-day neonatal mortality was 225 per 1000 livebirths for the intervention group and 232 per 1000 livebirths for the control group (relative risk [RR] 0·96, 95% CI 0·87–1·06, p = 0·65), and suspected maternal infection was reported in 236/2361 (10%) women in the intervention group and 133/2094 (6%) in the control group (odds ratio [OR] 1·67, 1·33–2·09, p < 0·0001).

Among the whole population, 28-day neonatal mortality was 27·4 per 1000 livebirths for the intervention group and 23·9 per 1000 livebirths for the control group (RR 1·12, 1·02–1·22, p = 0·0127), and suspected maternal infection was reported in 1207/48219 (3%) women in the intervention group and 867/51523 (2%) in the control group (OR 1·45, 1·33–1·58, p < 0·0001).

Despite the increased use of antenatal corticosteroids in low-birthweight infants in the intervention groups, neonatal mortality did not decrease in this group and increased in the population overall. For every 1000 women exposed to this strategy, an excess of 3·5 neonatal deaths occurred, and the risk of maternal infection seems to have been increased [12].

4.1. When and how to use corticosteroids for lung maturation

The treatment consists in betamethasone administration intramuscularly two 12 mg doses 24 hours apart or dexamethasone intramuscularly four 6 mg doses every 12 hours.

A single course of corticosteroids must be considered in twin pregnancy between 24th and 33rd week that have high risk of preterm delivery within 7 days, including for those with ruptured membranes and if the first course was administered previously more than 14 days. It also may be considered for pregnant women starting at 23 0/7 weeks of gestation who are at risk of preterm delivery within 7 days, based on a family's decision regarding resuscitation. A rescue course of corticosteroids can be considered before 7 days from the first dose if there is some clinical indication for that [51].

A new recommendation from the ACOG suggests that in pregnancy during the 34–37th week, the use of corticosteroids could be beneficial, even during this late period of pregnancy, regardless of the number of fetuses [7, 52].

Administration of corticosteroids can be considered in twin pregnancy between the 34th and 37th week which are in risk of preterm birth within 7 days and which have not received the previous course of betamethasone [52].

Unfortunately, according to the WHO, in Brazil only 30% of preterm birth received antenatal corticosteroids to lung maturation between 2010 and 2011 [53], whereas several pregnancies received unnecessary corticosteroids, without real indication for that [54].

5. Neuroprotection: the use of magnesium sulfate

In 1995, it was suggested that magnesium sulfate was a neuroprotector, decreasing the prevalence of cerebral palsy in very-low-birthweight newborns [55]. Since then, several studies have been conducted to elucidate this aspect.

Despite clinical trials have failed proving reduction of infant death, the use of antenatal magnesium sulfate for neuroprotection statistically diminished the risk of cerebral palsy in the survivors [56, 57]. Therefore, its use is recommended in cases of high risk of imminent preterm birth, in single and multiple pregnancies, in gestations <32nd week, and after viability [7, 34].

Many mechanisms were proposed to explain the neuroprotective effect of magnesium sulfate, but the exact one is actually unknown. Other questions about magnesium sulfate that are not yet clarified are best dose regimen, treatment duration, and risks or benefits of retreatment. An interesting point that were recently approached is that the exposure to magnesium proximal to delivery (<12 hours) seems to be related to more significant reduction of cerebral palsy when compared to the last infusion of this drug more than 12 hours before delivery [58].

In UNIFESP, this drug is administered intravenously, with a loading dose of 4 g in 20 minutes, followed by 1 g/h for up to 24 hours or until delivery [40]. Monitoring these pregnant women (by continuous evaluation of patellar reflex, respiratory frequency, urine output) is essential to prevent magnesium toxicity. Myasthenia gravis and myocardial compromise are contraindications for the use of magnesium sulfate, and adjusted dose should be used in patients with renal insufficiency [59].

6. Conclusion

The evaluation of the clinical history of the previous preterm birth and the presence of short cervix (≤25 mm) are the best predictors of preterm delivery in twin pregnancy. Transvaginal ultrasonography for evaluation of the uterine cervix between the 18th and 24th week should be indicated for its cost-effectiveness.

The use of isolated vaginal progesterone in multiple pregnancies with short cervix presents evidence that justifies its use; however, this evidence is to be confirmed by other clinical tests due to the potential bias of the most recent meta-analysis.

Most guidelines do not recommend the use of prophylactic cerclage in patients with short cervix; however, in selected cases of extreme severity, it can be considered.

The use of a cervical pessary does not present solid evidence; however, some studies point out, although with a low level of evidence, that it may be beneficial.

As the low index of complications and the absence of highly efficient intervention in twins justify the utilization of the association of progesterone and cervical pessary, for this author it seems to be better than observing the evolution of the clinical condition.

The use of corticosteroids, between 24th–25th and 34th week, must be indicated in pregnancy in the imminence of delivery or with a high risk of preterm birth and must be avoided in pregnancy with intermediate or low risk, as there are studies which point out undesired effects of this treatment in the short and medium term.

Tocolytics is to be used under the 34th week in order to gain time for carrying out corticosteroids. The first-option drugs in twin pregnancy are the calcium channel blockers.

The use of magnesium sulfate in deliveries under the 32nd week is recommended by the main scientific societies, for the purpose of neuroprotection in twin pregnancy.

Acknowledgements

We thank the Ingamed® and Dr. Carlos Gilberto Almodin for developing, manufacturing, and offering without cost the cervical pessaries used in this study. We also thank Mr. Rudolf Wiedemann for his help with the English language version of this article.

Author details

Marcelo Santucci Franca[1]*, Tatiana E. N. K. Hamamoto[1] and Antônio Fernandes Moron[2]

*Address all correspondence to: marcelosantucci.franca@gmail.com

1 Discipline of Fetal Medicine, Obstetrics Department, Federal University of São Paulo—UNIFESP, São Paulo, Brazil

2 Institute of Tropical Medicine, University of São Paulo (USP), São Paulo, Brazil

References

[1] Werner EF, Han CS, Pettker CM, Buhimschi CS, Copel JA, Funai EF, et al. Universal cervical-length screening to prevent preterm birth: A cost effectiveness analysis. Ultrasound in Obstetrics & Gynecology. 2011;**38**:32-37

[2] Roberts D, Brown J, Medley N, Dalziel SR. Antenatal corticosteroids for accelerating fetal lung maturation for women at risk of preterm birth. Cochrane Database of Systematic Reviews. 21 Mar 2017;(3):CD004454. DOI: 10.1002/14651858.CD004454.pub3

[3] Cahill AG, Odibo AO, Caughey AB, et al. Universal cervical length screening and treatment with vaginal progesterone to prevent preterm birth: A decision and economic analysis. American Journal of Obstetrics and Gynecology. 2010;**202**:548.e1-548.e8

[4] Brizot ML, Hernandez W, Liao AW, et al. Vaginal progesterone for the prevention of preterm birth in twin gestations: A randomized placebo-controlled double-blind study. American Journal of Obstetrics and Gynecology. 2015;**213**:82.e1-82.e9. DOI: 10.1016/j.ajog.2015.02.021

[5] Dudenhausen JW, Grunebaum A, Staudinger UM. Optimization of women's health before conception when pregnancy has been postponed. Journal of Perinatal Medicine. 2013;**41**:23-25. DOI: 10.1515/JPM.2011.115

[6] Tarter JG, Khoury A, Barton JR, Jacques DL, Sibai BM. Demographic and obstetric factors influencing pregnancy outcome in twin gestations. American Journal of Obstetrics and Gynecology. 2002;**186**(5):910-912

[7] American College of Obstetricians and Gynecologists. Practice bulletin No. 169. Multifetal gestation: Twin, triplet, and higher-order multifetal pregnancy. Obstetrics and Gynecology. 2016;**128**(4):131-146. DOI: 10.1097/AOG.0000000000001709

[8] Wisborg K, Henriksen TB, Secher NJ. Maternal smoking and gestational age in twin pregnancy. Acta Obstetricia et Gynecologica Scandinavica. 2001;**80**(10):926-930

[9] Rolnik DL, Wright D, Poon LCY, Syngelaki A, O'Gorman N, de Paco Matallana C, et al. ASPRE trial: Performance of screening for preterm pre-eclampsia. Ultrasound in Obstetrics & Gynecology. 2017;**50**(4):492-495. DOI: 10.1002/uog.18816

[10] Iams JD, Goldenberg RL, Meis PJ, Mercer BM, Moawad A, Das A, et al. The length of the cervix and the risk of spontaneous premature delivery. The New England Journal of Medicine. 1996;**334**(9):567-572

[11] Hatanaka AR, Mattar R, Kawanami TE, Franca MS, Rolo LC, Nomura RM, et al. Amniotic fluid "sludge" is an independent risk factor for preterm delivery. The Journal of Maternal-Fetal & Neonatal Medicine. 2016;**29**(1):120-125. DOI: 10.3109/14767058.2014.989202

[12] Althabe F, Belizán JM, McClure EM, Hemingway-Foday J, Berrueta M, Mazzoni A, et al. A population-based, multifaceted strategy to implement antenatal corticosteroid treatment versus standard care for the reduction of neonatal mortality due to preterm birth in low-income and middle-income countries: The ACT cluster-randomized trial. Lancet. 2015;**385**(9968):629-639. DOI: 10.1016/S0140-6736(14)61651-2

[13] Cooperstock MS, Bakewell J, Herman A, Schramm WF. Association of sociodemographic variables with risk for very preterm birth in twins. Obstetrics and Gynecology. 1998; **92**(1):53-56

[14] Fuchs F, Senat MV. Multiple gestations and preterm birth. Seminars in Fetal & Neonatal Medicine. 2016;**21**(2):113-120. DOI: 10.1016/j.siny.2015.12.010. Epub 2016 Jan 13

[15] Hofmeister C, Brizot ML, Liao A, Francisco RPV, Zugaib M. Two-stage transvaginal cervical length screening for preterm birth in twin pregnancy. Journal of Perinatal Medicine. 2010;**38**:479-484. DOI: 10.1515/JPM.2010.088

[16] Houlihan C, Poon LC, Ciarlo M, Kim E, Guzman ER, Nicolaides KH. Cervical cerclage for preterm birth prevention in twin gestation with short cervix: A retrospective cohort study. Ultrasound in Obstetrics & Gynecology. 2016;**48**(6):752-756. DOI: 10.1002/uog.15918

[17] Yang JH, Kuhlman K, Daly S, Berghella V. Prediction of preterm birth by second trimester cervical sonography in twin pregnancy. Ultrasound in Obstetrics & Gynecology. 2000;**15**(4):288-291

[18] Pires CR, Moron AF, Mattar R, Diniz AL, Andrade SG, Bussamra LC. Cervical gland area as an ultrasonographic marker for preterm delivery. International Journal of Gynaecology and Obstetrics. 2006;**93**(3):214-219. Epub 2006 Jan 26

[19] Dziadosz M, Bennett TA, Dolin C, West Honart A, Pham A, Lee SS, et al. Uterocervical angle: A novel ultrasound screening tool to predict spontaneous preterm birth. American Journal of Obstetrics and Gynecology. 2016;**215**(3):376.e1-376.e7. DOI: 10.1016/j.ajog.2016.03.033

[20] Honest H, Bachmann LM, Gupta JK, Kleijnen J, Khan KS. Accuracy of cervicovaginal fetal fibronectin test in predicting risk of spontaneous preterm birth: Systematic review. BMJ. 2002;**325**(7359):301. Review

[21] Berghella V, Hayes E, Visintine J, Baxter JK. Fetal fibronectin testing for reducing the risk of preterm birth. Cochrane Database of Systematic Reviews. 2008;**4**:CD006843. DOI: 10.1002/14651858.CD006843.pub2. Review. PubMed PMID: 18843732

[22] Oliveira T, de Souza E, Mariani-Neto C, Camano L. Fetal fibronectin as a predictor of preterm delivery in twin gestations. International Journal of Gynaecology and Obstetrics. 1998;**62**(2):135-139. PubMed PMID: 9749884

[23] Goldenberg RL, Iams JD, Miodovnik M, Van Dorsten JP, Thurnau G, Bottoms S, et al. The preterm prediction study: Risk factors in twin gestations. National Institute of Child Health and Human Development maternal-fetal medicine units network. American Journal of Obstetrics and Gynecology. 1996;**175**(4 Pt 1):1047-1053. PubMed PMID: 8885774

[24] El-refaie W, Abdelhafez MS, Badawy A. Vaginal progesterone for prevention of preterm labor in asymptomatic twin pregnancy with sonographic short cervix: A randomized clinical trial of efficacy and safety. Archives of Gynecology and Obstetrics. 2016;**293**(1): 61-67. DOI: 10.1007/s00404-015-3767-1

[25] Romero R, Conde-Agudelo A, El-Refaie W, Rode L, Brizot ML, Cetingoz E, et al. Vaginal progesterone decreases preterm birth and neonatal morbidity and mortality in women with a twin gestation and a short cervix: An updated meta-analysis of individual patient data. Ultrasound in Obstetrics & Gynecology. 2017;**49**(3):303-314. DOI: 10.1002/uog.17397

[26] Norman JE, Mackenzie F, Owen P, Mactier H, Hanretty K, Cooper S, et al. Progesterone for the prevention of preterm birth in twin pregnancy (STOPPIT): A randomized, double-blind, placebo-controlled study and meta-analysis. Lancet. 2009;**373**:2034-2040. DOI: 10.1016/S0140- 6736(09)60947-8

[27] Rafael TJ, Berghella V, Alfirevic Z. Cervical stitch (cerclage) for preventing preterm birth in multiple pregnancy. Cochrane Database of Systematic Reviews. 2014;**9**:CD009166. DOI: 10.1002/14651858.CD009166.pub2. Review

[28] Roman A, Rochelson B, Martinelli P, Saccone G, Harris K, Zork N, et al. Cerclage in twin pregnancy with dilated cervix between 16 to 24 weeks of gestation: Retrospective cohort study. American Journal of Obstetrics and Gynecology. 2016;**215**(1):98.e1-98.e11. DOI: 10.1016/j.ajog.2016.01.172. Epub 2016 Jan 28

[29] Tajik P, Monfrance M, van 't Hooft J, Liem SM, Schuit E, Bloemenkamp KW, et al. A multivariable model to guide the decision for pessary placement to prevent preterm birth in women with a multiple pregnancy: A secondary analysis of the ProTWIN trial. Ultrasound in Obstetrics & Gynecology. 2016;**48**(1):48-55. DOI: 10.1002/uog.15855

[30] Goya M, de la Calle M, Pratcorona L, Merced C, Rodó C, Muñoz B, et al. PECEP-twins trial group. Cervical pessary to prevent preterm birth in women with twin gestation and sonographic short cervix: A multicenter randomized controlled trial (PECEP-twins). American Journal of Obstetrics and Gynecology. 2016;**214**(2):145-152. DOI: 10.1016/j.ajog.2015.11.012.

[31] Fox NS, Rebarber A, Klauser CK, Peress D, Gutierrez CV, Saltzman DH. Prediction of spontaneous preterm birth in asymptomatic twin pregnancy using the change in cervical length over time. American Journal of Obstetrics and Gynecology. 2010;**202**(2):155.e1-155.e4. DOI: 10.1016/j.ajog.2009.09.004

[32] El-refaie W, Abdelhafez MS, Badawy A. Vaginal progesterone for prevention of preterm labor in asymptomatic twin pregnancies with sonographic short cervix: A randomized clinical trial of efficacy and safety. Archives of Gynecology and Obstetrics. 2016;**293**(1):61-67. DOI: 10.1007/s00404-015-3767-1

[33] Haas DM, Imperiale TF, Kirkpatrick PR, Klein RW, Zollinger TW, Golichowski AM. Tocolytic therapy: A meta-analysis and decision analysis. Obstetrics and Gynecology. 2009;**113**(3):585-594. DOI: 10.1097/AOG.0b013e318199924a

[34] American College of Obstetricians and Gynecologists. Practice bulletin No. 171 summary: Management of preterm labor. Obstetrics and Gynecology. 2016;**128**(4):931-933. DOI: 10.1097/AOG.0000000000001702

[35] Medley N, Poljak B, Mammarella S, Alfirevic Z. Clinical guidelines for prevention and management of preterm birth: A systematic review. BJOG. 2018;**125**(11):1361-1369. DOI: 10.1111/1471-0528.15173. Epub 2018 Mar 25. Review

[36] American College of Obstetricians and Gynecologists; Society for Maternal-Fetal Medicine. Obstetric care consensus No. 6: Periviable birth. Obstetrics and Gynecology. 2017; **130**(4):e187-e199. DOI: 10.1097/AOG.0000000000002352

[37] Simhan HN, Caritis S. Inhibition of Acute Preterm Labor. Post TW, ed. Waltham, MA: UpToDate Inc. Available from: http://www.uptodate.com [Accessed: 15-09-2018]

[38] Papatsonis DN, Kok JH, van Geijn HP, Bleker OP, Adèr HJ, Dekker GA. Neonatal effects of nifedipine and ritodrine for preterm labor. Obstetrics and Gynecology. 2000;**95**(4): 477-481

[39] Flenady V, Reinebrant HE, Liley HG, Tambimuttu EG, Papatsonis DN. Oxytocin receptor antagonists for inhibiting preterm labour. Cochrane Database of Systematic Reviews. 2014;**6**(6):CD004452. DOI: 10.1002/14651858.CD004452.pub3. Review

[40] Atualização Terapêutica de Prado. Ramos e Valle: urgências e emergências/ Presidente da comissão editorial. In: Emilia Inoue Sato. 3a ed. Vol. 2018. São Paulo: Artes Médicas. pp. 618-621

[41] Younger JD, Reitman E, Gallos G. Tocolysis: Present and future treatment options. Seminars in Perinatology. 2017;**41**(8):493-504. DOI: 10.1053/j.semperi.2017.08.008. Review

[42] Anotayanonth S, Subhedar NV, Garner P, Neilson JP, Harigopal S. Betamimetics for inhibiting preterm labour. Cochrane Database of Systematic Reviews. 2004;(4):CD004352. Review. Update in: Cochrane Database Syst Rev. 2014; 2:CD004352

[43] Vermillion ST, Scardo JA, Lashus AG, Wiles HB. The effect of indomethacin tocolysis on fetal ductus arteriosus constriction with advancing gestational age. American Journal of Obstetrics and Gynecology. 1997;**177**(2):256-259. Discussion 259-61

[44] Clive DM, Stoff JS. Renal syndromes associated with nonsteroidal antiinflammatory drugs. The New England Journal of Medicine. 1984;**310**(9):563-572. Review

[45] Liggins GC, Howie RN. A controlled trial of antepartum glucocorticoid treatment for prevention of the respiratory distress syndrome in premature infants. Pediatrics. 1972;**50**(4):515-525

[46] Crowley P. Prophylactic corticosteroids for preterm birth. Cochrane Database of Systematic Reviews. 2000;(2):CD000065. Review

[47] Crowther CA, Harding J. Repeat doses of prenatal corticosteroids for women at risk of preterm birth for preventing neonatal respiratory disease. Cochrane Database of Systematic Reviews. 2003;(3):CD003935. Review

[48] Paro-Panjan D, Kodri J, Sustersic B. Association between neurological signs and developmental outcome: Pilot results in preterm group. Croatian Medical Journal. 2009; **50**:345-350

[49] Soll R, Morley CJ. Prophylactic versus selective use of surfactant in preventing morbidity and mortality in preterm infants. Cochrane Database of Systematic Reviews. 2000; (2):CD000510

[50] França MS, Moron AF, Araujo Júnior E, Avedissian M, Pares DB, Nardozza LM, et al. Neonatal neuronal apoptosis after betamethasone administration in pregnant Wistar rats. The Journal of Maternal-Fetal & Neonatal Medicine. 2016;**29**(7):1089-1093

[51] American College of Obstetricians and Gynecologists. Committee on Obstetric Practice. Committee opinion No. 713: Antenatal corticosteroid therapy for fetal maturation. Obstetrics and Gynecology. 2017;**130**(2):e102-e109. DOI: 10.1097/AOG.0000000000002237

[52] Gyamfi-Bannerman C, Thom EA, Blackwell SC, Tita AT, Reddy UM, Saade GR, et al. NICHD maternal–fetal medicine units network. Antenatal betamethasone for women at risk for late preterm delivery. The New England Journal of Medicine. 2016;**374**(14):1311-1320. Epub 2016 Feb 4. DOI: 10.1056/NEJMoa1516783

[53] Vogel JP, Souza JP, Gümezoglu AM, Mori R, Lumbiganon P, Qureshi Z, et al. Use of antenatal corticosteroids and tocolytic drugs in preterm births in 29 countries: An analysis of the WHO multicountry survey on maternal and newborn health. Lancet. 2014;**384**(9957):1869-1877. DOI: 10.1016/S0140-6736(14)60580-8

[54] van Baaren GJ, Vis JY, Wilms FF, Oudijk MA, Kwee A, Porath MM, et al. Predictive value of cervical length measurement and fibronectin testing in threatened preterm labor. Obstetrics and Gynecology. 2014;**123**(6):1185-1192. DOI: 10.1097/AOG.0000000000000229

[55] Nelson KB, Grether JK. Can magnesium sulfate reduce the risk of cerebral palsy in very low birthweight infants? Pediatrics. 1995;**95**(2):263-269

[56] American College of Obstetricians and Gynecologists Committee on Obstetric Practice; Society for Maternal-Fetal Medicine. Committee opinion No. 455: Magnesium sulfate before anticipated preterm birth for neuroprotection. Obstetrics and Gynecology. 2010;**115**(3):669-671. DOI: 10.1097/AOG.0b013e3181d4ffa5

[57] Doyle LW, Crowther CA, Middleton P, Marret S. Magnesium sulphate for women at risk of preterm birth for neuroprotection of the fetus. Cochrane Database of Systematic Reviews. 2007;(3):CD004661. DOI: 10.1002/14651858.CD004661.pub2. Review. Update in: Cochrane Database Syst Rev. 2009;(1): CD004661

[58] Turitz AL, Too GT, Gyamfi-Bannerman C. Proximity of magnesium exposure to delivery and neonatal outcomes. American Journal of Obstetrics and Gynecology. 2016;**215**(4):508.e1-508.e6. DOI: 10.1016/j.ajog.2016.05.004. Epub 2016 May 10

[59] Simhan HN, Himes KP. Neuroprotective Effects of in Utero Exposure to Magnesium Sulfate. Post TW, ed. Waltham, MA: UpToDate Inc. Available from: http://www.uptodate.com [Accessed: 15-09-2018]

8

Clinical Trials in Pregnant Women with Preeclampsia

Leonel García Benavides, Diego Hernández Molina, Jessica L. Barajas Vega, Sylvia E. Totsuka Sutto, Fernando Grover Paéz, Francisco J. Hernández Mora, Ernesto J. Ramírez Lizardo, Sara Pascoe Gonzalez, David Cardona Müller and Ernesto G. Cardona Muñoz

Abstract

Preeclampsia (PE) is the leading cause of preterm birth by medical indication when associated with premature detachment of placenta normoinserta, and Intrauterine growth restriction (IUGR) is associated with high perinatal morbidity and mortality and long-term sequelae. The main problem of PE is threefold: the diagnostic difficulty, the complicated interrelationship of the pathophysiological processes, and the vulnerability of the maternal-fetal binomial to the therapeutic interventions. The approach for management with PE is preventing its late occurrence in pregnancy. The key to preventing PE is knowledge of the factors that trigger the pathophysiological processes that culminate in the presentation of PE. Understanding the developmental characteristics of the placenta in pregnancy at high risk for PE is essential for understanding the pathophysiology and developing strategies for prevention. When deciding that the population of study is a group of pregnant women, the first ethical criteria that need to be reviewed are those aimed at the protection of the fetus. There are no specific guidelines on how to assess fetal well-being during pregnancy routinely in the clinic, and this deficiency is shifted to clinical research with pregnant women.

Keywords: preeclampsia, eclampsia, pregnancy induced-hypertension, complications in pregnancy women

1. Introduction

Preeclampsia (PE) is the leading cause of preterm birth by medical indication when associated with premature detachment of placenta normoinserta, and IUGR is associated with high perinatal morbidity and mortality and long-term sequelae. It has been described that standardization in the management of health services and the use of clinical practice guidelines is associated with a reduction in adverse outcomes, and a fundamental part of the management of severe PE includes a complete evaluation of the mother and the fetus. Despite the advances in medicine, the frequency of this syndrome has not changed, and globally its incidence ranges between 2 and 10% of pregnancies. The World Health Organization (WHO) estimates that the incidence of PE is seven times higher in developing than in developed countries (2.8–0.4%). In Mexico, it is estimated that PE is a major cause of maternal and perinatal morbidity and mortality. In Jalisco alone, maternal deaths increased to 57.14% from 2011 to 2014, placing this state in fourth place at the national level in terms of maternal deaths, during 2015 [1]. Because it is a heterogeneous associated idiopathic syndrome to endothelial damage, so far there is no effective treatment that reduces the morbidity and mortality of this pathological entity, so it is necessary to reinforce prevention. In this area, only the use of calcium supplements and acetylsalicylic acid (ASA) appears to be a recommendation, albeit with controversial results [1, 2].

The main problem of PE is threefold, the diagnostic difficulty, the complicated interrelationship of the pathophysiological processes, and the vulnerability of the maternal-fetal binomial to the therapeutic interventions.

2. Pregnant women, scientifically complexed population

There are various concepts about the characteristics of vulnerable populations; however, it is generally accepted that a vulnerable group is one whose ability to protect their own interest or grant their consent is physically, psychologically, or socially compromised. Since the development of ethical principles in research, children, psychiatric patients, prisoners, and pregnant women have been included in this group; however, in recent years it has been intended to remove pregnant women from this group. The National Institutes of Health (NIH) through the Office of Research on Women's Health recommended as early as 2010 that pregnant women should be considered as a scientifically complex rather than vulnerable group, this being for the reason that this group has the same capacity and autonomy for decision making as its nonpregnant counterparts, including the decision of whether or not to participate in a clinical trial [3].

Scientific complexity arises from the special physiological conditions of pregnancy and from the ethical considerations of the balance between maternal well-being and fetal well-being.

Pregnancy is accompanied by important physiological changes and their knowledge is an element of great value for the proper management of the obstetric patient. Practically, all the body's system of the pregnant woman is adapted to house the product, among them are changes at the ocular, musculoskeletal, skin and mucous, hepatic, hematological, renal, and gastrointestinal levels. The most relevant changes occur at the uterine level, systemic vascular resistance is reduced due to high flow and low resistance circuit in the uteroplacental circulation. In pregnancy, uterine blood flow significantly increases to allow perfusion of intervillous placental spaces and fetal development. The trophoblast invades the uterine spiral arteries; vascular smooth muscle cells are lost and replaced by the fibrinoid material, converting them into large dilated blood vessels allowing greater perfusion of the placenta [4]. These changes pose a challenge for the researcher as they make it very difficult to define not only the possible therapeutic results of an intervention, but also to adapt the intervention to these new changes that are not present in nonpregnant women. In a pathological condition such as preeclampsia, this may represent a greater challenge, because of restrictions on research in a physiological pregnancy, ignorance or doubts about the effects of the intervention on the organism, or pathological adaptations that may affect the intervention that is intended to be performed are greater.

The ethical complexity is established in the possibility that the intervention applied in key phases causes a teratogenic risk or that affects the adaptation of the product to extrauterine life, and more worrying, the possibility of long-term toxicity. This is why it is necessary that preclinical teratogenicity studies have been completed prior to the intervention in pregnant women. Also, it is recommended to start the new interventions after the 12th week of gestation, when the organogenesis is finished and finally, it is recommended to follow the fetus and newborn [5]. However, these special considerations do not seem to be sufficient, as there are currently two forms of research in the group of pregnant women: the first consists of interventions unrelated to pregnancy that may benefit only the mother [3]. It seems that the previous recommendations were formulated with this type of research, since the use of thalidomide has contemplated the possibility of developing drugs that may attenuate different discomforts during pregnancy. The clinical investigation currently has to verify that the pharmacological interventions do not cause damage to the product and not only benefit the mother. The second type of research concerns interventions that may potentially benefit the mother and her fetus [3]. This aspect is more related to the development of pharmacological interventions for pathologies in pregnancy, specifically speaking of preeclampsia, the treatments are not indicated at the same time for the mother and for the fetus. Betamimetics used to prevent preterm birth are not intended to treat the mother and may even complicate maternal health. In contrast, depending on the severity of hypertension, the drugs could have a toxic effect on the fetus. These two aspects should be considered when deciding to experiment with a new therapeutic product or scheme [5].

3. Fetal well-being in the clinical trial

When deciding that the study population is the group of pregnant women, the first ethical criteria that need to be reviewed are those aimed at the protection of the fetus. Generally, investigations of pregnant women involving an intervention or experimental procedure such as in PE cases, should not expose the embryo or fetus to a greater risk than the minimum, except when the use of the intervention or procedure is justified for saving the life of the mother. However, in addition to a deep and sufficient knowledge of the intervention that is proposed to apply, there is no strategy to evaluate during the course of research the side effects on the product. Although maternal-fetal medicine is currently a fact, with several diagnostic imaging and biochemical resources, with established therapeutic procedures, there is no consensus on what tests are necessary to perform and monitor the product during investigations in pregnant women. Even experts do not dare to indicate any fetal diagnostic procedure, within the clinic in the management of pathological pregnancies, but it is at the discretion of the attending physician the use of some diagnostic or therapeutic techniques [6].

There are six most generalized methods to know and evaluate fetal well-being [7]:

1. Maternal evaluation of fetal activity. It consists of the count by the mother of the number of times fetal movement occurs. Although the fetal movement count is a recommendation that is made to every pregnant woman, there is no cutoff point when abnormal movement is considered abnormal, some clinicians mark the alarm in less than 10 fetal movements perceived per day, others when no movements are perceived within 2 h. This form of assessment of fetal well-being presents a false-positive rate, since it depends on the subjectivity of the mother.

2. Test without stress. It consists of the evaluation of fetal heart rate in relationship to uterine contractions. Although it has a low false-negative rate (0.19–1%), its high rate of false positives (55%) makes it a test with minimal benefits, and its counterpart, the stress test, in which it is administered by infusion intravenous oxytocin, is contraindicated in high-risk situations.

3. Biophysical profile. It is a test composed of the evaluation of five parameters, fetal heart activity, fetal respiratory movements, fetal thick movements, muscle tone, and volume of amniotic fluid. Although its false-negative rates are very low (0.07%), its false-positive rate is only lower than that of the stress-free test, and has not shown any difference in terms of fetal death, cesarean indication, and under Apgar score. In addition to being a dependent operator test, factors that may alter outcomes include hypoxemia, gestational age, steroid administration, magnesium sulfate administration, and labor; five factors that occur frequently in pregnant women with PE.

4. Modified biophysical profile. It is the combination of the stress-free test with the biophysical profile. Although it requires less time and experience for its realization, makes its result more reliable, its false-positive and -negative rates are similar to the two tests separately.

5. Fetal Doppler ultrasound. The evaluation consists in measuring by ultrasound the velocity of blood flow in the fetal vessels, usually the umbilical artery. Out of all of the above, Doppler has been evaluated with the most rigorous clinical trials and although it does not show a benefit in terms of fetal death in high-risk pregnancies, it has become an effective test in the reduction of fetal morbidity and mortality in high-risk pregnancies, being this an indication for its use. The use of Doppler in pregnant women with high risk of PE can be a predictive tool combined with serum biomarkers; this strategy is still being validated but promising.

6. Evaluation of fetal lung maturity. It consists the evaluating the presence of surfactant factor in the amniotic fluid. It is a useful evaluation when it is necessary to determine the best time to interrupt the pregnancy when the risk of continuing it is greater. Due to the fact

that in PE the treatment consists of the interruption of pregnancy, to be able to prolong it until reaching the fetal maturity, becomes one of the most difficult aspects of the management to avoid the fetal morbidity-mortality, reason why it is to make sure that the fetus counts with pulmonary maturity to resist extrauterine life has become essential.

Although these tests and diagnostic interventions are the most used in the clinic, the amount of imaging tests, serum markers, and procedures with maternal-fetal medicine is higher; however, many of the tests have not shown their value, they could be useful and applicable reason why they require to be studied, especially those that allow predicting the presentation of complications or diseases such as PE. Among the currently available tests are the evaluation of both fetal DNA and the cells that make up the placenta, even in an experimental way, it is possible to attenuate or increase gene expression through miRNAs, not only for diagnostic purposes, but also for possible therapeutic applications in the future.

The American Congress of Obstetricians and Gynecologists states that the evaluation of fetal well-being may be appropriate for pregnancies with an increased risk of fetal involvement; however, there are no comprehensive trials demonstrating the benefit of all tests and their potential indications. On the other hand, experts recommend carrying out tests of fetal well-being in cases of diabetes, uterine growth restriction, and hypertension [7].

As we can see that there are no specific guidelines on how to evaluate fetal well-being during pregnancy routinely in the clinic, and this deficiency is translated into clinical research with pregnant women. As mentioned before, although one of the principles of research in pregnancy is to maintain the integrity of the product, there are neither guidelines nor recommendations on which tests to apply and when to ensure the safety of the fetus. From the above, we can infer that most clinical trials involving pregnant women have not been able to guarantee or know with certainty the fetal well-being. So how is it possible to monitor fetal well-being in a clinical trial? How can we evaluate adverse effects on the product? And if there is no strategy to assess at least fetal well-being, is it ethical to allow the participation of pregnant women in clinical trials? It is up to the researcher to decide the degree of safety with which he plans to conduct his research, and in the absence of additional tests to ensure fetal well-being, using those available is the most reasonable. However, we should not be satisfied with the analysis of the structural function to guarantee the innocuousness of an intervention, it is necessary to find strategies that in fact allow to evaluate not only the welfare, structural integrity, and fetal vitality, but also to value the whole range of possible adverse effects, both acute and chronic, that may be occurring as a result of new pharmacological interventions or procedures.

4. Clinical research in women pregnant with PE

Pregnancy is a physiological condition inherent in almost all species and life; however, it is one of the lesser known states and a field of research that just begins to grow, because at the beginning of research with pregnant women, a series of events occurred that negatively marked research in this population.

Research is now making its way into the subject of pregnancy and its pathologies in order to have a better understanding of physiological processes and to reduce maternal-fetal morbidity and mortality. However, despite the intentions and efforts of researchers, little is known. In the context of PE, it has been possible to trace its origin to the inadequate invasion of the trophoblastic villi on the vascular bed of the uterine spiral arteries, little is known about the cause of this inadequate adaptation of the uteroplacental vascular system [8]. Moreover, we are in complete disbelief about why some women develop PE and others do not. There is no effective diagnostic test to predict who will have PE, the best biomarkers have poor predictive power, the best chance to achieve prevention so far arises from the combination of Doppler ultrasound with some of the serum markers, which have been implemented, nevertheless, only demonstrate efficacy once the first evident changes of PE are presented, when it is no longer possible to avoid the development of the disease [9]. A real opportunity for prevention of PE would arise from a marker that would allow us to know with great certainty, which women are at risk of having PE, even before the pregnancy is carried out. The best predictive tool we have are the risk factors that have been determined by both prospective and retrospective studies, but are only able to predict 30% of women who develop PE [9], there is even a larger group of the population that develops PE with no previous risk factors. On the other hand, from the group of women who develop PE, one part shows severe PE and another group develops eclampsia, and again it is not possible for the treating doctors to determine who and how they evolve to more serious stages.

In women with severe PE, who present it before fetal viability, maternal stabilization is recommended before interruption of pregnancy. Once treatment is established, close monitoring is required to identify the presence of serious complications of PE. Despite efforts to treat PE, treatment is symptom-based and focused on controlling blood pressure. In regard to the time of delivery, gestational age should transfer to the maximum possible. However, in severe PE, in addition to antihypertensive treatment, termination of pregnancy is recommended if it is greater than 34 weeks. If the pregnancy is less than 34 weeks and the mother and product are stable, the pregnancy should be continued with administration of corticosteroids. Currently, there are multiple criteria for better management of PE, but the only cure for PE is termination of pregnancy. This results in a difficult decision for the physician and the mother because of the psychological burden, and the social and economic morbidity [8].

The results of medical interventions have failed to significantly decrease the morbidity and mortality of PE. The main reason for this failure could be the multifactorial origin of pathogenic processes that lead to the development of PE. Therefore, the approach for management of patients with PE is preventing its late occurrence in pregnancy. The key to prevention of PE is knowledge of the factors that trigger pathophysiological processes that culminate in the presentation of the PE. However, efforts to understand the origin of these processes are still poorly or incompletely understood. There is a lack of knowledge because the approach to study this population may be unethical compared with diseases of nonpregnant women [10]. The multifactorial origin of PE and difficulty of carrying out an investigation in the early stages of pregnancy, because it can endanger the mother and fetus, have made research difficult. Understanding the developmental characteristics of the placenta in pregnancy at high risk for PE is essential for understanding the pathophysiology and for developing strategies of prevention [8].

5. Current state of research about PE

There are currently 236,008 clinical trials registered in clinicalTrials.gov, from which only 3% are focused on pregnancy, and among them 6.4% are about PE. Of all clinical trials dedicated to PE, 47.9% focus on strategies to improve treatment, 22.2% of the clinical trials aim to improve the diagnosis or its establishment in the early stages, and 16.7% aim to establish the utility of new biomarkers, for both diagnostic and monitoring. Finally, only 10.7% of the clinical trials registered until February 1, 2017 are focused on the prevention of PE (**Figure 1**).

Another aspect that should be taken under consideration is that more than half of the clinical trials directed to PE are carried out in regions classified as first world such as Europe and North America, whereas research in the rest of the world only constitutes 40%, despite the fact that developing countries are the ones that bear the greatest burden of morbidity and mortality caused by this disease (**Figure 2**).

In our times, PE has a worldwide relevance and it has been increasing over the years. Clinical trials with the objective of reducing the morbidity and mortality of this pathology have also increased over time. The previous chart denotes some of the terminated trials registered in clinicaltrials.gov, many of which have certain limitations that we were able to observe (**Table 1**).

In the study titled, "L-arginine and antioxidant vitamins during pregnancy to reduce preeclampsia", there is little coherence between the objective and the design of the study. Although

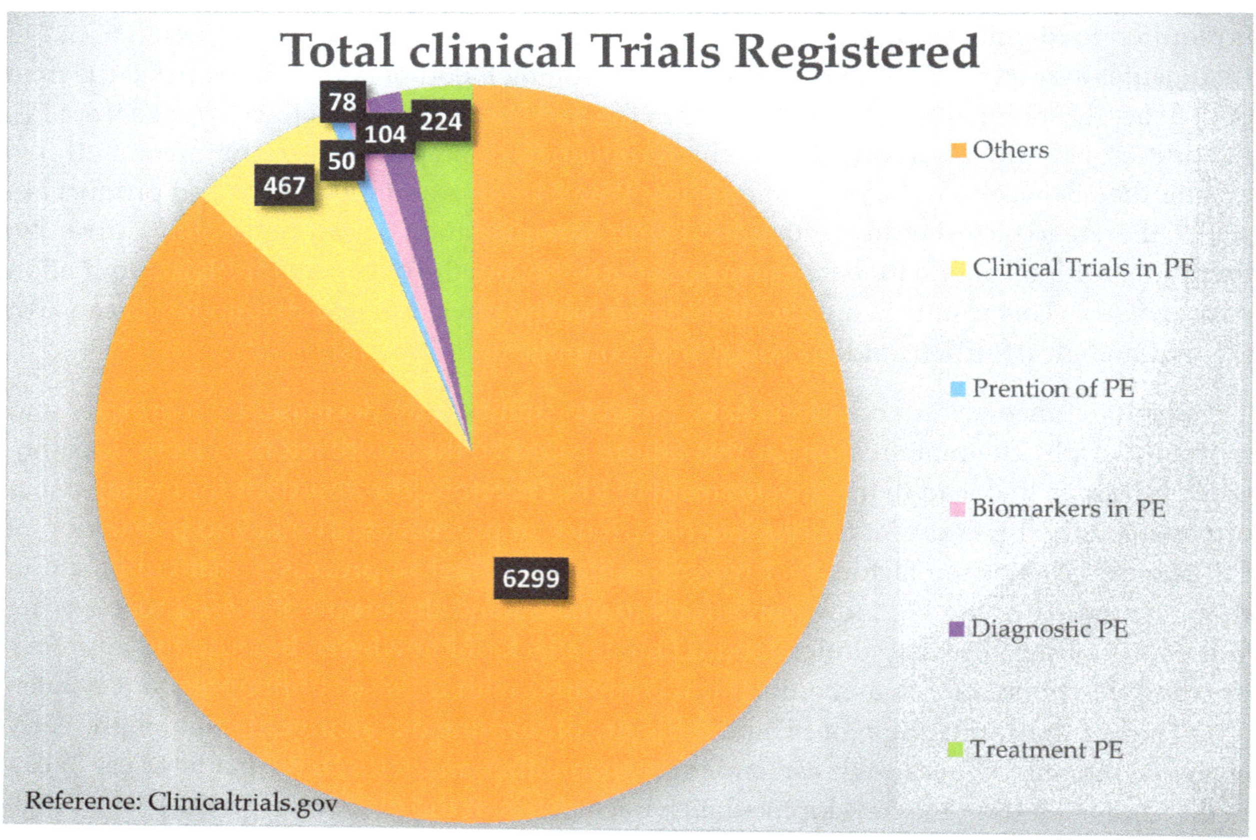

Figure 1. Clinical trials registered until February 1, 2017. Data from: clinicaltrials.gov.

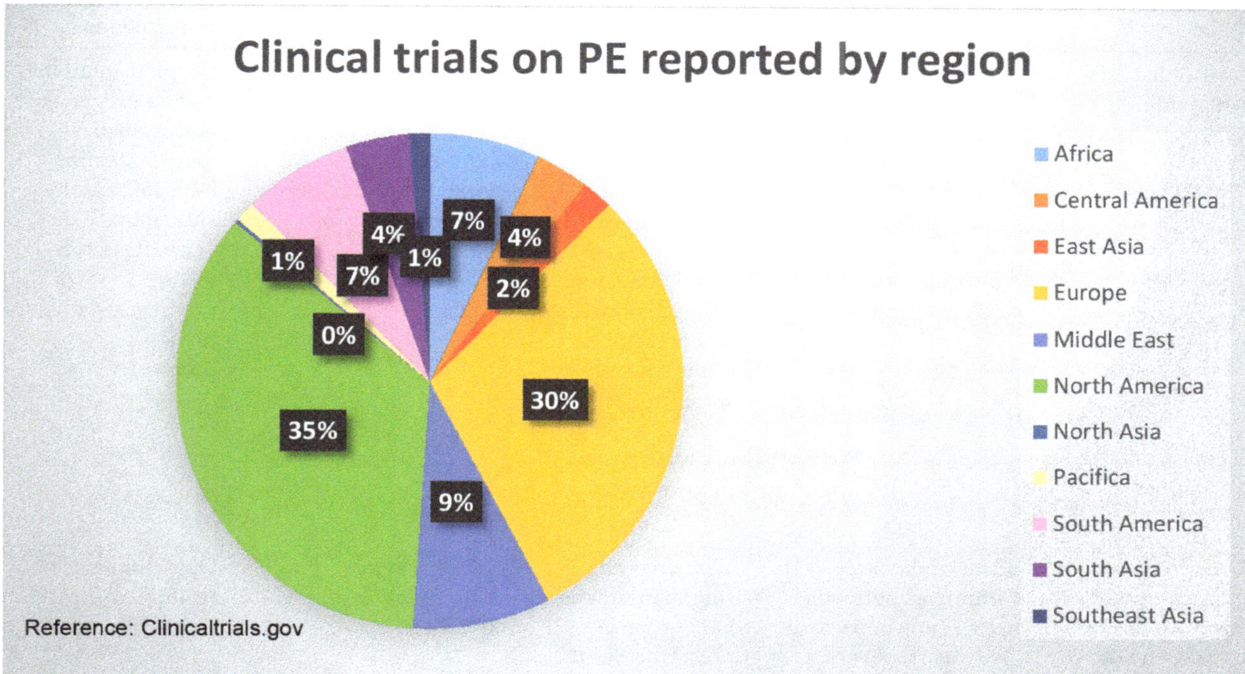

Figure 2. Clinical trials on PE reported by region.

it is known that the production of nitric oxide and L-arginine as the main substrate of nitric oxide synthase is involved in the pathophysiology of PE, the study design is directed at the effect of L-arginine that has on the development of PE; however, levels of L-arginine are not evaluated at any moment, neither its nitrates nor nitrites, being the reason why this design cannot help reach the hypothesis. In addition, the main inclusion criteria appeared to be having a high-risk profile for developing PE; however, high-risk factors such as diabetes, autoimmune diseases, and hypertension in pregnancy and kidney diseases are not considered as inclusion criteria, and these factors combined with a history of risk of developing PE in previous pregnancies, increase up to nine times the risk of developing PE. Another mistake that can be found in their design is noted when analyzing the main conclusion and the way the intervention was carried out, the conclusion states that the supplementation of L-arginine and vitamins reduces the incidence of PE; nevertheless, in the results it can appreciated that the group that only received the food-bar containing the vitamins did not have a significant reduction in the risk of developing PE. Meaning that the mayor contributing factor for the reduction of PE was indeed L-arginine and not the combination of L-arginine/vitamins, and these would have been more notorious if a supplementation group taking only L-arginine was added [11].

In the study titled "Usefulness of Extracorporeal Removal of sFLT-1 in Women with Very Early Severe Preeclampsia (ADENA)", at first instance we are lead to appreciate that the primary outcome of the study is about early severe PE; however, later, we appreciate that the intention is improving perinatal death as the primary outcome. The first comment worth mentioning is that using words such as "improving" in an investigation study may be to imprecise, it is better to use terms such as "reducing" for this instance. Moreover the levels of sFLT-1 are not per say an inclusion criteria for deciding whether or not to perform apheresis, even by being quantified before and after the intervention, those women with high levels of sFLT-1 could perhaps have a

Title	Hypothesis	Population	Intervention	Conclusions
L-Arginine and Antioxidant Vitamins during Pregnancy to Reduce Preeclampsia	To test that a relative deficiency of L-arginine, precursor of *nitric oxide* (NO) by the enzyme NO *synthase* (NOS), reduces the development of preeclampsia in high-risk pregnancies	Pregnant women with a history of a previous pregnancy complicated by preeclampsia, or preeclampsia in a first degree relative, whom are deemed to have an increased risk of recurrence of the disease, were studied from 14 to 32 weeks of gestation and followed until delivery	Supplementation with: medical food-bars containing L-arginine plus antioxidant vitamins, antioxidant vitamins alone or placebo	Supplementation during pregnancy with a medical food containing L-arginine and antioxidant vitamins reduced the incidence of preeclampsia in high-risk pregnancy
Usefulness of Extracorporeal Removal of sFLT-1 in women with very early severe Preeclampsia (ADENA)	The removal of s-Flt1 improves perinatal death in women with very early severe preeclampsia	Women with singleton pregnancy having severe preeclampsia at 23–25 6/7 weeks of gestation	Apheresis for extracorporal removal of sFlt-1	Does not have a result
Oral Progesterone and Low Dose Aspirin in the Prevention of Preeclampsia	Low-dose aspirin combined with progesterone will decrease the risk of preeclampsia in pregnant women with history of preeclampsia in a previous pregnancy	Pregnant patients with a previous history of preeclampsia in the immediate prior pregnancy	Aspirin 81 mg once a day orally, progesterone 200 mg twice daily	Does not have a result
Safety and Efficacy of RLX030 in Pregnant Women with Preeclampsia	Part 1: To assess the safety and tolerability of different doses of RLX030, when given to pregnant women with preeclampsia. Part 2: To assess whether an optimal dose of RLX030 can prolong pregnancy in women with preeclampsia	Pregnant women in 28 weeks (0 days) and 33 weeks (+4 days) of gestational age with a diagnosis of preeclampsia or superimposed preeclampsia requiring hospitalization	RLX030 15 μg/kg/day IV for 72 h	Not enough information was provided to analyze because the study was stopped after three patients were enrolled
CPAP in Preeclampsia	To assess the effects of nasal CPAP in pregnant women (24–37 gestational weeks) with preeclampsia	Women with 24–37 weeks of pregnancy with Singleton pregnancy, primiparous and primigravid diagnosis of preeclampsia	Continuous Positive Airway Pressure Ventilation (CPAP)	Does not have result

Source: Clinicaltrials.gov [11].

Table 1. Current state of clinical trials about PE.

greater benefit, reason why stabilizing grades at first instance could help the obstetrician make a better clinical decision. Finally, although its justifiable not using a control group, this type of design (before and after), not having a reference group, leads to a lower internal validity [11].

In the study titled "Oral Progesterone and Low Dose Aspirin in the Prevention of Preeclampsia", the main inclusion criterion is having a history with preeclampsia. Nevertheless, other factors of high risk were not taken account. Even though the study propounds that a deficiency of progesterone could lead to PE and in consequence, supplementation with progesterone could reduce the incidence of PE, serum values as an indicator to identify patients whom could benefit with progesterone supplementation were not taken into account. The comparison between before and after instead of vs the placebo group is also an inconvenient [11].

In the study titled "Oral Progesterone and Low-Dose Aspirin in Preeclampsia Prevention," the main inclusion criterion is the antecedent of PE in previous pregnancies; however, as in the previous study, other factors that increase the risk are not taken into account. The study assumes that a deficiency of progesterone could be the cause of PE, this argument seems to be the rationale to reduce the incidence of PE using supplementation with progesterone; but in the study, they did not take serum values in consideration as a marker to indicate which patients could benefit from supplementation. This study, as the previous one, also lacks the comparison against a placebo group, creating the same limitations [11].

In the study entitled "Safety and Efficacy of RLX030 in Pregnant Women with Pre-Eclampsia" proposed by the company NOVARTIS did not have sufficient information to perform an analysis, because of premature termination of the study [11].

In the study entitled "CPAP in Preeclampsia", the main objective is the evaluation of fetal well-being using nasal continuous positive airway pressure (CPAP) as a basis to increase fetal oxygenation; however, monitoring fetal movements is a scarce strategy to evaluate fetal well-being and it could be enhanced, according to the advances in fetal medicine to allow us to get closer to knowing the well-being of the fetus. The study did not make a distinction on the severity of PE, and if a clinical benefit of using CPAP is demonstrated, a distinction on the severity might be useful for clinical decisions. Therefore, the rationale to use CPAP is not clear [11].

In several studies, narrowing gestational age as inclusion criteria perhaps increases internal validity; however, the results cannot be extrapolated to other groups [11].

It is worth noting that the protocols registered in clinical trial go through variations during the study, which go unnoticed.

6. Transference of scientific knowledge to clinical practice persist in LAG

One of the most important advantages of basic research is the possibility to transfer knowledge to improve clinical practice. However, in the case of PE, new information regarding new biomarkers and new opportunities of intervention emerge every year, but these are not implemented by the treating physicians. Moreover, clinical practice guidelines are lagging too, and many years pass before a new intervention reaches the level of recommendation within them. On the one hand, this occurs because the information that is generated seems to be isolated and fragmented, there is no body or work team or expert committee that focus their efforts on trying to solve the problem or on generating a line of research on the subject. Another part of the transforming knowledge problem is that for this to be carried out it is necessary that the information obtained may be applicable to different populations at different times and with different characteristics, this is very complex to achieve in the first place because, as mentioned previously, there is no focus group to this and separated efforts generate a bias in the study population. Another bias that impedes transfer is that the risk factors presented by each population are different in the developed countries than those in the developing world, so information generated on the one side is not necessarily applicable in other parts of the world. Because the origin of PE is not well understood, the approaches with which the different studies are developed differ, while some may determine that the cause is oxidative stress, some others may argue that the cause is genetic. The truth is that so far it is considered multifactorial and because of this the international guidelines are more discreet about which recommendations to accept, in the sense of being able to verify which actions will have an evident weight in clinical practice.

Finally, one of the most worrying aspects that delay the transfer of knowledge is the lack of medical update on the subject. A very obvious example is that in practice, physicians do not intentionally seek pregnancies with a high risk of PE, and when a patient is classified with high risk, the first action of the doctor is an expectant management, without any intervention, although in the guidelines of clinical practice the administration of acetylsalicylic acid, calcium, and L-arginine is recommended, this happens because evidence of acetylsalicylic acid's efficacy in reducing the risk is contradictory, while calcium intake is reserved for those women with low risk and low calcium intake, and L-arginine, although it is part of the Canadian guide, no dosage or time is specified.

Other evidence in the lack of management of the subject in some specialists is the lack of communication they generate with patients who are at high risk. Patients are not informed of their situation and expectant management "poor surveillance" continues even after the patient develops PE, which is when the symptomatic management begins, and it seems that the physicians are waiting for a complication to occur, to make the decision of taking a more active management. It is true that during the 1st weeks of the PE, there are not many recommendations, and that most focus on the final stages in which fetal viability can be achieved, but this same reason should be what drives medical doctors to have a closer monitoring in research opportunities and new information to improve the outcome of the pregnancy, remembering that once PE is presented, there is no curative treatment, beyond the interruption of pregnancy. Efforts should be directed at preventing the occurrence of PE or, failing at that, occurring late in pregnancy.

Author details

Leonel García Benavides[1,2]*, Diego Hernández Molina[1], Jessica L. Barajas Vega[1], Sylvia E. Totsuka Sutto[1], Fernando Grover Paéz[1], Francisco J. Hernández Mora[2], Ernesto J. Ramírez Lizardo[1], Sara Pascoe Gonzalez[1], David Cardona Müller[1] and Ernesto G. Cardona Muñoz[1]

*Address all correspondence to: drleonelgb@hotmail.com

1 INTEC, Centro Universitario de Ciencias de la Salud, Universidad de Guadalajara, México

2 Hospital Civil de Guadalajara "Fray Antonio Alcalde", Guadalajara, Jalisco, México

References

[1] Atención integral de la preeclampsia en el segundo y tercer nivel de atención: secretaría de salud. 2008

[2] Campos A. O papel da AAS na prevenção da Pré-Eclâmpsia: Estado da Arte. Acta Médica Portuguesa. 2015;**28**(4):517-524

[3] American College of Obstetricians and Gynecologists. Ethical considerations for including women as research participants. Committee Opinion No. 646. Obstetrics and Gynecology. 2015;**126**:e 100-e107

[4] Ojeda-González JJ, Rodríguez-Älvarez M, Estepa Pérez JL, Piña-Loyola CN, Cabeza-Poblet BL. Cambios fisiológicos durante el embarazo. Su importancia para el anestesiólogo. Medisur. 2011;**9**(5):484-491

[5] Viada-González CE, Ballagas-Flores C, Blanco-López Y. Ética en la investigación con poblaciones especiales. Revista Cubana de Investigaciones Biomédicas. 2001;**20**(2):140-149

[6] Geaghan SM. Fetal laboratory medicine: On the frontier of maternal-fetal medicine. Clinical Chemistry. 2012;**58**(2):337-352

[7] O'Neill E. Thorp J. Antepartum evaluation of the fetus and fetal well being. Clinical Obstetrics and Gynaecology. 2012;**55**(3):722-730

[8] García Benavides L, Hernandez Molina D, Barajas Vega JL, Totsuka Sutto SE, Ramírez Lizardo EJ, et al. New pharmacological opportunities for prevention of preeclampsia. Journal of Clinical and Experimental Cardiology. 2016;**7**:457

[9] Duckitt K, Harrington D. Risk factors for pre-eclampsia at antenatal booking: Systematic review of controlled studies. British Medical Journal. 2005;**330**(7491):565

[10] Reglamento de la ley general de salud en materia de investigación para la salud [Internet]. 2014. Available from: http://www.ordenjuridico.gob.mx/leyes.php [Accessed: January 13, 2017

[11] https://clinicaltrials.gov

9

Quadruplets and Quintuplets

Stelios Fiorentzis, Styliani Salta, Michail Pargianas, Artemis Pontikaki, Dimitrios P. Koutsoulis, Christodoulos Akrivis, Dimitrios Akrivis and Ioannis Kosmas

Abstract

A high-order pregnancy is always a challenge not only for the couple but also for the obstetrician, the pediatricians, the midwives, and the whole stuff of an obstetric clinic. The breakthroughs of infertility treatments have made more couples to postpone the birth of their children until they feel professionally and financially safe, many times after the age of 40. The advanced age of the mother puts extra pressure to the clinician for immediate success, leading to a rise of high-order pregnancies until the introduction of regulations and laws in many countries. The cost of a quadruplet and quintuplet pregnancy can be unbearable, not only financially but also psychologically. The management of such a pregnancy is also challenging since its beginning and to the end. Modern techniques and methods can also be difficult to be implemented on a quadruplet of quintuplet pregnancy because of the fear of losing four or five embryos at once. At the same time, the limited number of cases makes it almost impossible for studies to be made and guidelines to be established for most of the cases.

Keywords: quadruplet, quintuplet, high-order, management

1. Introduction

"High-order pregnancy" is defined by the presence of three or more fetuses. Before the introduction and widespread of modern fertility methods, a high-order pregnancy was rare and unique. The first recording of quadruplets, the Smiths, was in 1750 [1]. In 2009, Samson described again the Gehri quadruplets, born in 1880, the first to have survived to adulthood.

In 1896, the Lyon quintuplets died within 15 days from birth while the Dionne quintuplets born in 1934 were the first to survive through infancy [2]. Nowadays, even with the galloping improvement in perinatal care, a high-order pregnancy still represents a challenge where outcome is not always favorable.

Dionys Hellin still since 1895 was trying to predict the occurrence of multiples in nature [3]. The "Hellin-Zeleny's rule" (after the publication of Zeleny's work in 1921 [4]) was a simple way to predict the occurrence of multiple births. Among others, Peller in 1946 [5] and Allen in 1960 [6] proposed new versions or improvements of this rule with various imitations [7, 8]. The incidence of multiple births has changed over time, presenting a decline until the late 1970s and an increase thereafter [9]. It is estimated that in the United States in 1980 there were 37 triplets or higher order births per 100,000 births, rising up to 1935 per 100,000 births in 1998 [10, 11]. Quadruplet and quintuplet or higher births raised from 229 and 40 in 1989 to 627 and 79, respectively, in 1998. Since 1999, a decline is observed, and in 2016, there were 1014 per 100,000 triplets or higher order births, 217 quadruplet and 31 quintuplet and other higher order births [12]. In France, the increase of triplets or high-order pregnancies reached 310% and in England and Wales 430% [13]. There is a difficulty to estimate accurately how many of these high-order pregnancies are a result of natural conception, estimates put this number around 20% [14].

Modern fertility treatments are the most important reason for the increase in multifetal pregnancies. Medical societies around the world have recognized the problem and have published guidelines in order to minimize the frequency of high-order pregnancies resulting from fertility treatment. The economic side of the matter is also of great importance. In 1996, there was a report concluding that the cost per woman who delivered singletons or twins was approximately $39,000, while the cost per woman who delivered triplets or quadruplets was up to $340,000 [15]. In 2006, the annual cost of each preterm neonate in the USA was estimated around $51,600 [16]. Since 90% of high-order pregnancies are born prematurely, considering that the average gestational age at delivery for quadruplets is 29.5 weeks and for quintuplets 29 weeks [17], it is easy to understand the impact of multifetal pregnancies to a tight health system budget. Aside the financial cost to the health system, a high-order pregnancy can wreck any family financial planning. The average costs per child is about $233,680 in the USA (for a child born in 2015, data published by the U.S. Department of Agriculture), without the college education. The birth of four, five, or more children can make the cost for the family unbearable.

Together with the progress in infertility treatment, a lot of progress is made in prenatal and neonatal care. Ultrasound has changed maternity care with the early diagnosis of fetal conditions. New techniques, such as fetal reduction, have made possible a favorable outcome from a pregnancy with normally poor outcome. Nevertheless, a high-order pregnancy still remains a challenge for both the clinician and the mother, not only during pregnancy but also after birth.

2. Pathophysiology of high-order pregnancy

A multiple gestation can either occur by a single fertilized ovum splitting (monozygotic), or by the fertilization of more than one ova at the same time (multizygotic), or even by the combination of the above. For monozygotic pregnancies, the timing of the fertilized ovum splitting dictates the pregnancy chorionicity. When the splitting occurs soon after the fertilization, it results in a diamniotic-dichorionic pregnancy. A diamniotic-monochorionic pregnancy occurs when the fertilized egg splits between the third and the eighth day after fertilization and a monoamniotic-monochorionic when the splitting occurs between the ninth and twelfth day. Conjoined twins are formed when the twinning process occurs after the formation of the yolk sac. A high-order pregnancy can harbor any of the above listed combinations [18]. Fetuses that result from the splitting of the same fertilized ovum are called monozygotic and the babies have the same genetic profile, physical characteristics, and sex, while fetuses that result from the fertilization of more eggs have different genetic background and can be of different sex.

A multiple pregnancy can occur as a consequence of a single ovum fertilization. Liu in 2010 [19] reported a case of a monozygotic quadruplet pregnancy as a result of IVF, although the pregnancy ended in the ninth week of gestation due to chromosomal abnormalities. Nnadi in 2013 [20] described a case of monozygotic quadruplet pregnancy conceived naturally that ended in an elective cesarean section of a set of monochorionic tetra-amniotic quadruplets at 37 weeks of gestation. Neubecker in 1962 [21] and Rau in 1940 [22] reported two cases of monozygotic quintuplet pregnancies, indicating the possibility of a quadruplet and quintuplet pregnancy arising from a single ovum.

The term superfecundation is used to denote the fertilization of a second or more ova within hours or days after a first fertilization, which can result in a multiple pregnancy. The two fertilizations can be either due to differed sexual intercourses or as a consequence to sexual intercourse in a context of in vitro fertilization and embryo transfer. Peigné in 2011 [23] reported a case of a multiple pregnancy as a result of intercourse 1 day after the oocyte pick-up, while Milki in 2001 [24] reported a case of multifetal pregnancy occurring after sexual intercourse 5 days prior to oocyte retrieval. Superfecundation raises the issue of paternity among separately fertilized ova. Wenk et al. in 1992 [25] reviewed a parentage test database of 39,000 records of parents involved in paternity suits and reported the percentage of heteropaternal superfecundation among dizygotic twins to be as high as 2.4%. In contrast to superfecundation, the term superfetation is used to describe a multiple pregnancy resulting after ovulation, and fertilization occurs during an established pregnancy. Superfetation has not yet been proven possible in humans, although it exists in animals [26].

3. Predisposing factors for a high-order pregnancy

There have been described several factors related to increased incidence of multiple pregnancy, in particular twin pregnancy. Factors predisposing to a multiple pregnancy differ between monozygotic and multizygotic pregnancies in nature. The difficulty to determine any predisposing factors for quadruplet and higher order pregnancies lies in the limited series of patients and the lack of available data. Therefore, many factors associated with twin pregnancies are also considered to have a possible influence on the incidence of high-order pregnancies.

Before the introduction of modern infertility treatments, the prevalence of monozygotic twinning was relatively constant among different origins, oscillating between 3 and 5 per 1000 live births [27]. On the other hand, the prevalence of dizygotic twinning differs concerning race, maternal age, and family history of twinning. Black women have the highest rate of dizygotic twins followed by Asian women and finally white women. Moreover, women with a family history for dizygotic twinning, such as a previous dizygotic pregnancy or being part of or related to a set of dizygotic twins, have greater probability to conceive dizygotic twins compared to women with no family history [14].

Since the early 1970s, maternal age was considered an important factor that could influence the conception of a multiple pregnancy, with a reported fourfold increase of dizygotic twinning rate between the ages of 15 and 37 [28]. Maternal age does not seem to affect monozygotic multiple pregnancy rates, as shown in multiple studies [29]. Women between the ages of 35 and 41 are more likely to have a multiple gestation. The increment in multifetal pregnancies is probably related to higher basal FSH levels for women over the age of 35 compared to younger women. Higher levels of FSH can be associated with the maturation of multiple follicles in natural cycles and consequently the occurrence of a multiple pregnancy [30].

There is evidence that a woman's somatometric parameters are associated with a multiple pregnancy. Women with a BMI over 30 are more likely to conceive more than one babies compared to women with normal BMI [31–34]. Noteworthy, a higher BMI increases the probability of multizygotic pregnancies but not monozygotic ones. Women's height has been associated with multiple pregnancies, even though its impact is less important than weight [34]. Women who are taller than 173 cm seem to have higher probability for dizygotic twinning compared to women shorter than 165 cm [31, 33].

Some lifestyle choices have also been proposed as predisposing factors for multiple pregnancy. Multivitamins and folic acid supplementation have been associated with an increased incidence of multiple gestation, even though the results were not statistically significant [35]. In order to confirm that the use of folic acid increases the rates of multiple pregnancies (up to 40%), more trials have to be performed [36]. Coffee consumption, smoking, and alcohol have also been evaluated for their possible positive correlation with multiple pregnancy without fertility treatments [37]. This observation is surprising, since smoking and alcohol are known to have negative effects on the fetus and the pregnancy outcome. Kapidaki in 1995 [38] showed that for each cup of coffee per day there was an increase in the odds for multifetal pregnancy. Parazzini in 1996 [37], on the other hand, found no relation between multiple pregnancy and the extent of coffee drinking. In the same study, however, they found that women who were drinking ≥15 alcohol units per week and those who were smoking ≥10 cigarettes per day were more likely to conceive a multifetal pregnancy. In any case, more studies are necessary in order to have results that are more reliable.

The use of contraceptive pill and the time after its discontinuation are associated with multiple pregnancy. The theory behind this affirmation is an increase in the secretion of gonadotropins shortly after the cessation of the pill that could result in multiple pregnancies. Many studies, since the 1970s [39–42], have denoted an increase in twin pregnancies after the cessation of oral contraceptive pills. A study by Campbell in 1987 [43], however, found no statistical significance between the cessation of oral contraceptives and the incidence of monozygotic or dizygotic twinning. In the same study, no significance was found between the time after cessation of contraceptives and the occurrence of twin pregnancy. As far as high-order pregnancies are concerned, there are no available data due to the limited number of cases.

Wen et al. in a study in 2004 [44] observed that women with high-order pregnancies were tended to be white (78.8% for twins, 89.4% for triplets, and 94.8% for quadruplets and more) and older (67.6% of mothers of triplets, 64.6% of quadruplets, and 46.3% of twins were older than 30 years). Moreover, they were more likely to be married (72% for twins, 90.6% for triplets, and 97.4% for quadruplets and more) and of higher education. Mothers of triplets, quadruplets, and more were less likely to have smoked during pregnancy and more likely to have received prenatal care earlier (93.6 and 94.6% for triplets and quadruplets in first trimester compared to the 85.4% for twin pregnancies). Finally, they were more likely to be women undergoing their first pregnancy (34.1% for twins, 51.2% for triplets, and 52.7% for quadruplets and higher). In a study by Luke and Brown in 2008 [45], which included the U.S. births from 1995 to 2000, the same demographic characteristics are evident among mothers of quadruplets, white, older women of higher education and at lower parity, married, and non-smokers.

Nowadays, the most important predisposing factor for multiple pregnancy is modern fertility techniques. Induction of ovulation, the transfer of more than one embryos, IVF, ICSI, assisted hatching, or even the culture media have all been associated with increased incidence of a multiple gestation [14]. Some of the above have been strongly associated with multiple pregnancy, and regulations have been established in many countries either by law or official guidelines in order to reduce the incidence and any eventual complications of a multiple pregnancy (for instance, there is a limitation of the number of embryos allowed to be transferred). Many studies exist in literature, including case reports, for quadruplet/quintuplet pregnancies after single/double blastocyst transfer. Quadruplet pregnancies have been reported after the transfer of only one [46] or two embryos [47–49], with variable chorionicity. There are also case reports of quintuplets originated from one fertilized egg (the Dionne quintuplets) and two [50, 51] or three blastocysts [52].

4. Diagnosis of a multifetal pregnancy

Early diagnosis of a multiple pregnancy is crucial for achieving the best outcome and for preventing as many complications as possible, either maternal or fetal [53]. The preferred method to diagnose a multifetal gestation is by ultrasonography. This method is accurate enough to reveal a multiple pregnancy by the fourth week of gestation, although the number of yolk or gestational sacs can be misleading as early in pregnancy [54].

The term "vanishing fetus" or "natural fetal reduction" is used to describe the loss, through miscarriage, of one or more fetuses during a multiple gestation. This phenomenon can be observed up to the 16th week of pregnancy, and it can be either asymptomatic or it can present with bleeding, pain, or abdominal cramps. Before the introduction of ultrasound, a vanishing fetus could only be diagnosed after delivery [55]. Dickey et al. estimated that the prevalence of a vanishing fetus before the 12th week of a quadruplet pregnancy could be as high as 65% with great variability among different researchers [56]. They also showed that the probability of a spontaneous absorption in a multiple pregnancy was directly related to the initial number of gestational sacs and to maternal age ($p < 0.001$ and $p < 0.01$, respectively). In the same study, they concluded that the average duration of reduced twin pregnancies with initially four sacs was 11 days shorter when compared to the duration of unreduced twin pregnancies (254 days–243 days, $p < 0.001$). In addition, the birth weight of naturally reduced twins was lower compared to the weight of unreduced twins (2024 ± 668 g compared to 2453 ± 575 gr, $p < 0.003$).

Ultrasonography plays an important role in the diagnosis of chorionicity and placentation of a pregnancy. Determining chorionicity is crucial, since twin and triplet pregnancies with at least one monochorionic pair have greater perinatal morbidity and mortality [57, 58]. Perinatal mortality in quadruplets tends to be five times higher when a monochorionic set is present compared to quadra-chorionic [57]. Adeghite et al. in 2007 [59] compared the differences in neonatal complications between quadra-chorionic quadramniotic and trichorionic newborns. There was statistically significant higher incidence for almost all complications considered within the trichorionic group. This group also had statistically significant higher rates in neonatal death when compared to the quadra-chorionic group. Furthermore, trichorionic infants were born much earlier and weighed less compared to the quadra-chorionic ones: 28 vs. 32 weeks and 69% <1000 g vs. 13% <1000 g ($p < 0.001$), respectively. There was no difference between the groups in regard to the mode of delivery. Some data suggest that the use of modern infertility treatment methods is associated with monozygotic twinning, although the data for some of these methods are conflicting [60]. Since 75% of monozygotic twins are also monochorionic [61], women who have undergone such treatments and have a multifetal gestation must be suspected for monochorionicity. Chow et al. in 2001 in a study of 464 multiple gestations showed that in multiple gestations arising from artificial reproduction treatments, there is a correlation between the number of fetuses and the rates of monochorionic pairs [62]. Monochorionic pairs were present in only 2.1% of twin pregnancies, while in quadruplet and quintuplet pregnancies the rates were as high as 25% ($p < 0.05$). Chow et al. finally confirmed the observation made in earlier studies that a monochorionic pair is more likely to be found in a naturally conceived gestation.

Early ultrasound evaluation can identify placentation correctly in over 90% of multiple gestations, and in case this is not possible, the gestation should be treated as monochorionic [17]. The data regarding the incidence of placenta previa in a multiple gestation are conflicting. Some of them suggest that placenta previa is up to 40% more common in twin pregnancies [63], probably due to limited space in the endometrial cavity [64], whereas others argue that the incidence of placenta previa is not correlated with the number of embryos [65].

5. Complications and management of quadruplet/quintuplet pregnancies

Women with quadruplets and higher-order pregnancies are at increased risk for obstetric complications compared to women with twin pregnancies. Moreover, a dose-response relationship can be found for certain complications of the pregnancy. Wen et al. [44] in 2004 compared the outcomes in women with twins, triplets, quadruplets, and high-order pregnancies from 1995 to 1997. They concluded that women with triplets and more were in greater risk for pregnancy associated hypertension, eclampsia, anemia, diabetes mellitus, placental abruption, premature rupture of the membranes, and cesarean delivery, even after the adjustment for important confounding factors. Wen also compared the maternal health outcomes. Women with triplets, quadruplets, and higher order are predisposed to develop pregnancy-associated hypertension and diabetes mellitus (7.68% for twins, 10.32% for triplets, and 11.57% for quadruplets and higher order for hypertension, while for diabetes mellitus the rates were 3.34% for twins, 5.97% for triplets, and 6.75% for quadruplets and higher order). Twins were less frequently delivered by cesarean section (51.21% compared to 86.78 and 84.87% for triplets and quadruplets or higher, respectively) and had less chances for a premature rupture of the membranes (6.66% for twins, 11.17% for triplets, and 10.65 for quadruplets and more). The rise in rates for cesarean delivery as the number of fetuses increases could also explain the low rates of induction of labor and use of forceps and vacuum among triplets and quadruplets compared to twin pregnancies. The study by Luke and Brown in 2008 [45] also came to the same results that quadruplet pregnancies have greater chances for pregnancy-associated complications when compared to twin pregnancies. In the study by Luke and Brown, the p-value was <0.0001 for diabetes mellitus, incompetent cervix, induction of labor, stimulation of labor, tocolysis, cesarean delivery, premature rupture of the membranes, infant death of ≥ 1 baby, birth at ≤ 29 weeks of pregnancy, and <0.05 for pregnancy-associated hypertension and eclampsia.

Multiple pregnancies present increased spontaneous loss rates, and these rates increase in parallel with the increase of the number of the fetuses. The authors estimate that a quadruplet pregnancy has a 25% chance for a spontaneous loss, while a quintuplet has three times more, up to 75%. This rise is more obvious when these rates are compared with the ones for a twin and a triplet pregnancy (8 and 15 respectively) [66].

Preterm labor has been proven the most common maternal complication in high-order pregnancies [67], and it is directly associated with the increased perinatal morbidity and mortality observed in these pregnancies, while the rates of pregnancy complications seem to be raised alongside the increase of the number of fetuses [14]. More than 90% of high-order pregnancies are born prematurely, with the approximate gestational age at delivery for quadruplets to be estimated around 29.5 weeks, while for quintuplets this point is up to 29 weeks of gestation [17]. In USA, in 2016, the 93% of quadruplets (217 cases) and the 100% of quintuplets and higher order pregnancies (31 cases) have been born before the 34th week of gestation [12].

In order to prolong the pregnancy, several methods have been used. Bed rest, either hospitalization or home rest, is a method still widely used. Although some researchers considered bed rest the most important mode of treatment and it was used to be advised to all patients [53], Crowther in 2001 [68] for a Cochrane review synthesized seven controlled trials including twin and triplet gestations. Bed rest has been proven ineffective to reduce preterm labor, while on the same time it was psychologically distressing.

Another method widely used for reduction of preterm labor in high-order pregnancies was prophylactic cervical cerclage. In the 1970s, it was suggested that prophylactic cervical cerclage could be beneficial in the prevention of preterm labor for multiple pregnancies [69]. More than 40 years after that, prophylactic placement of cervical cerclage—transabdominal or transvaginal—is considered of undetermined value [70] or of no significance regardless of the indication [71]. Straus in 2002 compared a group of quadruplet and quintuplet pregnancies with cerclage and one without and found that the birth weight was higher in the cerclage group ($p < 0.001$). Despite the higher birth weight in the cerclage group, it was also evident that the perinatal morbidity and mortality were higher (69 vs. 32% for the non-cerclage group for morbidity and 10.26 vs. 5.55% for mortality), although the results due to the small number of cases were of no statistical significance. Strauss concluded that in order to see if prophylactic placement of cervical cerclage has anything to offer to multiple pregnancies, randomized controlled studies have to be made, something difficult due to the limited number of multiple pregnancies.

Tocolysis is also another method for the prevention or delay of preterm labor. Several researchers and clinicians used several different medicines, as prophylactic treatment. Prophylactic tocolysis is not recommended since the data show no effect on risk reduction for preterm birth and further studies are needed [72]. Prolonged use of these medicines is also not recommended since tocolysis does not seem to have a significant result to extend the pregnancy for more than 7 days [73].

Cervical pessary is another widely used strategy to prevent preterm labor. Research has been made for singleton and twin pregnancies, with conflicting results [74]. For multiple pregnancies, Liem et al. [75] in a randomized controlled trial, cervical pessaries were not effective in preventing preterm birth, but showed some success for cases with a cervical length of less than the 25th percentile, but further research is needed with more patients. The researchers also noted the low cost of a pessary and the fact that it was well tolerated by the women in the trial, making it a choice to consider in developing countries.

Another strategy used to prolong a multiple pregnancy is the use of progesterone, with vaginal distribution to be preferred than the intramuscular one in terms of fewer maternal side effects [76]. Although for singleton pregnancies, progesterone is considered an effective choice, for multiple pregnancies there is insufficient evidence for the recommendation of its use, with or without a short cervical length, despite the use of 17-alpha-hydroxy-progesteronecaproate by some experts in women with multiple pregnancy and prior spontaneous preterm birth [77].

It is estimated that about 25–30% of preterm labor is the result of preterm premature rupture of the membranes [78]. Luke and Brown in 2008 [65] published a study in which they compared risk rates for maternal and neonatal complications among high-order pregnancies. According to their results, quadruplet pregnancies are more likely to be diagnosed with preterm premature rupture of the membranes (10.64% compared to 9.61% for triplets and 6.17% for twin pregnancies, $p < 0.001$). In another retrospective cohort study of more than 290,000 live births, premature rupture of the membranes complicated 19.6% for quadruplet and 100% for higher order (>4) pregnancies compared to 19.3% for triplets, 11.2% for twins, and 3.1% for singletons [79]. In the same study, the proportion of preterm birth attributable to premature rupture of the membranes for extremely preterm gestational ages (before 28 weeks of pregnancy) was 50% for quadruplets and 100% for higher order pregnancies compared to 26.9, 34.6, and 26.5% for triplets, twins, and singletons, respectively ($p < 0.001$). On the other hand, premature rupture of the membranes for late preterm gestational ages (34–37 weeks of gestation) contributed to 10% of quadruplets, 12.2% of triplets, 11% of twins, 10.2% of singletons, while no high-order pregnancies could reach that gestational age ($p < 0.001$). Finally, for quadruplets and high-order pregnancies, Caucasian race was a common aggravating factor, and premature rupture of the membranes in multifetal gestations increased with gestational plurality and occurred at earlier gestational age.

Hypertensive disorders of pregnancy are more common among multiple pregnancies, in particular quadruplet pregnancies have a reported incidence of pregnancy-associated hypertension up to 40% with earlier and more severe onset [80]. Day in 2005 [81] showed that the rate of mild and severe preeclampsia is similar for triplets and quadruplets, with the exclusion of women who delivered before 28 weeks. The rates for development of any pregnancy-associated hypertensive disorder were 19.6% for quadruplets, 20% for triplet pregnancies, 12.7% for twins, and 6.5% for singleton pregnancies. The same study showed that the rates for severe pregnancy-associated hypertensive disorders were 1.1, 3.1, 1.6, and 0.5% for quadruplet, triplet, twin, and singleton pregnancies, respectively. When comparing quadruplet with singleton pregnancies, quadruplets were strongly associated with severe pregnancy hypertension disorders ($p < 0.01$). The studies by Wen in 2004 [64] and Luke and Brown in 2008 [65] also showed that women with quadruplets are more likely to develop pregnancy-associated hypertension compared to twins. Since placenta plays an important role in preeclampsia [82], the increased mass of the placenta in multifetal pregnancies is probably associated with the occurrence of preeclampsia. Preeclampsia is often atypical, with hypertension not always present, but with abnormal laboratory values. Hardardottir in 1996 [83] reported that in a series of three cases delivered for preeclampsia among eight quadruplet pregnancies, only one developed hypertension, none proteinuria, one had edema, and two had elevated uric acid >5 mg/dl. In the same study, the mean age for women with quadruplets and preeclampsia was 34 years and without preeclampsia was 28.6 years, with no statistical significance. Despite the progress in understanding the pathogenesis of preeclampsia, little progress has been made in terms of treatment [84].

Molar pregnancy coexisting with live fetuses is a rare condition, with cases resulting to the delivery of a live fetus to be even scarcer. There are reports of quadruplet pregnancies with coexisting mole with different management and outcomes. The outcome does not usually include viable fetuses [85]. No guidelines for the management of a multiple pregnancy coexisting with a complete hydatidiform mole and live fetuses occur. Therapeutic abortion is always an option to consider, since the chances for delivering a live fetus are very low and the maternal risks are very high [86]. Tariq in 2014 [87] published a case report of a molar pregnancy diagnosed at 22 weeks where continuation of the pregnancy with close surveillance was decided. The mother was under close monitoring and went into preterm labor at 33 weeks. Three viable fetuses were delivered.

Gestational diabetes can be expected to be more common among women with multifetal pregnancy. It has been shown that women with twins have higher rate of gestational diabetes than women with singleton pregnancies [88] and women with triplets tend to have higher rates than twins [89]. Wen in 2004 [64] showed a direct relationship between the number of fetuses and the rates of gestational diabetes. Luke and Brown [65] in 2008 confirmed these results by comparing twin and quadruplet pregnancies (p-value < 0.0001). The rarity of quadruplet and quintuplet pregnancies makes further research necessary in order to confirm that the rise in gestational diabetes rates continues among quadruplet and quintuplet pregnancies.

Women carrying multiples are at increased risk for urinary tract infection, with the rates for multiple pregnancies to be up to 4.6% compared to 3.7% for singleton pregnancies [90], possibly because of the larger size of the uterus or the levels of progesterone in the maternal circulation.

Nutrition and weight gain are of great importance in a multifetal pregnancy. Unfortunately, there are no recommendations available for quadruplet and quintuplet pregnancies. What is expected, is that weight gain might be faster than with triplets and twins, and although there are recommendations for singletons, twins and triplets, that has not yet been possible for higher-order pregnancies [91]. Multivitamin supplements such as folic acid, calcium, and vitamins are recommended, due to the high nutrient needs of the mother and the fetuses. Anemia and iron deficiency are the most common pregnancy-related complications [92, 93] and are associated with a series of maternal and neonatal complications, such as preterm delivery [94], low birth weight [95], birth asphyxia [92], and iron deficiency in high-risk infants [96]. Anemia and iron deficiency are more prevalent among women with a multifetal pregnancy compared to women carrying singletons, so nutriments and supplements containing iron are highly recommended [93]. Vitamin D and calcium through supplements, essential fatty acids through fresh or canned oil-rich fish, and additional energy and macronutrients are advised but there no studies estimating the exact daily requirements [91].

The positive effect of corticosteroid administration in singleton pregnancies is well established. In multifetal gestations however, the datas are still limited. There have been reports suggesting that betamethasone administration in quadruplet births is associated with increased uterine contractions, preterm labor with cervical change, and preterm labor requiring tocolysis [97]. Despite that, a single course of corticosteroids is recommended for all multifetal pregnant women at risk of preterm delivery between 24 and 0/7 weeks and 33 and 6/7 weeks of gestation. In addition, a single repeat dose should be administered to women less than 34 weeks of gestation, at risk of preterm delivery within 7 days, and whose prior dose of corticosteroids was administered more than 14 days before [98].

Quadruplets and quintuplets have higher neonatal and perinatal mortality compared to triplets. Skrablin et al. in 2000 [99] published a study of 51 quadruplet and quintuplet pregnancies compared to 156 triplet pregnancies. They found no significant difference when compared the two groups for stillborns and neonatal mortality ≥28 weeks. On the other hand, they observed a statistically significant difference when they compared neonatal deaths (p = 0.02), the "Discharged Alive" (76.3% for triplets, 54.9% for quadruplets and quintuplets, p = 0.003), early neonatal mortality for ≥1000 g (p = 0.04), and perinatal mortality for >24 and ≥28 weeks of pregnancy (both p = 0.005). Mortality and morbidity seem to be related with preterm delivery, and high-order infants have comparable rates compared to singletons and twins of the same gestational age [70, 100]. In a retrospective study by Hernandez in 2009 [101], 26% of multiple pregnancies had at least one death (including triplets). In particular, 54% of quadruplet and 100% of quintuplet pregnancies had at least one death, while the average weight at birth was 750 g for dead quadruplets and 1341 g for surviving quadruplets ($p < 0.0007$). Chibber in 2003 [102] in a study including 100 triplet, 27 quadruplets, and 10 quintuplet pregnancies showed that low birth weight is crucial for perinatal mortality and morbidity, with low birth weight complicating most of the 34 neonatal deaths in the quadruplet and quintuplet groups. Multiples are at increased risk of growth problems compared to singletons, with the degree of intrauterine growth restriction to increase as the number of fetuses increase. In the USA, in 2016, 77.1% of quadruplets were below 1500 g and 96.2% below 2500 g. When considering quintuplets and more, these rates rise up to 80.7 and 100%, respectively. The limited space in uterus and the limited nutrient supply might be responsible for low birth weight [103]. Unfortunately, there are no specific data for quadruplets and quintuplets.

A low Apgar score at birth is a common concern for neonatologists when a high-order pregnancy ends. Chibber in 2003 [102] highlighted the differences between triplet and higher pregnancies when the Apgar scores of the first and fifth minute were compared. The mean first-minute Apgar score for triplets was 7.8, while for quadruplets and quintuplets was only 6.2 ($p < 0.01$). When compared the five-minute Apgar score, this was 8.8 for triplets and 7.2 for quadruplets and quintuplets ($p < 0.05$). Skrablin et al. in 2000 [99] also observed statistical significances in their study, with the mean first-minute Apgar score for triplets to be 6.4 and for quadruplets-quintuplets 4.9 ($p = 0.003$) and the five-minute Apgar score to be 7.6 for triplets and 6 for quadruplets and quintuplets ($p = 0.01$).

There are also some rare complications which have been reported in high-order pregnancies, but due to the limited number of cases, no guidelines are available. Fetofetal transfusion has been reported in quadruplet pregnancies [104–106] as well as quadruplet pregnancies with conjoined twins [107, 108]. Another complication that has been described in a quadruplet pregnancy was the rupture of an unscarred uterus, raising the debate of the ideal delivery time for a high-order pregnancy [109]. High-order pregnancies have significant higher rates of peripartum hysterectomy compared to singleton pregnancies [110], although the data from quadruplet and quintuplet pregnancies are limited.

6. Multifetal pregnancy reduction

High-order pregnancies hold a significant risk of miscarriage as well as neonatal and maternal morbidity and mortality. Fetal reduction, since its introduction in 1988 by Evans and his associates [111], has shown encouraging results in regard to the outcome of a multiple pregnancy [66]. Antsaklis et al. in 2004 [112] in a series of 313 multiple pregnancies showed that fetal reduction can reduce the risk of pregnancy loss and severe prematurity in quadruplets and higher order pregnancies and result, in most cases, in at least one live neonate. In particular, he compared the two largest groups, that is triplets and quadruplets reduced to twins, as for miscarriage (8.25 vs. 8.96%), preterm delivery defined as <33 weeks (11.18 vs. 19.67%), and total fetal loss rate (15.41 vs. 14.93%). Altogether, the reduction of a high-order pregnancy with more than four fetuses to twins holds the best outcome. When the median gestational age at delivery was compared, this was higher for >4 fetuses reduced to twins rather than triplets (36 vs. 31 weeks respectively) and for quadruplets reduced to singletons rather than twins (38 vs. 36 weeks respectively). Evans in 2014 [66] showed a 25% decrement of fetal loss when quadruplet pregnancies were reduced to either twins or singletons. In the same line, when quintuplets were reduced to twins, the risk of fetal loss was decreased by 50%.

Fetal reduction can be done either transabdominally or transvaginally. When the transabdominal approach is used, the proposed time frame is between the 10th and 16th week of gestation, although the optimal timing is often arbitrary (Davis in 2014 [113] cited four different time frames suggested by four different researchers). Fetal reduction using the transvaginal approach can be performed earlier in the pregnancy when the placenta and the embryo are smaller. There is some skepticism concerning the transvaginal approach and the possibility of introducing vaginal bacteria [114]. Therefore, each center follows the practice they are more experienced in, since it has been shown to affect significantly pregnancy outcomes in terms of fetal loss and prematurity. Evans et al. in 2001 [115] studied the evolution of pregnancy outcomes across time: before 1991, from 1991 to 1994, and after 1994. Loss rates decreased from 13.2 to 9.7 to 6.4%, respectively. More specifically, loss rates for quadruplets reduced to twins were 13% before 1994 and only 6.6% thereafter, although it is difficult to identify whether experience, better ultrasonography techniques, or both played the most important role.

Fetal reduction is usually done by directly injecting KCL as a cardiotoxic agent, although aspiration of the embryonic parts has also been used [116]. Another reduction method used is thermocoagulation [117], either bipolar cord coagulation or radiofrequency ablation with similar results [118, 119]. Ligation of the cord as well as suture and compression of the cord on the uterine wall have also been used for fetal reduction [120].

First trimester reduction is a relatively simple and safe procedure with good results [121]. Nevertheless, many authors propose to perform fetal reduction in the second trimester after prenatal screening and possible detection of fetal abnormalities. Geva et al. in 2000 [122] published a series of 38 multifetal reduction procedures in the second trimester compared to 70 fetal reduction procedures in the first trimester. He included four quadruplet gestations in the first group and 18 in the second. The mean gestational age for quadruplets reduced to twins in the second trimester was higher compared to quadruplets reduced to twins in the first trimester (36.7 ± 1.2 vs. 33.6 ± 3.9 weeks respectively, $p = 0.01$). Accordingly, the mean birth weight of quadruplets reduced to twins in the second trimester was higher compared to the mean birth weight of quadruplets reduced to twins in the first trimester (2111 ± 3089 g vs. 1762 ± 503 g respectively) (statistically significant). When all pregnancy complications were compared, no statistically significant difference was found between the two groups, except for premature labor ($p = 0.046$). The authors concluded that when the second trimester is chosen for reduction, detection of fetal abnormalities and selection of an affected fetus can improve the outcome to similar results as for a first trimester reduction. This observation motivated several authors to propose the 15th–16th week of pregnancy as the optimal moment for fetal reduction [113].

Fetal reduction has shown to be a valuable option for high-order pregnancies (≥4) [123, 124]. Antsaklis et al. in 1999 [125] compared the outcomes of reduced twins (from quadruplets and triplets) to unreduced twins. There was no difference in regard to perinatal or obstetric complications. When he compared the outcomes of reduced twins between the 10th and 11th week of gestation from triplet or quadruplet pregnancies, there were still no significant differences between the two groups. Wang in 2007 [126] studied 37 multifetal pregnancies reduced between the 12th + 1 and 25th week of gestation. He concluded that the incidence of preeclampsia is decreased after reduction. Boulot in 1993 [124], from a series of 61 multifetal pregnancies, concluded that the rate of miscarriage is lower when the aim of the reduction is twins rather than singletons. However, he found that the miscarriage rate was significantly lower when one fetus was reduced compared to 2 fetuses (6 vs. 24% respectively, $p < 0.05$). In another study by Timor-Tritsch in 2004 [127], the total pregnancy loss (at less than 24 weeks) for reduced quadruplets was at 1.8% (2.4% for the transabdominal route and 0% for the transvaginal route, $p = 0.56$). In the same study, the total pregnancy loss (at less than 24 weeks) for reduced quintuplets was at 14.3% (15.4% for the transabdominal route and 12.5% for the transvaginal route, $p = 0.65$). Multiple studies have concluded that the birth weight, gestational age at delivery, and perinatal mortality rate were directly correlated with the final number of fetuses [112, 128, 129]. Reductions of more than one fetus can be done in one session; however, when 5 or more fetuses need to be reduced to a singleton, two sessions seem to have better results than one, with 1 week interval between the sessions [66].

Another point to consider when counseling a couple about fetal reduction is the possibility of one of the remaining fetuses to develop intrauterine growth restriction. There is evidence that fetal reduction is not associated with an increased risk of intrauterine growth restriction, unless it is performed on a high-order pregnancy [130]. Depp et al. in 1996 [131] have shown that when quadruplet and higher order pregnancies were reduced to twins the incidence of one or more IUGR among fetuses was greater compared to non-reduced twins. The frequency of discordance was directly linked to the pre-reduction fetal number. The frequency in the non-reduced twin cohort was at 16.3%, and the rate of discordance for quadruplets reduced to twins was at 26.1%,while for higher order reductions reduced to twins was at 34.2%.

When discussing with a couple about the risks of multifetal pregnancy and the option for fetal reduction, the psychological strain needs to be addressed and properly managed. The first reaction of a couple when a multiple pregnancy is diagnosed is generally favorable, although parents need to be counseled about the risks of a multifetal pregnancy. A proposed fetal reduction can cause anxiety to the couple, but eventually the majority of patients accept to abort some fetuses in order to preserve the lives of the others [132]. Specifically, when quadruplets or more fetuses are involved, couples are more inclined to go through a reduction procedure [133], and in some cases, they consider reduction as mandatory [121], although ethical issues may always be a concern.

7. Delivery of a quadruplet or quintuplet pregnancy

The delivery of high-order pregnancies is challenging for the mother, the obstetricians, and pediatricians. Malpresentations are common, while the babies often require intensive care and special treatment, considering that more than 90% of high-order pregnancies are born prematurely. Average gestational age at delivery is estimated around 29.5 weeks for quadruplets and 29 weeks for quintuplets [17], although term delivery has also been reported, mostly as case reports [20, 134, 135]. The rates of preterm birth in the USA at <37 weeks of gestation are estimated at 96.77% for quadruplets and 100% for quintuplets and more. When it comes at <34 weeks, the estimated rates are at 93.09% for quadruplets and 100% for quintuplets [12].

Cord prolapse, hemorrhage, and abruption of the placenta are undesirable possible complications for any vaginal delivery, but in a high-order pregnancy where the mother and the fetuses are more vulnerable are even more undesirable. While there are many reviews about the mode of delivery for twin and triplet gestations, this is not possible for quadruplet and quintuplet pregnancies. For quadruplet pregnancies, vaginal delivery has been reported [136]. Cesarean section is preferred if the obstetrician is not confident enough with vaginal delivery maneuvers [137], while on the same time when an elective cesarean is selected, it allows the optimal preparation and logistic conditions [138]. The time of the elective delivery is also to be considered, with Elliot reporting choosing the 34 + 0 weeks for quadruplets [17]. Finally, further research is needed in order to safely determine whether cesarean or vaginal delivery can affect the Apgar score of the newborns [139].

The most challenging cases of quadruplet and quintuplet pregnancies are the cases where preterm labor of at least one fetus has occurred and delayed interval delivery is considered an option in order to improve the chances of survival for the remaining fetuses. Such cases with at least one newborn surviving have been published, both for quadruplet [140, 141] and for quintuplet pregnancies [142]. For twin and triplet gestations, some authors consider delayed internal delivery a viable option [143, 144], while for quadruplet and quintuplet pregnancies, there are still not enough data.

8. Conclusion

In cases of a quadruplet, quintuplet, or any high-order pregnancy, early diagnosis is crucial for the further management and treatment. The international literature concerning pregnancies with more than three fetuses is still limited, and it is not going to be any better in the future. The prevalence of high-order pregnancies after the rise until 1996 is tending to normalize, making—again—unique and rare such cases. The lack of cases and the diversity of these cases make it difficult to manage the complications, which will probably arise during a high-order pregnancy. New treatments used for singleton or twin pregnancy complications cannot always be considered as options for treating a high-order pregnancy, especially when no data are available. Beside the scientific interest for these cases and the challenge they pose to anyone dealing with them, it is always important to remember that the couple suffers the greater burden. The psychology of the couple should never be underestimated. Even by the beginning of the pregnancy, the possibility of a result not favorable is always in mind, so additional support is necessary. Fetal reduction is a method that improves the outcome of these pregnancies and could be offered as an option when there is experience with the procedure and no other limitations are present (e.g. religious).

Author details

Stelios Fiorentzis[1], Styliani Salta[2,3], Michail Pargianas[4], Artemis Pontikaki[5], Dimitrios P. Koutsoulis[6], Christodoulos Akrivis[7], Dimitrios Akrivis[7] and Ioannis Kosmas[7*]

*Address all correspondence to: kosmasioannis@gmail.com

1 Agios Nikolaos Crete, Greece

2 Cancer Biology and Therapeutics, Centre de Recherche Saint-Antoine, Institut National de la Santé et de la Recherche Médicale (INSERM) U938 and Institut Universitaire de Cancérologie, Faculté de Médecine, Sorbonne Université, Paris, France

3 Service d'Hématologie Biologique Hôpital Tenon, Hôpitaux Universitaires Est Parisien, Assistance Publique Hôpitaux de Paris (AP-HP), Paris, France

4 Medical School, University of Ioannina, Obstetrics and Gynecology, Ioannina, Greece

5 Department of Obstetrics and Gynecology, University Hospital of Heraklion, Greece

6 General Panarcadian of Tripolis, Greece

7 Department of Obstetrics and Gynecology, Ioannina State General Hospital G. Chatzikosta, Ioannina, Greece

References

[1] Aldwell A. Jane Smith, a fisherman's wife in Kinsale, had four boys at a birth. Cork Post Office General Directory. 1884-5. F. Jackson. p. 156. Available from: http://www.corkpastandpresent.ie/places/streetandtradedirectories/1844-5aldwellscountycitypo-generaldirectory/1844-5pages132to191/GeneralDirectory1844Pages156%20to%20161.pdf

[2] Wright C. They Were Five: The dionne quintuplets revisited. Journal of Canadian Studies. 1995;**29**(4):5-14. DOI: 10.3138/jcs.29.4.5

[3] Hellin D. Die Ursache der Multiparität der Uniparen Tiere überhaupt und Zwillingsschwangerschaft beim Menschen insbesondere. Edinburgh Medical Journal. 1895; **41**:241

[4] Zeleny C. The relative numbers of twins and triplets. Science. 1921;**53**(1368):262-263. Available from: http://science.sciencemag.org/content/53/1368/262.abstract

[5] Peller S. A new rule for predicting the occurrence of multiple births. American Journal of Physical Anthropology. 2005;**4**(1):99-106. DOI: 10.1002/ajpa.1330040110

[6] Allen G. A differential method for estimation of type frequencies in triplets and quadruplets. American Journal of Human Genetics. 1960;**12**:210-224. Available from: http://www.ncbi.nlm.nih.gov/pubmed/13792733

[7] Fellman J, Eriksson AW. Statistical analyses of Hellin's Law. Twin Research and Human Genetics. 2009;**12**(2):191-200. Available from: https://www.cambridge.org/core/article/statistical-analyses-of-hellins-law/A6CF905FE383DEB83FC7D2A39CA4D317

[8] Fellman J, Eriksson AW. On the history of Hellin's Law. Twin Research and Human Genetics. 2009;**12**(2):183-190. Available from: https://www.cambridge.org/core/article/on-the-history-of-hellins-law/DBD48A06374EFA1F33894ADD09A1C0FF

[9] Pison G, D'Addato AV. Frequency of twin births in developed countries. Twin Research and Human Genetics. 2006;**9**(2):250-259. Available from: https://www.cambridge.org/core/article/frequency-of-twin-births-in-developed-countries/26A0B60A621D3BE5B7AEB664010D822E

[10] Martin JA, Park MM. Trends in twin and triplet births: 1980-97. National Vital Statistics Reports. 1999;**47**(24):1-16. Available from: http://www.ncbi.nlm.nih.gov/pubmed/11968567

[11] Ventura SJ, Martin JA, Curtin SC, Mathews TJ, Park MM. Births: Final data for 1998. National Vital Statistics Reports. 2000;**48**(3):1-100. Available from: http://www.ncbi.nlm.nih.gov/pubmed/10761414

[12] Martin JA, Hamilton Brady E, MJK O, Driscoll AK, Drake P. Births: Final data for 2016. National Vital Statistics Reports. 2018;**67**(1):p.9, p.49-50. Available from: https://www.cdc.gov/nchs/data/nvsr/nvsr67/nvsr67_01.pdf

[13] Blondel B, Kaminski M. Trends in the occurrence, determinants, and consequences of multiple births. Seminars in Perinatology. 2002;**26**(4):239-249. Available from: http://www.ncbi.nlm.nih.gov/pubmed/12211614

[14] Practice Committee of American Society for Reproductive Medicine. Multiple gestation associated with infertility therapy: An American Society for Reproductive Medicine Practice Committee opinion. Fertility and Sterility. 2012;**97**(4):825-834 Available from: http://www.ncbi.nlm.nih.gov/pubmed/22192352

[15] Goldfarb JM, Austin C, Lisbona H, Peskin B, Clapp M. Cost-effectiveness of in vitro fertilization. Obstetrics and Gynecology. 1996;**87**(1):18-21. Available from: http://www.ncbi.nlm.nih.gov/pubmed/8532258

[16] Bromer JG, Ata B, Seli M, Lockwood CJ, Seli E. Preterm deliveries that result from multiple pregnancies associated with assisted reproductive technologies in the USA: A cost analysis. Current Opinion in Obstetrics & Gynecology. 2011;**23**(3):168-173. Available from: http://www.ncbi.nlm.nih.gov/pubmed/21372712

[17] Elliott JP. High-order multiple gestations. Seminars in Perinatology. 2005;**29**(5):305-311. Available from: http://linkinghub.elsevier.com/retrieve/pii/S0146000505000832

[18] Smith-Levitin M, Skupski Daniel W, Frank AC. Multifetal pregnancies: Epidemiology, clinical characteristics, and management. In: Clinical Obstetrics. USA: Blackwell Publishing, Inc.; 2008. pp. 177-202. Available from: https://onlinelibrary.wiley.com/doi/abs/10.1002/9780470753293.ch13

[19] Liu F, He L, Long X, Sun X, Zhang W, Zeng X, et al. Monozygotic quadruplets after in vitro fertilization and embryo transfer. Fertility and Sterility. 2010;**94**(6):2301-2302. Available from: http://www.ncbi.nlm.nih.gov/pubmed/20466362

[20] Nnadi D, Nwobodo E, Ibrahim A. Spontaneous monochorionic tetra-amniotic quadruplet pregnancy at term. Journal of Basic and Clinical Reproductive Sciences. 2013;**2**(1):57. Available from: http://www.jbcrs.org/text.asp?2013/2/1/57/112597

[21] Neubecker RD, Blumberg JM, Townsend FM. A human monozygotic quintuplet placenta: Report of a specimen. The Journal of Obstetrics and Gynaecology of the British Empire. 1962;**69**:137-139. Available from: http://www.ncbi.nlm.nih.gov/pubmed/14479143

[22] Rau RK, Aiyar AA, Mathew TV. Quintuplets: Record of a premature delivery. British Medical Journal. 1940;**1**(4125):127-128. Available from: http://www.ncbi.nlm.nih.gov/pubmed/20782923

[23] Peigné M, Andrieux J, Deruelle P, Vuillaume I, Leroy M. Quintuplets after a transfer of two embryos following in vitro fertilization: A proved superfecundation. Fertility and Sterility. 2011;**95**(6):2124.e13-2124.e16. Available from: http://www.sciencedirect.com/science/article/pii/S0015028211000392

[24] Milki AA, Hinckley MD, Grumet FC, Chitkara U. Concurrent IVF and spontaneous conception resulting in a quadruplet pregnancy. Human Reproduction. 2001;**16**(11): 2324-2326. Available from: http://www.ncbi.nlm.nih.gov/pubmed/11679513

[25] Wenk RE, Houtz T, Brooks M, Chiafari FA. How frequent is heteropaternal superfecundation? Acta Geneticae Medicae et Gemellologiae. 1992;**41**(1):43-47. Available from: http://www.ncbi.nlm.nih.gov/pubmed/1488855

[26] Cunningham F, Leveno K, Bloom S, et al. Multifetal gestation. In: Williams Obsetrics. 22nd ed. NY: McGraw-Hill; 2005. pp. 911-948

[27] Gill P, Van Hook JM. Pregnancy, twins. In: StatPearls. Treasure Isl: StatPearls Publ; 2018

[28] Benirschke K. The biology of twinning in man. By M. G. Bulmer. Clarendon Press, Oxford. 205 pp. 1970. Teratology. 1971;**4**(2):213-213. Available from: http://doi.wiley.com/10.1002/tera.1420040214

[29] Bortolus R. The epidemiology of multiple births. Human Reproduction Update. 1999;**5**(2): 179-187. Available from: https://academic.oup.com/humupd/article-lookup/doi/10.1093/humupd/5.2.179

[30] Beemsterboer SN, Homburg R, Gorter NA, Schats R, Hompes PGA, Lambalk CB. The paradox of declining fertility but increasing twinning rates with advancing maternal age. Human Reproduction. 2006;**21**(6):1531-1532. Available from: http://www.ncbi.nlm.nih.gov/pubmed/16497698

[31] Nilsen T, Ørstavik R. Maternal body composition in relation to twinning. Norsk Epidemiologi. 2016;**26**(1-2):77-81. Available from: http://www.ntnu.no/ojs/index.php/norepid/article/view/2019

[32] Hoekstra C, Willemsen G, van Beijsterveldt CEMT, Lambalk CB, Montgomery GW, Boomsma DI. Body composition, smoking, and spontaneous dizygotic twinning. Fertility and Sterility. 2010;**93**(3):885-893. Available from: http://www.ncbi.nlm.nih.gov/pubmed/19061995

[33] Basso O, Nohr EA, Olsen J, Christensen K. Relationship of maternal body mass index and height to twinning. Obstetrics and Gynecology. 2005;**106**(2):411. Available from: http://content.wkhealth.com/linkback/openurl?sid=WKPTLP:landingpage&an=00006250-200508000-00048

[34] Reddy UM, Branum AM, Klebanoff MA. Relationship of maternal body mass index and height to twinning. Obstetrics and Gynecology. 2005;**105**(3):593-597. Available from: http://www.ncbi.nlm.nih.gov/pubmed/15738030

[35] Lumley J, Watson L, Watson M, Bower C. Periconceptional supplementation with folate and/or multivitamins for preventing neural tube defects. Cochrane Database of Systematic Reviews. 2001;(3). Article No.: CD001056. DOI: 10.1002/14651858.CD001056. Available from: http://www.ncbi.nlm.nih.gov/pubmed/11686974

[36] Collins J. Global epidemiology of multiple birth. Reproductive Biomedicine. 2007; **15**(Suppl 3):45-52. Available from: http://www.ncbi.nlm.nih.gov/pubmed/18598609

[37] Parazzini F, Chatenoud L, Benzi G, Di Cintio E, Pino DD, Tozzi L, et al. Pregnancy: Coffee and alcohol intake, smoking and risk of multiple pregnancy. Human Reproduction. 1996;**11**(10):2306-2309. Available from: http://dx.doi.org/10.1093/oxfordjournals.humrep.a019094

[38] Kapidaki M, Roupa Z, Sparos L, Tzonou A, Olsen J, Trichopoulos D. Coffee intake and other factors in relation to multiple deliveries: A study in Greece. Epidemiology. 1995;**6**(3):294-298. Available from: http://www.ncbi.nlm.nih.gov/pubmed/7619939

[39] Rothman KJ. Fetal loss, twinning and birth weight after oral-contraceptive use. The New England Journal of Medicine. 1977;**297**(9):468-471. Available from: http://www.ncbi.nlm.nih.gov/pubmed/887128

[40] Harlap S. Multiple births in former oral contraceptive users. British Journal of Obstetrics and Gynaecology. 1979;**86**(7):557-562. Available from: http://www.ncbi.nlm.nih.gov/pubmed/476022

[41] Murphy MF, Campbell MJ, Bone M. Is there an increased risk of twinning after discontinuation of the oral contraceptive pill? Journal of Epidemiology and Community Health. 1989;**43**(3):275-279. Available from: http://www.ncbi.nlm.nih.gov/pubmed/2607308

[42] Kotb MM, El-Ghannam MA. Oral contraceptive and twinning: Case-control study. The Journal of the Egyptian Public Health Association. 1993;**68**(3-4):265-275. Available from: http://www.ncbi.nlm.nih.gov/pubmed/17265648

[43] Campbell D, Thompson B, Pritchard C, Samphier M. Does the use of oral contraception depress DZ twinning rates? Acta Geneticae Medicae et Gemellologiae. 1987;**36**(3):409-415. Available from: http://www.ncbi.nlm.nih.gov/pubmed/3451649

[44] Wen SW, Demissie K, Yang Q, Walker MC. Maternal morbidity and obstetric complications in triplet pregnancies and quadruplet and higher-order multiple pregnancies. American Journal of Obstetrics and Gynecology. 2004;**191**(1):254-258. Available from: http://www.ncbi.nlm.nih.gov/pubmed/15295375

[45] Luke B, Brown MB. Maternal morbidity and infant death in twin vs triplet and quadruplet pregnancies. American Journal of Obstetrics and Gynecology. 2008;**198**(4):401.e1-401.10. Available from: http://www.ncbi.nlm.nih.gov/pubmed/18177828

[46] Saravelos SH, Zhang T, Chung JPW, Sun L-M, Sun Y, Li T-C, et al. Monochorionic quadramniotic and triamniotic pregnancies following single embryo transfers: Two case reports and a review of the literature. Journal of Assisted Reproduction and Genetics. 2016;**33**(1):27-32. Available from: http://www.ncbi.nlm.nih.gov/pubmed/26564016

[47] Carrillo-Vadillo R, García-Lozano JC, Lozano Arana MD, Moliní Rivera JL, Sánchez Martín P, Antiñolo G. Two sets of monozygotic twins after intracytoplasmic sperm injection and transfer of two embryos on day 2. Fertility and Sterility. 2007;**88**(6):1676.e3-1676.e5. Available from: http://www.ncbi.nlm.nih.gov/pubmed/17481624

[48] Cahill DJ, Jenkins JM, Soothill PW, Whitelaw A, Wardle PG. Quadruplet pregnancy following transfer of two embryos: Case report. Human Reproduction. 2003;**18**(2):441-443. Available from: http://www.ncbi.nlm.nih.gov/pubmed/12571187

[49] Grgic O, Ivanisevic M, Djelmis J, Lucinger D, Krile L. Successful pregnancy and delivery of two sets of monozygotic twins after intracytoplasmic sperm injection and embryo transfer: Case report and literature review. Fertility and Sterility. 2009;**92**(1):392.e5-392.e8. Available from: http://www.ncbi.nlm.nih.gov/pubmed/19439292

[50] Zikopoulos K, Platteau P, Kolibianakis E, Albano C, Van Steirteghem A, Devroey P. Quintuplet pregnancy following transfer of two blastocysts: Case report. Human Reproduction. 2004;**19**(2):325-327. Available from: http://www.ncbi.nlm.nih.gov/pubmed/14747174

[51] Unger S, Hoopmann M, Bald R, Foth D, Nawroth F. Monozygotic triplets and monozygotic twins after ICSI and transfer of two blastocysts: Case report. Human Reproduction. 2004;**19**(1):110-113. Available from: http://www.ncbi.nlm.nih.gov/pubmed/14688167

[52] Yakín K, Kahraman S, Cömert S. Three blastocyst stage embryo transfer resulting in a quintuplet pregnancy. Human Reproduction. 2001;**16**(4):782-784. Available from: http://www.ncbi.nlm.nih.gov/pubmed/11278234

[53] Schenker JG, Laufer N, Weinstein D, Yarkoni S. Quintuplet pregnancies. European Journal of Obstetrics, Gynecology, and Reproductive Biology. 1980;**10**(4):257-268. Available from: http://www.ncbi.nlm.nih.gov/pubmed/6769719

[54] Arabin B, van Eyck J. The role of ultrasound in multiple pregnancy. Twin Research. 2001;**4**(3):141-145. Available from: http://www.ncbi.nlm.nih.gov/pubmed/11665312

[55] Goldman GA, Dicker D, Feldberg D, Ashkenazi J, Yeshaya A, Goldman JA. The vanishing fetus. A report of 17 cases of triplets and quadruplets. Journal of Perinatal Medicine. 1989;**17**(2):157-162. Available from: http://www.ncbi.nlm.nih.gov/pubmed/2681669

[56] Dickey RP, Taylor SN, Lu PY, Sartor BM, Storment JM, Rye PH, et al. Spontaneous reduction of multiple pregnancy: Incidence and effect on outcome. American Journal of Obstetrics and Gynecology. 2002;**186**(1):77-83. Available from: http://www.ncbi.nlm.nih.gov/pubmed/11810089

[57] Sebire NJ, Snijders RJ, Hughes K, Sepulveda W, Nicolaides KH. The hidden mortality of monochorionic twin pregnancies. British Journal of Obstetrics and Gynaecology. 1997;**104**(10):1203-1207. Available from: http://www.ncbi.nlm.nih.gov/pubmed/9333002

[58] Adegbite AL, Ward SB, Bajoria R. Perinatal outcome of spontaneously conceived triplet pregnancies in relation to chorionicity. American Journal of Obstetrics and Gynecology. 2005;**193**(4):1463-1471. Available from: http://www.ncbi.nlm.nih.gov/pubmed/16202741

[59] Adegbite AL, Ward BS, Bajoria R. Perinatal outcome of quadruplet pregnancies in relation to chorionicity. Journal of Perinatology. 2007;**27**(1):15-21. Available from: http://www.ncbi.nlm.nih.gov/pubmed/17180127

[60] Mateizel I, Santos-Ribeiro S, Done E, Van Landuyt L, Van de Velde H, Tournaye H, et al. Do ARTs affect the incidence of monozygotic twinning? Human Reproduction. 2016;**31**(11):2435-2441. Available from: http://www.ncbi.nlm.nih.gov/pubmed/27664211

[61] Shulman LS, van Vugt JMG. Prenatal Medicine. Washington, DC: Taylor & Francis; 2006. 447 p

[62] Chow JS, Benson CB, Racowsky C, Doubilet PM, Ginsburg E. Frequency of a monochorionic pair in multiple gestations: Relationship to mode of conception. Journal of Ultrasound in Medicine. 2001;**20**(7):757-760; quiz 761. Available from: http://www.ncbi.nlm.nih.gov/pubmed/11444734

[63] Weis MA, Harper LM, Roehl KA, Odibo AO, Cahill AG. Natural history of placenta previa in twins. Obstetrics and Gynecology. 2012;**120**(4):753-758 Available from: http://www.ncbi.nlm.nih.gov/pubmed/22996091

[64] Benirschke K. The biology of the twinning process: How placentation influences outcome. Seminars in Perinatology. 1995;**19**(5):342-350. Available from: http://www.ncbi.nlm.nih.gov/pubmed/8821022

[65] Francois K, Johnson JM, Harris C. Is placenta previa more common in multiple gestations? American Journal of Obstetrics and Gynecology. 2003;**188**(5):1226-1227. Available from: http://www.ncbi.nlm.nih.gov/pubmed/12748486

[66] Evans MI, Andriole S, Britt DW. Fetal reduction: 25 years' experience. Fetal Diagnosis and Therapy. 2014;**35**(2):69-82. Available from: http://www.ncbi.nlm.nih.gov/pubmed/24525884

[67] Abu-Heija AT. Maternal and neonatal outcome of high order gestation. Archives of Gynecology and Obstetrics. 2003;**268**(1):15-18. Available from: https://doi.org/10.1007/s00404-002-0322-7

[68] Crowther CA, Han S. Hospitalisation and bed rest for multiple pregnancy. Cochrane Database of Systematic Reviews. 2010;(7). Article No.: CD000110. DOI: 10.1002/14651858.CD000110.pub2. Available from: http://www.ncbi.nlm.nih.gov/pubmed/20614420

[69] Zakut H, Insler V, Serr DM. Elective cervical suture in preventing premature delivery in multiple pregnancies. Israel Journal of Medical Sciences. 1977;**13**(5):488-492. Available from: http://www.ncbi.nlm.nih.gov/pubmed/873765

[70] Strauss A, Heer IM, Janssen U, Dannecker C, Hillemanns P, Müller-Egloff S. Routine cervical cerclage in higher order multiple gestation—Does it prolong the pregnancy? Twin Research. 2002;**5**(2):67-70. Available from: http://www.ncbi.nlm.nih.gov/pubmed/11931683

[71] Rafael TJ, Berghella V, Alfirevic Z. Cervical stitch (cerclage) for preventing preterm birth in multiple pregnancy. Cochrane Database of Systematic Reviews. 2014;(9). Article No.: CD009166. DOI: 10.1002/14651858.CD009166.pub2. Available from: http://www.ncbi.nlm.nih.gov/pubmed/25208049

[72] Crowther CA. Prevention of preterm birth in multiple pregnancy. Baillière's Clinical Obstetrics and Gynaecology. 1998;**12**(1):67-75. Available from: http://www.ncbi.nlm.nih.gov/pubmed/9930290

[73] Haram K, Mortensen JHS, Morrison JC. Tocolysis for acute preterm labor: Does anything work. The Journal of Maternal-Fetal & Neonatal Medicine. 2015;**28**(4):371-378. Available from: http://www.ncbi.nlm.nih.gov/pubmed/24990666

[74] Boelig RC, Berghella V. Current options for mechanical prevention of preterm birth. Seminars in Perinatology. 2017;**41**(8):452-460. Available from: http://www.ncbi.nlm.nih.gov/pubmed/29033106

[75] Liem S, Schuit E, Hegeman M, Bais J, de Boer K, Bloemenkamp K, et al. Cervical pessaries for prevention of preterm birth in women with a multiple pregnancy (ProTWIN): A multicentre, open-label randomised controlled trial. Lancet (London, England). 2013;**382**(9901): 1341-1349. Available from: http://www.ncbi.nlm.nih.gov/pubmed/23924878

[76] Kuon R-J, Abele H, Berger R, Garnier Y, Maul H, Schleußner E, et al. Progesterone for prevention of preterm birth—Evidence-based indications. Zeitschrift für Geburtshilfe und Neonatologie. 2015;**219**(3):125-135. Available from: http://www.ncbi.nlm.nih.gov/pubmed/26114408

[77] Society for Maternal-Fetal Medicine Publications Committee with Assistance of VB. Progesterone and preterm birth prevention: Translating clinical trials data into clinical practice. American Journal of Obstetrics and Gynecology. 2012;**206**(5):376-386. Available from: http://www.ncbi.nlm.nih.gov/pubmed/22542113

[78] Goldenberg RL, Culhane JF, Iams JD, Romero R. Epidemiology and causes of preterm birth. Lancet (London, England). 2008;**371**(9606):75-84. Available from: http://www.ncbi.nlm.nih.gov/pubmed/18177778

[79] Pakrashi T, Defranco EA. The relative proportion of preterm births complicated by premature rupture of membranes in multifetal gestations: A population-based study. American Journal of Perinatology. 2013;**30**(1):69-74. Available from: http://www.ncbi.nlm.nih.gov/pubmed/22773281

[80] Gibbs RS, Karlan S, Beth Y, Haney AF, Nygaard IE. Multiple gestation. In: Danforth's Obstetrics and Gynecology. 10th ed. United States, Philadelphia: Wolters Kluwer Lippincott Williams & Wilkins; 2008

[81] Day MC, Barton JR, O'Brien JM, Istwan NB, Sibai BM. The effect of fetal number on the development of hypertensive conditions of pregnancy. Obstetrics and Gynecology. 2005;**106**(5 Pt 1):927-931. Available from: http://www.ncbi.nlm.nih.gov/pubmed/16260508

[82] Al-Jameil N, Aziz Khan F, Fareed Khan M, Tabassum H. A brief overview of preeclampsia. Journal of Clinical Medical Research. 2014;**6**(1):1-7. Available from: http://www.ncbi.nlm.nih.gov/pubmed/24400024

[83] Hardardottir H, Kelly K, Bork MD, Cusick W, Campbell WA, Rodis JF. Atypical presentation of preeclampsia in high-order multifetal gestations. Obstetrics and Gynecology. 1996;**87**(3):370-374. Available from: http://www.ncbi.nlm.nih.gov/pubmed/8598957

[84] English FA, Kenny LC, McCarthy FP. Risk factors and effective management of preeclampsia. Integrated Blood Pressure Control. 2015;**8**:7-12. Available from: http://www.ncbi.nlm.nih.gov/pubmed/25767405

[85] Chao AS, Tsai TC, Soong YK. Clinical management of a quadruplet pregnancy combining a triplet pregnancy with a classical hydatidiform mole: Case report and review of literature. Prenatal Diagnosis. 1999;**19**(11):1073-1076. Available from: http://www.ncbi.nlm.nih.gov/pubmed/10589065

[86] Amano T, Takahashi K, Kita N, Kimura F, Hirose M, Noda Y. A case of quadruplet pregnancy with a complete hydatidiform mole. Prenatal Diagnosis. 2005;**25**(8):718-721. Available from: http://www.ncbi.nlm.nih.gov/pubmed/16049994

[87] Tariq N, Ghazali U, Uddin Z, Rasheed K, Tariq H. Complete hydatidiform mole coexisting with three viable fetuses in a quadruplet pregnancy. Journal of the College of Physicians and Surgeons–Pakistan. 2016;**26**(4):326-328. Available from: http://www.ncbi.nlm.nih.gov/pubmed/27097708

[88] Rauh-Hain JA, Rana S, Tamez H, Wang A, Cohen B, Cohen A, et al. Risk for developing gestational diabetes in women with twin pregnancies. The Journal of Maternal-Fetal & Neonatal Medicine. 2009;**22**(4):293-299. Available from: http://www.ncbi.nlm.nih.gov/pubmed/19340713

[89] Sivan E, Maman E, Homko CJ, Lipitz S, Cohen S, Schiff E. Impact of fetal reduction on the incidence of gestational diabetes. Obstetrics and Gynecology. 2002;**99**(1):91-94. Available from: http://www.ncbi.nlm.nih.gov/pubmed/11777517

[90] Conde-Agudelo A, Belizán JM, Lindmark G. Maternal morbidity and mortality associated with multiple gestations. Obstetrics and Gynecology. 2000;**95**(6 Pt 1):899-904. Available from: http://www.ncbi.nlm.nih.gov/pubmed/10831988

[91] Roem K. Nutritional management of multiple pregnancies. Twin Research. 2003;**6**(6): 514-519. Available from: http://www.ncbi.nlm.nih.gov/pubmed/14965462

[92] Suryanarayana R, Chandrappa M, Santhuram AN, Prathima S, Sheela SR. Prospective study on prevalence of anemia of pregnant women and its outcome: A community based study. Journal of Family Medicine and Primary Care;**6**(4):739-743. Available from: http://www.ncbi.nlm.nih.gov/pubmed/29564255

[93] Ru Y, Pressman EK, Cooper EM, Guillet R, Katzman PJ, Kent TR, et al. Iron deficiency and anemia are prevalent in women with multiple gestations. The American Journal of Clinical Nutrition. 2016;**104**(4):1052-1060. Available from: http://www.ncbi.nlm.nih.gov/pubmed/27581469

[94] Scholl TO, Hediger ML, Fischer RL, Shearer JW. Anemia vs iron deficiency: Increased risk of preterm delivery in a prospective study. The American Journal of Clinical Nutrition. 1992;**55**(5):985-988. Available from: http://www.ncbi.nlm.nih.gov/pubmed/1570808

[95] Sangeetha V, Pushpalatha S. Severe maternal anemia and neonatal outcome. Scholars Journal of Applied Medicine Sciences. 2014;**2**:303-309

[96] Geltman PL, Meyers AF, Mehta SD, Brugnara C, Villon I, Wu YA, et al. Daily multivitamins with iron to prevent anemia in high-risk infants: A randomized clinical trial. Pediatrics. 2004;**114**(1):86-93. Available from: http://www.ncbi.nlm.nih.gov/pubmed/15231912

[97] Elliott JP, Radin TG. The effect of corticosteroid administration on uterine activity and preterm labor in high-order multiple gestations. Obstetrics and Gynecology. 1995;**85**(2):250-254. Available from: http://www.ncbi.nlm.nih.gov/pubmed/7824240

[98] Committee on Obstetric Practice. Committee Opinion No. 713: Antenatal corticosteroid therapy for fetal maturation. Obstetrics and Gynecology. 2017;**130**(2):e102-e109. Available from: http://www.ncbi.nlm.nih.gov/pubmed/28742678

[99] Skrablin S, Kuvacić I, Pavicić D, Kalafatić D, Goluza T. Maternal neonatal outcome in quadruplet and quintuplet versus triplet gestations. European Journal of Obstetrics, Gynecology, and Reproductive Biology. 2000;**88**(2):147-152. Available from: http://www.ncbi.nlm.nih.gov/pubmed/10690673

[100] Suri K, Bhandari V, Lerer T, Rosenkrantz TS, Hussain N. Morbidity and mortality of preterm twins and higher-order multiple births. Journal of Perinatology;**21**(5):293-299. Available from: http://www.ncbi.nlm.nih.gov/pubmed/11536022

[101] Hernández Herrera RJ, del Rayo Rivas Ortiz Y, Alcalá Galván LG, Ramos González R, Flores Santos R, Torcida González ME. Perinatal mortality in multiple pregnancies. Ginecología y Obstetricia de México. 2009;**77**(3):147-150. Available from: http://www.ncbi.nlm.nih.gov/pubmed/19400518

[102] Chibber R, Fouda M, Shishtawy W, Al-Dossary M, Al-Hijji J, Amen A, et al. Maternal and neonatal outcome in triplet, quadruplet and quintuplet gestations following ART: A 11-year study. Archives of Gynecology and Obstetrics. 2013;**288**(4):759-767. Available from: http://www.ncbi.nlm.nih.gov/pubmed/23543239

[103] Blickstein I, Keith L. Intrauterine growth. In: Multiple Pregnancy: Epidemiology, Gestation and Perinatal Outcome. 2nd ed. Abingdon: Taylor and Francis; 2005. pp. 505-513

[104] Berg C, Baschat AA, Geipel A, Germer U, Smrcek J, Krapp M, et al. First trimester twin-to-twin transfusion syndrome in a trichorionic quadruplet pregnancy—A diagnostic challenge. Fetal Diagnosis and Therapy;**17**(6):357-361. Available from: http://www.ncbi.nlm.nih.gov/pubmed/12393966

[105] O'Brien BM, Feltovich HM, Carr SR, Luks FI. Feto-fetal transfusion syndrome in monochorionic quadruplets. Obstetrics and Gynecology. 2010;**115**(2 Pt 2):470-472. Available from: http://www.ncbi.nlm.nih.gov/pubmed/20093884

[106] Tul N, Bricelj K, Ravnik D, Diehl W, Hecher K. Successful laser treatment in monochorionic quadruplets affected by fetofetal transfusion syndrome. Ultrasound in Obstetrics & Gynecology. 2015;**46**(6):749-750. Available from: http://www.ncbi.nlm.nih.gov/pubmed/26411739

[107] Mendilcioglu I, Simsek M. Conjoined twins in a trichorionic quadruplet pregnancy after ovulation induction with clomiphene citrate. Fetal Diagnosis and Therapy. 2008;**24**(1):51-54. Available from: http://www.ncbi.nlm.nih.gov/pubmed/18504382

[108] Rohilla S, Dahiya K, Rathee S, Yadav RK, Dhaulakhandi DB. Conjoined twins in a spontaneous trichorionic quadruplet pregnancy: A case report. The Journal of Reproductive Medicine;**56**(7-8):351-355. Available from: http://www.ncbi.nlm.nih.gov/pubmed/21838168

[109] Tarney CM, Whitecar P, Sewell M, Grubish L, Hope E. Rupture of an unscarred uterus in a quadruplet pregnancy. Obstetrics and Gynecology. 2013;**121**(2 Pt 2 Suppl 1):483-485. Available from: http://www.ncbi.nlm.nih.gov/pubmed/23344417

[110] Francois K, Ortiz J, Harris C, Foley MR, Elliott JP. Is peripartum hysterectomy more common in multiple gestations? Obstetrics and Gynecology. 2005;**105**(6):1369-1372. Available from: http://www.ncbi.nlm.nih.gov/pubmed/15932831

[111] Evans MI, Fletcher JC, Zador IE, Newton BW, Quigg MH, Struyk CD. Selective first-trimester termination in octuplet and quadruplet pregnancies: Clinical and ethical issues. Obstetrics and Gynecology. 1988;**71**(3 Pt 1):289-296. Available from: http://www.ncbi.nlm.nih.gov/pubmed/3347412

[112] Antsaklis A, Souka AP, Daskalakis G, Papantoniou N, Koutra P, Kavalakis Y, et al. Pregnancy outcome after multifetal pregnancy reduction. The Journal of Maternal-Fetal & Neonatal Medicine. 2004;**16**(1):27-31. Available from: http://www.ncbi.nlm.nih.gov/pubmed/15370079

[113] Davis C, Douglas H. Selective reduction of fetuses in multiple pregnancies and the law in Australia. Journal of Law and Medicine. 2014;**22**(1):155-173. Available from: http://www.ncbi.nlm.nih.gov/pubmed/25341325

[114] Berkowitz RL, Lynch L, Chitkara U, Wilkins IA, Mehalek KE, Alvarez E. Selective reduction of multifetal pregnancies in the first trimester. The New England Journal of Medicine. 1988;**318**(16):1043-1047. Available from: http://www.ncbi.nlm.nih.gov/pubmed/3352698

[115] Evans MI, Berkowitz RL, Wapner RJ, Carpenter RJ, Goldberg JD, Ayoub MA, et al. Improvement in outcomes of multifetal pregnancy reduction with increased experience. American Journal of Obstetrics and Gynecology. 2001;**184**(2):97-103. Available from: http://www.ncbi.nlm.nih.gov/pubmed/11174487

[116] Mansour RT, Aboulghar MA, Serour GI, Sattar MA, Kamal A, Amin YM. Multifetal pregnancy reduction: Modification of the technique and analysis of the outcome. Fertility and Sterility. 1999;**71**(2):380-384. Available from: http://www.ncbi.nlm.nih.gov/pubmed/9988416

[117] Rodeck C, Deans A, Jauniaux E. Thermocoagulation for the early treatment of pregnancy with an acardiac twin. The New England Journal of Medicine. 1998;**339**(18):1293-1295. Available from: http://www.ncbi.nlm.nih.gov/pubmed/9791145

[118] Yinon Y, Ashwal E, Weisz B, Chayen B, Schiff E, Lipitz S. Selective reduction in complicated monochorionic twins: Prediction of obstetric outcome and comparison of techniques. Ultrasound in Obstetrics & Gynecology. 2015;**46**(6):670-677. Available from: http://www.ncbi.nlm.nih.gov/pubmed/25867754

[119] Peng R, Xie H-N, Lin M-F, Yang J-B, Zhou Y, Chen H-Q, et al. Clinical outcomes after selective fetal reduction of complicated monochorionic twins with radiofrequency ablation and bipolar cord coagulation. Gynecologic and Obstetric Investigation. 2016;**81**(6):552-558. Available from: http://www.ncbi.nlm.nih.gov/pubmed/27035917

[120] Gallot D, Laurichesse H, Lemery D. Selective feticide in monochorionic twin pregnancies by ultrasound-guided umbilical cord occlusion. Ultrasound in Obstetrics & Gynecology. 2003;**22**(5):484-488. Available from: http://www.ncbi.nlm.nih.gov/pubmed/14618661

[121] Vauthier-Brouzes D, Lefebvre G. Selective reduction in multifetal pregnancies: Technical and psychological aspects. In: Presented at the 7th World Congress of In Vitro Fertilization and Assisted Procreations, Paris, France, June 30 to July 3, 1991. Fertility and Sterility. 1992;**57**(5):1012-1016. Available from: http://www.sciencedirect.com/science/article/pii/S0015028216550183

[122] Geva E, Fait G, Yovel I, Lerner-Geva L, Yaron Y, Daniel Y, et al. Second-trimester multifetal pregnancy reduction facilitates prenatal diagnosis before the procedure. Fertility and Sterility. 2000;**73**(3):505-508. Available from: http://www.ncbi.nlm.nih.gov/pubmed/10689003

[123] Donner C, de Maertelaer V, Rodesch F. Multifetal pregnancy reduction: Comparison of obstetrical results with spontaneous twin gestations. European Journal of Obstetrics, Gynecology, and Reproductive Biology. 1992;**44**(3):181-184. Available from: http://www.ncbi.nlm.nih.gov/pubmed/1607057

[124] Boulot P, Hedon B, Pelliccia G, Lefort G, Deschamps F, Arnal F, et al. Multifetal pregnancy reduction: A consecutive series of 61 cases. British Journal of Obstetrics and Gynaecology. 1993;**100**(1):63-68. Available from: http://www.ncbi.nlm.nih.gov/pubmed/8427841

[125] Antsaklis AJ, Drakakis P, Vlazakis GP, Michalas S. Reduction of multifetal pregnancies to twins does not increase obstetric or perinatal risks. Human Reproduction. 1999;**14**(5):1338-1340. Available from: http://www.ncbi.nlm.nih.gov/pubmed/10325290

[126] Wang X, Li H, Feng H, Zuo C, Chen Y, Li L, et al. Clinical study of selective multifetal pregnancy reduction in second trimester. Zhonghua Fu Chan Ke Za Zhi. 2007;**42**(3): 152-156. Available from: http://www.ncbi.nlm.nih.gov/pubmed/17537297

[127] Timor-Tritsch IE, Bashiri A, Monteagudo A, Rebarber A, Arslan AA. Two hundred ninety consecutive cases of multifetal pregnancy reduction: Comparison of the transabdominal versus the transvaginal approach. American Journal of Obstetrics and Gynecology. 2004;**191**(6):2085-2089. Available from: http://www.ncbi.nlm.nih.gov/pubmed/15592295

[128] Brambati B, Tului L, Baldi M, Guercilena S. Genetic analysis prior to selective fetal reduction in multiple pregnancy: Technical aspects and clinical outcome. Human Reproduction. 1995;**10**(4):818-825. Available from: http://www.ncbi.nlm.nih.gov/pubmed/7650128

[129] Timor-Tritsch IE, Peisner DB, Monteagudo A, Lerner JP, Sharma S. Multifetal pregnancy reduction by transvaginal puncture: Evaluation of the technique used in 134 cases. American Journal of Obstetrics and Gynecology. 1993;**168**(3 Pt 1):799-804. Available from: http://www.ncbi.nlm.nih.gov/pubmed/8456883

[130] Torok O, Lapinski R, Salafia CM, Bernasko J, Berkowitz RL. Multifetal pregnancy reduction is not associated with an increased risk of intrauterine growth restriction, except for very-high-order multiples. American Journal of Obstetrics and Gynecology. 1998;**179**(1):221-225. Available from: http://www.ncbi.nlm.nih.gov/pubmed/9704791

[131] Depp R, Macones GA, Rosenn MF, Turzo E, Wapner RJ, Weinblatt VJ. Multifetal pregnancy reduction: Evaluation of fetal growth in the remaining twins. American Journal of Obstetrics and Gynecology. 1996;**174**(4):1233-1238, 40. Available from: http://www.ncbi.nlm.nih.gov/pubmed/8623851

[132] Schreiner-Engel P, Walther VN, Mindes J, Lynch L, Berkowitz RL. First-trimester multifetal pregnancy reduction: Acute and persistent psychologic reactions. American Journal of Obstetrics and Gynecology. 1995;**172**(2 Pt 1):541-547. Available from: http://www.ncbi.nlm.nih.gov/pubmed/7856683

[133] Goldfarb J, Kinzer DJ, Boyle M, Kurit D. Attitudes of in vitro fertilization and intrauterine insemination couples toward multiple gestation pregnancy and multifetal pregnancy reduction. Fertility and Sterility. 1996;**65**(4):815-820. Available from: http://www.ncbi.nlm.nih.gov/pubmed/8654645

[134] Ogunnowo T, Oluwole O, Aimakhu C, Ilesanmi A, Omigbodun A. Term quadruplet pregnancy: A case report. Nigerian Journal of Surgical Research. 2004;**6**(1-2):56-58. Available from: http://www.ajol.info/index.php/njsr/article/view/54796

[135] Edris FE. Trichorionic quadruplet delivered beyond 36 weeks of gestation: A case report and literature review. Case Reports in Obstetrics and Gynecology. 2011;**2011**:181034. Available from: http://www.ncbi.nlm.nih.gov/pubmed/22567493

[136] Atlay RD, Pennington GW. The use of clomiphene citrate and pituitary gonadotropin in successive pregnancies: The Sheffield quadruplets. American Journal of Obstetrics and Gynecology. 1971;**109**(3):402-407. Available from: http://www.ncbi.nlm.nih.gov/pubmed/5549182

[137] Loucopoulos A, Jewelewicz R. Management of multifetal pregnancies: Sixteen years' experience at the Sloane hospital for women. American Journal of Obstetrics and Gynecology. 1982;**143**(8):902-905. Available from: http://www.sciencedirect.com/science/article/pii/0002937882904719

[138] Strauss A, Paek BW, Genzel-Boroviczény O, Schulze A, Janssen U, Hepp H. Multifetal gestation—Maternal and perinatal outcome of 112 pregnancies. Fetal Diagnosis and Therapy;**17**(4):209-217. Available from: http://www.ncbi.nlm.nih.gov/pubmed/12065948

[139] Ron-El R, Mor Z, Weinraub Z, Schreyer P, Bukovsky I, Dolphin Z, et al. Triplet, quadruplet and quintuplet pregnancies: Management and outcome. Acta Obstetricia et Gynecologica Scandinavica. 2018;**71**(5):347-350. Available from: https://doi.org/10.3109/00016349209021071

[140] Olatunbosun OA, Turnell RW, Sankaran K, Ninan A. Delayed interval delivery in quadruplets. International Journal of Gynaecology and Obstetrics. 1995;**50**(3):287-290. Available from: http://www.ncbi.nlm.nih.gov/pubmed/8543113

[141] Flynn A, Scott F, Birrell W, Evans N. Delayed-interval delivery in a quadruplet pregnancy: The use of transperineal ultrasound and cervical cerclage. The Australian & New Zealand Journal of Obstetrics & Gynaecology. 1995;**35**(3):280-282. Available from: http://www.ncbi.nlm.nih.gov/pubmed/8546643

[142] Elias M, Heimrath J, Zimmer M, Woytoñ J, Goluda M. Delayed interval delivery in a quintuplet pregnancy. Human Reproduction. 1998;**13**(1):224-226. Available from: http://www.ncbi.nlm.nih.gov/pubmed/9580192

[143] Poeschmann PP, van Oppen CA, Bruinse HW. Delayed interval delivery in multiple pregnancies: Report of three cases and review of the literature. Obstetrical & Gynecological Survey. 1992;**47**(3):139-147. Available from: http://www.ncbi.nlm.nih.gov/pubmed/1741099

[144] Wittmann BK, Farquharson D, Wong GP, Baldwin V, Wadsworth LD, Elit L. Delayed delivery of second twin: Report of four cases and review of the literature. Obstetrics and Gynecology. 1992;**79**(2):260-263. Available from: http://www.ncbi.nlm.nih.gov/pubmed/1731296

10

Multiple Pregnancy in Women of Advanced Reproductive Age

Laura Pérez Martín and Duna Trobo Marina

Abstract

Assisted reproduction techniques (ARTs) allow women of advanced reproductive age to become pregnant. One of the most frequent complications of ART is twin pregnancy. Cases where both factors are present represent a specially vulnerable population for obstetric complications and medical perinatal and post-partum consequences for both the mother and babies. Pre-existing medical conditions are more frequent at advanced age, and the pregnancy physiological changes and the high metabolic demand associated with a twin pregnancy may reveal or worsen any previous disease. A careful counselling process is very important in this population and certain obstetric interventions might be particularly addressed to it. Single embryo transfer should be strongly enforced in advanced age women to minimise risk for the mother and children.

Keywords: twin pregnancy, advanced maternal age, ART, obstetric complications, reproductive counselling, oocyte donation, obstetric care

1. Introduction

Dizygotic twin pregnancies are known to increase with age of the mother. Naturally conceived twins are thought to occur in a 0.3% rate in women under 25 years, 1.4% between 25 and 34, 3% between 34 and 39, and 4.1% in women in their 40s or over [1]. We also know that at least 50% of all twin pregnancies are conceived through ART and that this proportion is probably higher for women in their 40s. International guidelines affirm that maternal mortality associated with multiple births is 2.5 times that for singleton births [2]. Since obstetric and obstetric-related medical complications are amplified in the case of women of advanced reproductive age and also in twin gestations, the combination represents a particularly vulnerable group.

In Spain, for example, according to the 2013th ESHRE registry [3], a total of 56,704 treatments were performed, 18,113 consisting in egg donation, which makes almost 32% of all treatments. The percentage of women older than 40 years undergoing treatment and arriving to egg aspiration was 15.7%, with a pregnancy rate of 29.9%, but a delivery rate of 9.5%. For egg donation programmes, the percentage of women over 40 increased to 66.9%, with a pregnancy rate of 48.4 and a delivery rate of 30.5%. This means that in 2013–2014, 4272 women over 40 carried and delivered a baby in Spain. The proportion of double embryo transfers was 71.5%, with 20.9% of twin deliveries in FIV/ICSI treatments and 24.6% in egg donation: around 982 twin deliveries in women over 40 in Spain in 2013. And this only counts for the pregnancies achieved through ART. This same registry suggests that the overall preterm birth rate for twins was 51%.

But, which age is "too old"? Can we set a threshold? Can we legislate against advanced reproductive age? And, would this legislation only account for women seeking reproductive care? If we already know all these, why is it still happening? Can we, as a society, deny maternity to any woman? Can we afford this? What if maternity age continues to increase in the world? Should not this evolve with society? This chapter will raise many questions that, sorry, we would not probably able to answer.

2. Ethical issues in the reproduction clinic

2.1. Setting a threshold for treatment

In most countries, there is no legislation restricting maternal age. Some countries would not include women of advanced age in their public reproduction schemes, but the same restrictions usually do not apply to the private sector. And more importantly, in many countries, there is no restriction in the number of embryos being transferred to these women. Not only access cannot be denied but two and three embryos can also be transferred freely.

Classically, advanced maternal age has been defined as any woman conceiving after 35 years of age. Given the late reproductive trends, this threshold should now be reconsidered, as in developed countries it might include a high percentage of the pregnant population. Advanced maternal age nowadays might be considered as a woman conceiving after 40–43 years of age, which is the approximate age in which ovary ageing may have almost completely prevented spontaneous conception. However, although rare, spontaneous conception over 40s is possible, so is it fair to deny reproductive treatment to a woman whose same-age neighbour might have conceived spontaneously?

In this environment, most clinics set their own thresholds (or not at all) without much governmental support. Very few clinics would accept to perform reproductive treatment on a woman older than 50, which represents an age in which more or less half of the female population is menopausal. However, peri- and postnatal risk for the mother and the babies start increasing progressively much earlier than that. But when a clear guidance does not exist, decision making becomes somehow subjective, mainly considering our previous experiences. Can we impose our own personal opinion over a woman's family desire?

2.2. Counselling advanced reproductive age mothers

Autonomy principle involves that appropriately informed patients can decide whether they want to undergo or refuse a diagnostic test or treatment, accepting the benefits and risks of their decision. Following this principle, any woman seeking reproductive treatment after the age of 35, or more appropriately, after the age of 40, should be carefully informed about obstetrical complications and the health implication for them and the child. They should also be informed about preventive and treatment strategies that may be put in place to avoid them. When counselling women with pre-existing medical conditions, their head specialist should review the case and advise for or against pregnancy. It is very important to remember that certain medical conditions do contraindicate pregnancy, as they might lead to a life-threatening situation.

2.3. Fertility in older mothers' children

Although most causes of infertility are not genetic, it has been observed in a US population study that daughters from mothers older than 40 years are more likely to remain childless in their lifetime [4]. However, it is difficult to discern whether this is a "learnt" pattern or a true "inherited" infertility trait. In the same population, daughters from "old" mothers were at double risk for delivering twins than daughters from "young" mothers (OR = 2.1, 95% CI: 0.8–5.4), although this difference was not statistically significant. This may suggest that delaying childbirth might be perpetuated and worsen with time in our current society.

2.4. Oocyte donation programmes

Oocyte donation restores pregnancy possibility in women of advanced reproductive age and reduces the chances for implantation failure found among them. Most women seeking this treatment are happily married women, well-educated and high-income, and physically and psychologically healthy [5]. However, oocyte donation recipients experienced a higher risk of pregnancy complications largely due to advanced maternal age, particularly hypertensive disorders and diabetes, and the risk increases with age [6]. The Ethics Committee of the American Society for Reproductive Medicine recommends women of advanced reproductive age undergo a comprehensive medical test to ascertain fitness for pregnancy in order to prevent the rise of obstetric complications during pregnancy [7]. Multiple pregnancy is known to increase obstetrical and neonatal risks in women of all ages; therefore, it is particularly important to avoid a twin gestation in older mothers.

3. Reproduction treatment and advanced maternal age

3.1. Low ovarian reserve

The effect of age in the ovarian reserve is unavoidable. Although menopause is considered the end of the reproductive age in women, changes in the ovarian cycle take place many years prior to menopause. These changes may lead to a fertility dysfunction in women that decide to get pregnant at an advanced age. The primary mechanism behind this process is the decrease of primordial follicle count in the ovary susceptible to developing a good-quality ovule. Classically, follicle count during menstrual cycle has been assessed using ultrasound. In addition, numerous studies have reported changes in the hormone patterns associated with reproductive ageing, such as shortened follicular phase, elevated follicular phase oestrogen, and decreased luteal phase progesterone [8–13]. During the last decade, anti-Müllerian hormone (AMH) has emerged as an early biochemical marker able to predict the decrease in the ovarian reserve. Low AMH serum levels predict an altered folliculogenesis by inhibiting the recruitment of primordial follicles and its sensitivity to FSH [14]. The reduction of AMH serum levels appears to be more strongly and more consistently correlated with age than the decrease number of antral follicles observed in the ovary by ultrasound, inhibin B levels, or FSH levels [15, 16].

3.2. Ageing uterus

In addition to changes observed in the ovarian reserve and quality of the oocytes, the uterus is an essential organ to achieve pregnancy. As in any other human organ, ageing also has an effect on the uterus of fertile women. Even though it is difficult to evaluate these changes in humans, animal studies indicate that older mice show an impaired artificially induced decidual response, probably due to reduced progesterone secretion [17–19]. Microscopic changes have also been confirmed, with more hyperaemia and higher vascular development and growth of the myometrium and stroma of young hamsters in comparison with the older ones [20]. Older mothers are also more likely to experience intrapartum complications and the rate of caesarean delivery is higher, suggesting that myometrial function is impaired by advanced maternal age [21]. The risk of stillbirth in mothers over the age of 40 is twice as high as younger mothers due to foetal chromosomal abnormalities, multiple pregnancy, obesity, pre-eclampsia, insulin-dependent diabetes, and multiple pregnancy [21, 22]. These evidences suggest that changes in the uterus in older women may have a reflection on fertility and the ability of maintaining a pregnancy.

3.3. Chromosomal abnormalities

Women who delay childbearing are at an increased risk of foetal chromosomal abnormalities. This occurs as a consequence of an error in chromosomal disjunction during maternal meiosis I or II, which has been reported as more frequent in advanced age women [23–25]. Among them, numeric chromosomal abnormalities seem to be more frequent than structural chromosomal abnormalities. Chromosomal aneuploidies related to maternal age include trisomy 21, trisomy 18, trisomy 13, triple X syndrome, and Klinefelter syndrome [26]. A recent study highlights that trisomy 21 showed an incidence rate of 11.34 out of 1000 cases at the age of 35 years, 15.41 cases at the age of 40, and 37.04 cases at the age of 45. In addition, trisomy 18 showed an incidence rate of 1.89 out of 1000 cases at the age of 35 years, 5.14 cases at the age of 40, and 37.04 cases at the age of 45. Nowadays, prenatal diagnostic techniques such as ultrasound and cell-free foetal DNA test allow professionals to make an early screening for foetal aneuploidy. However, invasive techniques remain the gold standard for definitive diagnosis, with a risk of miscarriage *per se* of 0.35% (CI 95%: 0.07 to 0.63) following amniocentesis and 0.35% (95% CI: -0.31 to 1.00) following chorionic villus sampling [27].

3.4. Oocyte donation

The use of donor oocytes in assisted reproduction techniques (ARTs) during the last decades has been a great advance for women whose reproductive dysfunction could not be treated otherwise. It was initially addressed for young women with premature ovarian failure. But this technique provides a valuable weapon to avoid age-related changes in the ovary, allowing premenopausal and menopausal women to get pregnant and fulfil their reproductive desire with acceptable success rates [28–30]. Moreover, the use of oocytes from donors has numerous advantages, as it reduces the rate of aneuploidies and stillbirth in women of advanced age. Case reports of successful pregnancy and delivery in a 70-year-old patient with donated oocytes demonstrate that the uterus may be able to maintain pregnancy far beyond the age of menopause [21]. Women are delaying childbearing; it is likely that the percentage of women looking for donor oocytes will increase, as it has been in the last decade.

3.5. Strategies to reduce twin pregnancies in the elderly mother

Twins occur spontaneously, and we still do not understand the causes or the conditions under which an embryo decides to split in two. However, the vast majority of twin pregnancies, particularly in women of advanced reproductive age, happened as a result of ART. Women seeking reproductive treatment usually have been trying to conceive spontaneously for a long period of time, and many have undergone previous unsuccessful treatments. Frustration, impatience, and economic costs are probably the main reasons why transfer of two and even three embryos is still a common practice in many countries [1]. This practice increases the chances of achieving pregnancy per embryo-transfer but also increases the chances of obtaining a multiple pregnancy. Multiple pregnancies have an important impact on the mothers' and babies' health as a consequence of medical and obstetric complications, and this carries an important economic burden for society, mainly due to preterm delivery, long hospital stay of the premature babies, and treatment of subsequent disabilities in the long term [31].

For obvious reasons, the main strategy to reduce the number of twin pregnancies in all women is the widespread use of the single embryo transfer (sET) during a fertility treatment. Our target should be to resemble the spontaneous twinning rate of embryos. Thanks to the development of vitrification, a fast freezing technique that increases post-thawed embryo survival rate, a single embryo can be transferred in a fresh cycle, while the rest will be transferred posteriorly in vitrified-thawed cycles without any loss of implantation potential [32]. The latest studies show the promising potential of sET to markedly reduce the risk of multiple pregnancy without affecting pregnancy outcomes. Even though sET might increase the time to pregnancy, minimising the risk of twin pregnancy becomes a huge advantage for public and individual health, particularly for elderly mothers.

4. Physiological homeostasis changes that may affect elderly mothers' health

During pregnancy, a series of physiological homeostatic changes take place in a woman's body that activate numerous adaptive mechanisms, mainly cardiovascular, respiratory, and hemodynamic. These changes are essential for the evolution and progress of a normal pregnancy. Adaptive mechanisms can be compromised as a consequence of underlying diseases, which appear more frequently in women of advanced age.

The increase in cardiac output, extracellular volume, and arterial compliance and the decrease in arterial blood pressure (BP) and peripheral resistance are some of the cardiovascular changes that occur in pregnant mothers [33]. Mean BP decreases during pregnancy presenting its lower values in the middle of the second trimester and then it starts to increase reaching values comparable to non-pregnant women at the end of pregnancy. In addition, redistribution of blood flow to different organs is essential in order to cover for the higher metabolic requirements, and so venous return and cardiac output raise dramatically [34]. There are also hormonal factors that favour these changes to appear. Oestrogens and relaxin are both involved in the production of nitrous oxide (NO), which produces vasodilatation during pregnancy and facilitates the distribution of blood to key organs [35, 36]. Ageing is associated with structural changes in the vascular wall, which leads to loss of arterial elasticity and reduced arterial compliance. Cardiovascular adaptive mechanisms could be impaired in elderly mothers due to pre-existing hypertensive disorders or venous insufficiency; therefore, they are at high risk of suffering from complications such as preeclampsia and placental insufficiency, increasing morbidity and mortality for both the mother and the baby.

Modifications in the respiratory system also take place during pregnancy. Pulmonary function is affected by location and orientation changes of the airway and configuration of the thorax due to the presence of the gravid uterus as well as hormonal effects. The elevation of the diaphragm decreases the lung's vertical diameter and subsequently enlarges the transversal and anteroposterior diameters. The displacement of the diaphragm produces a progressive decline in expiratory reserve volume and residual volume. Progesterone, cortisol, and relaxin produce dilatation of the airway in pregnant women reducing pulmonary resistance [37]. Ageing is associated with structural changes not only in the chest bones and diaphragm but also in the lung tissue. The dilatation of the alveoli decreases the exchange surface increasing the residual volume and functional residual capacity. These physiological changes added to those typical from pregnancy can cause alterations in the ventilation-perfusion ratio in elderly mothers.

Dilatation of the renal pelvis and ureters is characteristic during pregnancy on account of the growth of the uterus and the effect of hormones, such as progesterone, that cause relaxation of the smooth muscle. This predisposes women to suffer from urinary tract infections during pregnancy. Renal function is also modified during this period with an increased blood flow and glomerular filtration up to 60% [38]. Precisely for that reason, we should be aware of any medical pre-existing renal dysfunction that can worsen during pregnancy. For example, diabetes mellitus type 2 appears more often after the fourth decade of life and affects directly the renal function. Renal function–affected women need to be closely monitored during pregnancy.

These are only some of the major adaptive mechanisms in a woman's body during pregnancy, but there are many more subtle changes that occur in this period. We should pay attention to any minimal sign of hemodynamic decompensation especially in pregnant women of advanced age who are more likely to suffer from diseases, previously undiagnosed, as a result of ageing of their organs.

5. Obstetric complications in twin pregnancy related to age

There are not many studies specifically evaluating obstetric outcomes in twin pregnancies in advanced maternal age, and most of them are retrospective. These studies usually set the threshold for advanced maternal age at the "classic" 35 years, but in current times, this threshold should probably be reconsidered. A recent study by Zhu et al. [39] showed that, in twin pregnancies, advanced maternal age was associated with a higher risk of post-partum haemorrhage, gestational diabetes, and preterm delivery. However, other studies do not demonstrate any significantly increased risk over controls [40].

Much more attention has been paid to the obstetric complications in twins resulting from ART. Particularly, they are at increased risk of placenta praevia, caesarean section birth, preterm birth, and low birth weight [41]. Again, other studies showed no significant differences [42]. What we can be sure of is that twin pregnancies represent a huge demand for the body and that they do come with a higher obstetrical risk. Advanced age mothers' physical fitness necessarily cannot be the same to compensate for this fact.

5.1. Preterm delivery

We defined preterm delivery as birth prior to 37 weeks of gestation. Preterm birth complicates 5–18% of pregnancies and is the leading cause of neonatal death and the second cause of childhood death below the age of 5 years [43]. We should distinguish between preterm deliveries medically indicated secondary to foetal or maternal complications during pregnancy, such as preeclampsia, intrauterine growth restriction, or gestational diabetes, from those that occur after spontaneous onset of labour. Many studies have described multiple risk factors for preterm birth [44–47], although others propose this entity is a syndrome caused by multiple pathologic processes [43].

Twin pregnancy has been classically described as one of the risk factors associated with preterm birth. Although multiple gestation accounts for only 2–3% of all births, this type of gestation constitute 17% of births before 37 weeks of gestation and 23% of birth before 32 weeks [48]. The mechanism for preterm birth in multiple gestations may be related to the increased uterine distension; however, some studies suggest that the increased amount of oestrogen, progesterone, and sex steroids compared with singleton pregnancies could play an important role in the physiopathology of the syndrome [49, 50].

The effect of maternal age also influences the risk of preterm birth. Some studies suggest that even after adjusting for cofounders such as hypertension, diabetes, race, and mode of conception, maternal age over 40 years is an independent risk factor for preterm delivery [47, 51].

The widespread availability of reproductive technology has increased the percentage of multiple gestations and preterm delivery as an aftermath. Therefore, it is our duty to inform women of the risk of this type of pregnancies and enforce the use of the different strategies in order to achieve singleton pregnancy.

5.2. Preeclampsia

As we have seen before, mean BP decreases during the first and second trimesters secondary to the reduction of peripheral resistances and starts to increase reaching values similar to non-pregnant women in the third trimester.

Preeclampsia (PE) is a hypertensive disorder that appears during pregnancy. PE is a major obstetric complication that causes 15–20% of maternal mortality worldwide, especially in developing countries [52]. It is characterised by the presence of high BP (> 140/90 mmHg) and proteinuria (> 300 mg/dL) beyond 20 weeks of pregnancy. The finding of higher values of BP before this stage of pregnancy is considered chronic hypertension, which can also worsen in the second half of pregnancy, with what we call superimposed preeclampsia. The physiopathology of this multisystemic disorder still remains unknown.

In the last decades, several aetiologies have been described. Some authors suggest that it appears secondary to an abnormal vascular response of the uterine blood vessels to trophoblast invasion, causing platelet aggregation and endothelial dysfunction [52–54]. The increase of BP during pregnancy can also have an effect on the foetus, developing complications such as low birth weight, oligoamnios, and intrauterine growth restriction [54, 55]. In addition, preeclampsia is considered severe when it affects multiple organs, finally producing pulmonary oedema, renal failure, seizures, thrombocytopenia, elevation of liver enzymes, and disseminated intravascular coagulation [54].

The rate of preeclampsia ranges between 2 and 7% in healthy nulliparous women [54, 56, 57]. These rates increase to 14% in twin pregnancies [58]. Preeclampsia is regarded as typical of the first pregnancy. In spite of this, the risk of developing preeclampsia in subsequent pregnancies raises till 18% [58].

Numerous studies proposed several risk factors to classify a specific group of women who are at a high risk of developing preeclampsia, including nulliparity, older age, chronic hypertension, and diabetes mellitus [59–61]. Other studies indicate that, after adjusting for other cofounders, women of advanced maternal age are 1.5 times more likely to have preeclampsia compared to those under 35 years of age [62]. Multiple pregnancy is a moderate risk factor for the development of pre-eclampsia during pregnancy. Women with multiple pregnancy, who have any of the other moderate risk factors for pre-eclampsia (first pregnancy, age 40 years or older, pregnancy interval of more than 10 years, BMI of 35 kg/m^2 or more at first visit, or family history of preeclampsia), should receive a daily aspirin dose [63].

As we have seen before, single-embryo transfer is the main technique to reduce the rate of twin pregnancies. We should focus our effort on identifying those women with pre-existing medical conditions who are predisposed to suffer PE and, if applying ART, enforce the importance of achieving a singleton gestation to avoid adverse perinatal outcomes.

5.3. Gestational diabetes

Gestational diabetes mellitus (GDM) is a diabetic state diagnosed for the first time in pregnancy. It is one of the most common metabolic disorders in pregnancy. GDM complicates 3–5% of pregnancies and it is considered a risk factor for adverse perinatal outcomes, such as macrosomia, shoulder dystocia, cerebral palsy, and foetal death [64–66]. It is defined as basal glucose ≥126 mg/dl (7.0 mmol/l), HbA1c ≥ 6.5% (47.5 mmol/mol), or glucose levels ≥200 mg/dl (11.1 mmol/l) at any time of the day or screen positive for any of the GDM tests available [67].

Diabetes predisposes pregnant women to suffer urine infections, hypertensive disorders, and prematurity. It is well known that pregestational diabetes can cause foetal malformations, intrauterine growth restriction, stillbirth, and congenital heart disease probably due to vascular alterations in mothers. Both gestational and pregestational diabetes have effects on the foetus secondary to hyperinsulinemia, such as macrosomia, polyhydramnios, and foetal lung immaturity that may cause foetal neonatal distress.

Women of advanced maternal age are at a higher risk of developing GDM [68]. Twin pregnancies have also been related to GDM [69]. The development of GDM usually indicates a reduced pancreatic reserve in the pregnant mother and is a marker of pre-diabetes, putting them at a higher risk of developing diabetes mellitus type 2 in the future. It is essential to highlight the importance of adopting healthy habits during pregnancy in order to avoid consequences for the future health of both the mother and the baby.

Gestational diabetes in twins is also associated with an increased risk of hypertensive disorders, macrosomia, and preterm birth, but it reduces the risk for low birth weight [70]. Furthermore, it has been suggested that gestational diabetes could potentially benefit twin pregnancies, as low 5-min Apgar score and neonatal death are reduced in twins compared to singletons when this maternal complication is present, maybe due to the increased birth weight of the twin pairs [71, 72]. However, growth in the twin pair tends to be asymmetric when GDM or glucose intolerance is present [73].

Early diagnosis and treatment are essential in order to avoid complications during pregnancy. Nowadays, guidelines from different countries recommend the screening for gestational diabetes in women with risk factors such as previous history of gestational diabetes, obesity (body mass index over 30 kg/m^2), and previous delivery of a macrosomic baby [74–76]. Some of them support the use of a universal screening test in the second trimester and also in the first trimester in every woman over the age of 35 [77]. However, the increase in maternal age over the last years implies offering this diagnostic test to a very high percentage of the pregnant population [70]. Given the importance of early treatment, all twin pregnancies, as well as in the case of advanced maternal age, first trimester screening should be considered, although there is no international agreement [78].

5.4. Growth abnormalities

In mothers older than 40, small and large for gestational age babies and intrauterine growth restriction (IUGR) are increased [79, 80]. Small-for-gestational-age babies (SGA) and IUGR are assumed to be due to placental dysfunction, whose incidence increases with age.

One study found in a very large twin cohort that advanced maternal age was indirectly associated with SGA babies. However, when SGA was present in an older mother, neonatal mortality increased compared to appropriate-for-gestational-age twins in the same age range [81], maybe suggesting an increased severity of the syndrome in this women.

Although it may look as a contradiction, foetal macrosomia also seems to increase with age. It has been suggested that this increased incidence in large-for-gestational-age babies might be due to an overall increase in the body mass index with age [82] and an increased risk of gestational diabetes. However, as we previously mentioned, the increased birth weight in twin pregnancies associated with gestational diabetes could be beneficial for the twin pair, or at least not as detrimental as it could be in singletons.

5.5. Post-partum haemorrhage

Most protocols worldwide recognise maternal age as an independent risk factor for >10,000 mL blood loss during delivery and for post-partum haemorrhage, in both vaginal and caesarean births. Mechanisms behind this increased risk are not well established. Most doctors working in a labour ward are persuaded that uterine atony is somehow more common among older mothers, although there is no evidence for that. Age is associated with certain obstetric complications, such as hypertensive disorders, placental abnormalities, or preterm birth. On the other hand, advanced maternal age increases the risk of induction of labour, large foetuses for gestational age, prolonged labour, oxytocin augmentation, or caesarean delivery. All of the above are well known risk factors of post-partum haemorrhage [83, 84]. So age may not act as a completely independent factor for post-partum haemorrhage. Results from the WOMAN trial showed an adjusted odds ratio of peripartum hysterectomy of 5.98 (95% CI: 3.34–10.70) for women between 30 and 39 years and of 11.73 (95% CI: 6.30–21.85) for women aged ≥40 [85]. This is a trend shown to be repeated worldwide [86]. Advanced maternal age does not only increase the risk of excessive bleeding but also its severity and the risk of needing aggressive treatment strategies, such as hysterectomy.

Again, twin pergnancy is also associated with a higher risk of post-partum haemorrhage. At the same time, twin pregnancy is often associated with other post-partum haemorrhage risk factors, such as preeclampsia, caesarean delivery, and the use of a caesarean delivery for a preterm delivery [87]. Delivery in this group of patients should be undertaken in tertiary hospitals by trained staff.

5.6. Venous thrombosis

The incidence of deep venous thrombosis is increased three times during pregnancy. Pulmonary embolism may occur in 1 in every 1000 pregnancies and represents the leading non-obstetrical cause of maternal death [88]. Both age older than 35 years and multiple pregnancy are listed as risk factors for venous thromboembolism. If we consider that the presence of thrombophilia is more common in women undergoing IVF and that deep venous thrombosis is also more common in these women [89, 90], we could conclude that women of advanced maternal age and carrying a multiple pregnancy definitely represent a high-risk group for venous thromboembolism. Under any other risk factor, thromboprophylaxis should be considered carefully.

5.7. Stillbirth

Advanced maternal age has been associated with an increased incidence of stillbirth [91]. A mechanism under this increase is placental dysfunction, which accounts for around 65% of stillbirths, and it has been observed more frequently in mice models and humans with age. Placentas from older mothers (35–39 and ≥ 40 years old) are less efficient in the sense that foetal/placenta weight ratio was lower than placentas from controls under 30 years old. They seem to be bigger in size and display mechanisms to ameliorate function, like increased relaxation of myometrium arteries and increased amino acid transport, but this does not correlate with a higher birth weight in the offspring. The hypothesis is that an increased size could be an adaptive mechanism trying to make up for placental dysfunction [92]. It has also been suggested that the greater contribution to stillbirth in older mothers could arise from their increased risk of chromosomal abnormalities [80].

Twin pregnancies are also high risk for stillbirth and neonatal death, increasing thirteenfold in monochorionic and fivefold in dichorionic pregnancies compared to singletons [93, 94].

Although this is not under the scope of this chapter, advanced paternal age has also been associated with stillbirth and death of the child before 5 years of age [95, 96]. The risk might be linked to a higher rate of sperm chromatin or chromosomal aberrations. Interestingly, this association dissolves when adjusting for paternal education level, when the association between advanced maternal age and the risk of stillbirth is independent of socioeconomic and educational levels.

6. Delivery and post-partum care in twin pregnancies in advanced maternal age

6.1. Delivery mode and time of delivery

Advanced maternal age is associated with a high frequency of caesarean delivery. Many factors participate in this. For instances, a more frequent prolonged labour due to worse myometrial function and decreased flexibility of pelvic joints [97], increased frequency of large babies

[98, 99], and the presence of coexisting obstetrical or medical complications associated with poorer obstetric outcomes. However, most women over 40 have a successful vaginal delivery even after induction of labour without an increased risk for operative vaginal delivery or perineal trauma [100].

In dichorionic twin pregnancies, the perinatal risks are balanced with the risks associated with iatrogenic prematurity until 37 + 0–6 weeks' gestation and until 36 + 0–6 in monochorionic pregnancies, with higher risks of stillbirths than neonatal deaths beyond this gestation [94].

Pre-labour caesarean delivery may be beneficial in pregnancies with the first twin in non-cephalic presentation or when any or both the twins have a low weight, but evidence for both statements is not strong [100].

6.2. Post-partum care

When obstetric complications such as preeclampsia or diabetes mellitus presented during pergnancy, persistence of medical conditions such as chronic hypertension and type 2 diabetes (T2DM) should be monitored after delivery. Chronic hypertension in women affected by gestational hypertension or preeclampsia is a common event, usually developing years after delivery [101]. Age at pregnancy might reduce this time interval, but this has not been studied before. Likewise, age does not increase the odds of post-partum eclampsia [102]. Age at pregnancy is a risk factor for the development of T2DM when GDM is present [103]. Anyhow, advanced maternal age is a risk factor for developing cardiovascular complications during pregnancy and for developing severe morbidity due to cardiovascular disease [104], so strict and long-term follow-up strategies should be put in place.

Secondary post-partum haemorrhage is increased in women affected by primary post-partum haemorrhage and in women ≥35 years old, both risk factors being independently associated with the event [105].

Maternal age at delivery >35 years has been indicated as a risk factor for venous thromboembolism in the post-partum period and later in life [106]. However, its contribution is probably small when compared to other factors, such as caesarean delivery [107].

Twin pregnancies are also associated with all the complications mentioned above. Again, this specific population is particularly vulnerable for developing post-partum complications.

Various studies suggest that advanced maternal age at the time of delivery is associated with a higher risk of developing stress urinary incompetence (SUI) in the post-partum period [108, 109]. Suspected aetiological mechanisms are many and they are thought to start developing during pregnancy. Some studies suggest that vaginal delivery may worsen SUI, particularly in elderly women, and advise a caesarean delivery in this population when SUI is already present during pregnancy [108]. However, this protective effect is not consistent in literature, so currently, such a recommendation is controversial [110]. Of course, pelvic floor changes are greater in twin pregnancies, as abdominal pressure on it is irredeemably higher [111]. Anyhow, elderly mothers carrying a twin pregnancy are at higher risk of developing pelvic floor disorders, so preventive strategies should be enforced during pregnancy and early investigation and proper treatment in the post-partum period.

Advanced maternal age is considered to be a risk factor for post-partum depression [112]. This is a poorly studied condition, which can be devastating for the mothers, children, and family. On the other hand, parents of twins frequently experience higher levels of anxiety and depression and are at higher risk for post-partum depression and for marital decline [113, 114]. Post-partum depression has also been linked to preterm birth, so common among twins, due to a lesser mother-infant interaction and parents' concern for both medical and economic subsequent issues [115]. Sleeping disorders 3 months post-partum are more frequent in mothers older than 35 years old [116]. Psychosocial and physical support should be provided.

7. Long-term disabilities due to advanced maternal age

Several neurological disorders have been shown to be more frequent in children born from elderly mothers, particularly cerebral palsy [117, 118] and autism spectrum disorders [119]. In terms of learning disabilities, one study found that developmental vulnerability decreases with the mother's age from 15 to 30 years, but starts to increase when the mother is older than 35, this increase being independent from the socioeconomic status [120]. Interestingly, children born from old parents show a poorer neurocognitive performance in childhood [121]. However, environment might make up for the "biological disadvantage", as older parents are usually in a better financial state, are more highly educated, and usually have reached a more stable couple/marriage situation. All this may give them certain emotional maturity and life experience that improves child-rearing abilities. Compared to singletons, twins exhibited higher rates of cerebral palsy and mental retardation and showed more pronounced speech delays, motor development, and behavioural problems. However, the main explaining factor is the higher frequency for preterm delivery that results in low and very low birth weight children [122]. Maternal age contributes by increasing the risk for preterm delivery, but the same way in singletons and twins.

Trisomy 21 is very well known to increase with maternal age due to meiotic non-disjunction errors. More recently, mitochondrial dysfunction and epigenetic changes associated with oocyte ageing can be inherited by the descendant and may predispose also to chromosome segregation errors in grandchildren [123].

8. Conclusions

Twin pregnancy in advanced reproductive age represents a very vulnerable population for obstetric and medical complication during and after pregnancy. Most of these pregnancies are a result of assisted reproduction. Counselling prior to treatment is essential, particularly to discern whether the woman is fit for pregnancy and to enforce specific preventive strategies, such as single embryo transfer. Both conditions, advanced maternal age and twin pregnancy, are risk factors for many obstetric and medical complications. During pregnancy, early diagnosis and treatment of the issues discussed in this chapter can reduce risks and sequelae to the minimum.

Author details

Laura Pérez Martín[1]* and Duna Trobo Marina[2]

*Address all correspondence to: laurapmar@gmail.com

1 HM Fertility Center Puerta del Sur, Móstoles, Spain

2 Gregorio Marañón University Hospital, Madrid, Spain

References

[1] Bateman BT, Simpson LL. Higher rate of stillbirth at the extremes of reproductive age: A large nationwide sample of deliveries in the United States. American Journal of Obstetrics and Gynecology. 2006;**194**:840-845

[2] National Institute for Clinical Excellence. Multiple Pregnancy: Antenatal Care for Twin and Triplet Pregnancies. Clinical Guideline 129. National Collaborating Centre for Women's and Children's Health. London, UK: NICE; 2011

[3] Calhaz-Jorge C, De Geyter C, Kupka MS, de Mouzon J, Erb K, Mocanu E, et al. The European IVF-monitoring (EIM) Consortium for the European Society of Human Reproduction and Embryology (ESHRE). Assisted reproductive technology in Europe, 2013: Results generated from European registers by ESHRE. Human Reproduction. 2017;**32**(10):1957-1973

[4] Basso O, Weinberg CR, D'Aloisio AA, Sandler DP. Maternal age at birth and daughters' subsequent childlessness. Human Reproduction. 2018;**33**(2):311-319

[5] Bracewell-Milnes T, Saso S, Bora S, Ismail AM, Al-Memar M, Hamed AH, et al. Investigating psychosocial attitudes, motivations and experiences of oocyte donors, recipients and egg sharers: A systematic review. Human Reproduction Update. 2016;**22**(4):450-465

[6] Sauer MV, Paulson RJ, Lobo RA. Oocyte donation to women of advanced reproductive age: Pregnancy results and obstetrical outcomes in patients 45 years and older. Human Reproduction. 1996;**11**(11):2540-2543

[7] Ethics Committee of the American Society for Reproductive Medicine. Oocyte or embryo donation to women of advanced reproductive age: An ethics committee opinion. Fertility and Sterility. 2016;**106**(5):e3-e7

[8] Klein NA, Battaglia DE, Fujimoto VY, Davis GS, Bremner WJ, Soules MR. Reproductive aging: Accelerated ovarian follicular development associated with a monotropic follicle-stimulating hormone rise in normal older women. The Journal of Clinical Endocrinology and Metabolism. 1996;**81**:1038-1045

[9] Lenton EA, Landgren BM, Sexton L, Harper R. Normal variation in the length of the follicular phase of the menstrual cycle: Effect of chronological age. British Journal of Obstetrics and Gynaecology. 1984;**91**:681-684

[10] Reyes FI, Winters JS, Faiman C. Pituitary-ovarian relationships preceding the menopause. A cross-sectional study of serum follice-stimulating hormone, luteinizing hormone, prolactin, estradiol, and progesterone levels. American Journal of Obstetrics and Gynecology. 1977;**129**:557-564

[11] Santoro N, Brown JR, Adel T, Skurnick JH. Characterization of reproductive hormonal dynamics in the perimenopause. The Journal of Clinical Endocrinology and Metabolism. 1996;**81**:1495-1501

[12] Shideler SE, DeVane GW, Kalra PS, Benirschke K, Lasley BL. Ovarian-pituitary hormone interactions during the perimenopause. Maturitas. 1989;**11**:331-339

[13] Santoro N, Isaac B, Neal-Perry G, Adel T, Weingart L, Nussbaum A, et al. Impaired folliculogenesis and ovulation in older reproductive aged women. The Journal of Clinical Endocrinology and Metabolism. 2003;**88**(11):5502-5509

[14] Gruijters MJ, Visser JA, Durlinger AL, Themmen AP. Anti-Mullerian hormone and its role in ovarian function. Molecular and Cellular Endocrinology. 2003;**211**:85-90

[15] Barad DH, Weghofer A, Gleicher N. Comparing anti-Mullerian hormone (AMH) and follicle-stimulating hormone (FSH) as predictors of ovarian function. Fertility and Sterility. 2009;**91**:1553-1555

[16] Yang YS, Hur MH, Kim SY, Young K. Correlation between sonographic and endocrine markers of ovarian aging as predictors for late menopausal transition. Menopause. 2011;**18**:138-145

[17] Shapiro M, Talbert GB. The effect of maternal age on decidualization in the mouse. Journal of Gerontology. 1974;**29**:145-148

[18] Holinka CF, Finch CE. Age-related changes in the decidual response of the C57BL/6J mouse uterus. Biology of Reproduction. 1977;**16**:385-393

[19] Holinka CF, Tseng Y-C, Finch CE. Reproductive ageing in C57BL/6J mice: Plasma progesterone, viable embryos and resorption frequency throughout pregnancy. Biology of Reproduction. 1979;**20**:1201-1211

[20] Sorger T, Soderwall A. The aging uterus and the role of edema in endometrial function. Biology of Reproduction. 1981;**24**:1135-1144

[21] Nelson SM, Telfer EE, Anderson RA. The ageing ovary and uterus: New biological insights. Human Reproduction Update. 2013;**19**(1):67-83

[22] Fretts RC, Schmittdiel J, McLean FH, Usher RH, Goldman MB. Increased maternal age and the risk of fetal death. The New England Journal of Medicine. 1995;**333**:953-957

[23] Kwon JY, Park IY, Kwon SM, Kim CJ, Shin JC. The quadruple test for down syndrome screening in pregnant women of advanced maternal age. Archives of Gynecology and Obstetrics. 2012;**285**:629-633

[24] Dailey T, Dale B, Cohen J, Munne S. Association between nondisjunction and maternal age in meiosis-II human oocytes. American Journal of Human Genetics. 1996;**59**:176-184

[25] Freeman SB, Allen EG, Oxford-Wright CL, Tinker SW, Druschel C, Hobbs CA, et al. The National down Syndrome Project: Design and implementation. Public Health Reports. 2007;**122**:62-72

[26] Ferguson-Smith MA, Yates JR. Maternal age specific rates for chromosome aberrations and factors influencing them: Report of a collaborative European study on 52 965 amniocenteses. Prenatal Diagnosis. 1984;**4**:5-44

[27] Beta J, Lesmes-Heredia C, Bedetti C, Akolebar R. Risk of miscarriage following amniocentesis and chorionic villus sampling: A systematic review of the literature. Minerva Ginecologica. 2018;**70**:215-219

[28] Sauer MV, Paulson RJ, Lobo RA. Reversing the natural decline in human fertility: An extended clinical trial of oocyte donation to woman of advanced reproductive age. JAMA. 1992;**268**:1275-1279

[29] Pantos K, Meimeti-Damianaki T, Vaxevanoglou T, Kapetanakis E. Oocyte donation in menopausal women aged over 40 years. Human Reproduction. 1993;**8**:488-491

[30] Paulson RJ, Hatch IE, Lobo RA, Sauer MV. Cumulative conception and live birth rate after oocyte donation: Implications regarding endometrial receptivity. Human Reproduction. 1997;**12**:835-839

[31] Callahan T, Hall J, Ettner S, Christiansen C, Greene M, Crowley W. The economic impact of multiple-gestation pregnancies and the contribution of assisted-reproduction techniques to their incidence. The New England Journal of Medicine. 1994;**331**(4):244-249

[32] Cobo A, Diaz C. Clinical application of oocyte vitrification: A systematic review and meta-analysis of randomized controlled trials. Fertility and Sterility. 2011;**96**:277-285

[33] Christianson RE. Studies on blood pressure during pregnancy. I. Influence of parity and age. American Journal of Obstetrics and Gynecology. 1976;**125**:509-513

[34] Meah VL, Cockcroft JR, Backx K, Shave R, Stöhr EJ. Cardiac output and related haemodynamics during pregnancy: A series of meta-analyses. Heart. 2016;**102**(7):518-526

[35] Sladek SM, Magness RR, Conrad KP. Nitric oxide and pregnancy. The American Journal of Physiology. 1997;**272**:R441-R463

[36] Conrad KP, Novak J. Emerging role of relaxin in renal and cardiovascular function. American Journal of Physiology. Regulatory, Integrative and Comparative Physiology. 2004;**287**:R250-R261

[37] Wise RA, Polito AJ, Krishnan V. Respiratory physiologic changes in pregnancy. Immunology and Allergy Clinics of North America. 2006;**26**(1):1-12

[38] Gulmi F, Felsen D, Vaughan E. Pathophysiology of urinary tract obstruction. In: Campbell's Urology. 11th ed. Philadelphia: Saunders; 2002. pp. 1089-1103

[39] Zhu C, Wang M, Niu G, Yang J, Wang Z. Obstetric outcomes of twin pregnancies at advanced maternal age: A retrospective study. Taiwanese Journal of Obstetrics & Gynecology. 2018;**57**(1):64-67

[40] Prapas N, Kalogiannidis I, Prapas I, Xiromeritis P, Karagiannidis A, Makedos G. Twin gestation in older women: Antepartum, intrapartum complications, and perinatal outcomes. Archives of Gynecology and Obstetrics. 2006;**273**(5):293-297

[41] Qin JB, Wang H, Sheng X, Xie Q, Gao S. Assisted reproductive technology and risk of adverse obstetric outcomes in dichorionic twin pregnancies: A systematic review and meta-analysis. Fertility and Sterility. 2016;**105**(5):1180-1192

[42] Geisler ME, O'Mahony A, Meaney S, Waterstone JJ, O'Donoghue K. Obstetric and perinatal outcomes of twin pregnancies conceived following IVF/ICSI treatment compared with spontaneously conceived twin pregnancies. European Journal of Obstetrics, Gynecology, and Reproductive Biology. 2014;**181**:78-83

[43] Romero R, Dey SK, Fisher SJ. Preterm labor: One syndrome, many causes. Science. 2014;**345**(6198):760-765

[44] Esplin MS, O'Brien E, Fraser A, Kerber RA, Clark E, Simonsen SE, et al. Estimating recurrence of spontaneous preterm delivery. Obstetrics and Gynecology. 2008;**112**(3):516-523

[45] Köck K, Köck F, Klein K. Diabetes mellitus and the risk of preterm birth with regard to the risk of spontaneous preterm birth. The Journal of Maternal-Fetal & Neonatal Medicine. 2010;**23**(9):1004-1008

[46] Di Renzo GC, Giardina I, Rosati A, Clerici G, Torricelli M, Petraglia F, et al. Maternal risk factors for preterm birth: A country-based population analysis. European Journal of Obstetrics, Gynecology, and Reproductive Biology. 2011;**159**(2):342-346

[47] Fuchs F, Monet B, Ducruet T, Chaillet N, Audibert F. Effect of maternal age on the risk of preterm birth: A large cohort study. PLoS One. 2018;**13**(1):e0191002

[48] Kiely JL. What is the population-based risk of preterm birth among twins and other multiples? Clinical Obstetrics and Gynecology. 1998;**41**(1):3

[49] TambyRaja RL, Ratnam SS. Plasma steroid changes in twin pregnancies. Progress in Clinical and Biological Research. 1981;**69A**:189

[50] Muechler EK, Huang KE. Plasma estrogen and progesterone in quintuplet pregnancy induced with menotropins. American Journal of Obstetrics and Gynecology. 1983;**147**(1):105

[51] Delbaere I, Verstraelen H, Goetgeluk S, Martens G, De Backer G, Temmerman M. Pregnancy outcome in primiparae of advanced maternal age. European Journal of Obstetrics, Gynecology, and Reproductive Biology. 2007;**135**(1):41-46

[52] Report of the National High Blood Pressure Education Program. Working group report on high blood pressure in pregnancy. American Journal of Obstetrics and Gynecology. 2000;**183**:S1-S22

[53] Duley L. Pre-eclampsia and the hypertensive disorders of pregnancy. British Medical Bulletin. 2003;**67**:161-176

[54] Sibai BM. Diagnosis and management of gestational hypertension and preeclampsia. Obstetrics and Gynecology. 2003;**102**:181-192

[55] Ness RB, Roberts JM. Heterogeneous causes constituting the single syndrome of preeclampsia: A hypothesis and its implications. American Journal of Obstetrics and Gynecology. 1996;**175**(5):1365-1370

[56] Hauth JC, Ewell MG, Levine RL, Esterlitz JR, Sibai BM, Curet LB. Pregnancy outcomes in healthy nulliparous women who subsequently developed hypertension. Obstetrics and Gynecology. 2000;**95**:24-28

[57] Vatten LJ, Skjaerven R. Is pre-eclampsia more than one disease? BJOG. 2004;**111**:298-302

[58] Sibai BM, Caritis S, Hauth J, Lindheimer MD, MacPherson C, Klebanoff M, et al. Hypertensive disorders in twin versus singleton gestations. National Institute of Child Health and Human Development Network of Maternal-Fetal Medicine Units. American Journal of Obstetrics and Gynecology. 2000;**182**:938-942

[59] Ruano R, Fontes RS, Zugaib M. Prevention of preeclampsia with low-dose aspirin – A systematic review and meta-analysis of the main randomized controlled trials. Clinics (São Paulo, Brazil). 2005;**60**(5):407-414

[60] Cnossen JS, ter Riet G, Mol BW, et al. Are tests for predicting pre-eclampsia good enough to make screening viable? A review of reviews and critical appraisal. Acta Obstetricia et Gynecologica Scandinavica. 2009;**88**(7):758-765

[61] Bartsch E, Medcalf KE, Park AL, Ray JG, High Risk of Pre-eclampsia Identification Group. Clinical risk factors for pre-eclampsia determined in early pregnancy: Systematic review and meta-analysis of large cohort studies. BMJ. 2016;**353**:i1753

[62] Lamminpää R, Vehviläinen-Julkunen K, Gissler M, Heinonen S. Preeclampsia complicated by advanced maternal age: A registry-based study on primiparous women in Finland 1997-2008. BMC Pregnancy and Childbirth. 2012;**11**:12-47

[63] National Institute for Clinical Excellence. Hypertension in Pregnancy: The Management of Hypertensive Disorders during Pregnancy. Clinical Guideline. National Collaborating Centre for Women's and Children's Health. London, UK: NICE; 2010

[64] Crowther CA, Hiller JE, Moss JR, McPhee AJ, Jeffries WS, Robinson JS, et al. Effect of treatment of gestational diabetes mellitus on pregnancy outcomes. The New England Journal of Medicine. 2005;**352**:2477-2486

[65] Shand AW, Bell JC, McElduffs A, Morris J, Roberts CL. Outcomes of pregnancies in women with pre-gestational diabetes mellitus and gestational diabetes mellitus; a

population-based study in New South Wales, Australia, 1998-2002. Diabetic Medicine. 2008;**5**:708-715

[66] Mohammadbeigi A, Farhadifar F, Soufi Zadeh N, Mohammadsalehi N, Rezaiee M, Aghaei M. Fetal macrosomia: Risk factors, maternal, and perinatal outcome. Annals of Medical and Health Sciences Research. 2013;**3**(4):546-550

[67] International Association of Diabetes and Pregnancy Study Groups. International association of diabetes and pregnancy study groups recommendations on the diagnosis and classification of hyperglycemia in pregnancy. Diabetes Care. 2010;**33**:676-682

[68] Makgoba M, Savvidou MD, Steer PJ. An analysis of the interrelationship between maternal age, body mass index and racial origin in the development of gestational diabetes mellitus. BJOG : An International Journal of Obstetrics and Gynaecology. 2012;**119**(3):276-282

[69] Rauh-Hain JA, Rana S, Tamez H, Wang A, Cohen B, Cohen A, et al. Risk for developing gestational diabetes in women with twin pregnancies. The Journal of Maternal-Fetal & Neonatal Medicine. 2009;**22**(4):293-299

[70] González González NL, Goya M, Bellart J, Lopez J, Sancho MA, Mozas J, et al. Obstetric and perinatal outcome in women with twin pregnancy and gestational diabetes. The Journal of Maternal-Fetal & Neonatal Medicine. 2012;**25**(7):1084-1089

[71] Luo ZC, Simonet F, Wei SQ, Xu H, Rey E, Fraser WD. Diabetes in pregnancy may differentially affect neonatal outcomes for twins and singletons. Diabetic Medicine. 2011;**28**(9):1068-1073

[72] Guillén MA, Herranz L, Barquiel B, Hillman N, Burgos MA, Pallardo LF. Influence of gestational diabetes mellitus on neonatal weight outcome in twin pregnancies. Diabetic Medicine. 2014;**31**(12):1651-1656

[73] Tward C, Barrett J, Berger H, Kibel M, Pittini A, Halperin I, et al. Does gestational diabetes affect fetal growth and pregnancy outcome in twin pregnancies? American Journal of Obstetrics and Gynecology. 2016;**214**(5):653.e1-8

[74] National Institute for Clinical Excellence. Diabetes in Pregnancy: Full Guideline. Clinical Guideline 63. National Collaborating Centre for Women's and Children's Health. London, UK: NICE; 2008

[75] Grupo Español de Diabetes y Embarazo (GEDE). Care of pregnancies complicated by diabetes. Clinical Practice Guidelines: 2014 update. Avances en Diabetología. 2015;**31**:45-59

[76] Committee on Practice Bulletins—Obstetrics. ACOG Practice Bulletin No. 190: Gestational diabetes mellitus. Obstetrics and Gynecology. 2018;**131**(2):e49-e64

[77] Scott DA, Loveman E, McIntyre L, Waugh N. Screening for gestational diabetes: A systematic review and economic evaluation. Health Technology Assessment. 2002;**6**:1-161

[78] Caissutti C, Berghella V. Scientific evidence for different options for GDM screening and management: Controversies and review of the literature. BioMed Research International. 2017;**2017**:2746471

[79] Zapata-Masias Y, Marqueta B, Gómez Roig MD, Gonzalez-Bosquet E. Obstetric and perinatal outcomes in women ≥40years of age: Associations with fetal growth disorders. Early Human Development. 2016;**100**:17-20

[80] Lean SC, Derricott H, Jones RL, Heazell AEP. Advanced maternal age and adverse pregnancy outcomes: A systematic review and meta-analysis. PLoS One. 2017;**12**(10):e0186287

[81] Kristensen S, Salihu HM, Keith LG, Kirby RS, Pass MA, Fowler KB. Impact of advanced maternal age on neonatal survival of twin small-for-gestational-age subtypes. The Journal of Obstetrics and Gynaecology Research. 2007;**33**(3):259-265

[82] Weng YH, Yang CY, Chiu YW. Risk assessment of adverse birth outcomes in relation to maternal age. PLoS One. 2014;**9**(12):e114843

[83] Kramer MS, Berg C, Abenhaim H, Dahhou M, Rouleau J, Mehrabadi A, et al. Incidence, risk factors, and temporal trends in severe postpartum hemorrhage. American Journal of Obstetrics and Gynecology. 2013;**209**(5):449.e1-7

[84] Ekin A, Gezer C, Solmaz U, Taner CE, Dogan A, Ozeren M. Predictors of severity in primary postpartum hemorrhage. Archives of Gynecology and Obstetrics. 2015;**292**(6):1247-1254

[85] Hugue S, Roberts I, Fawole B, Chaudhri R, Arulkumaran S, Shakur-Still H. Risk factors for peripartum hysterectomy among women with postpartum haemorrhage: Analysis of data from the WOMAN trial. BMC Pregnancy and Childbirth. 2018;**18**(1):186

[86] Sheldon WR, Blum J, Vogel JP, Souza JP, Gülmezoglu AM, Winikoff B, et al. Postpartum haemorrhage management, risks, and maternal outcomes: Findings from the World Health Organization Multicountry Survey on Maternal and Newborn Health. BJOG. 2014;**121**(Suppl 1):5-13

[87] Young BC, Wylie BJ. Effects of twin gestation on maternal morbidity. Seminars in Perinatology. 2012;**36**(3):162-168

[88] Gray G, Nelson-Piercy C. Thromboembolic disorders in obstetrics. Best Practice & Research. Clinical Obstetrics & Gynaecology. 2012;**26**(1):53-64

[89] Petukhova NL, Tsaturova KA, Vartanian EV, Schigoleva AV, Markin AV. Study of the frequency of occurrence of genetic and acquired thrombophilia in infertile women prior IVF. Gynecological Endocrinology. 2014;**30**(Suppl 1):32-34

[90] Hansen AT, Kesmodel US, Juul S, Hvas AM. Increased venous thrombosis incidence in pregnancies after in vitro fertilization. Human Reproduction. 2014;**29**(3):611-617

[91] Huang L, Sauve R, Birkett N, Fergusson D, van Walraven C. Maternal age and risk of stillbirth: A systematic review. CMAJ. 2008;**178**(2):165-172

[92] Lean SC, Heazell AEP, Dilworth MR, Mills TA, Jones RL. Placental dysfunction underlies increased risk of fetal growth restriction and stillbirth in advanced maternal age women. Scientific Reports. 2017;**7**(1):9677

[93] Peter C, Wenzlaff P, Kruempelmann J, Alzen G, Bueltmann E. Perinatal morbidity and early neonatal mortality in twin pregnancies. Open Journal of Obstetrics and Gynecology. 2013;**3**:78-89

[94] Cheong-See F, Schuit E, Arroyo-Manzano D, Khalil A, Barrett J, Joseph KS, et al. Prospective risk of stillbirth and neonatal complications in twin pregnancies: Systematic review and meta-analysis. BMJ. 2016;**354**:i4353

[95] Urhoj SK, Andersen PK, Mortensen LH, Davey Smith G, Nybo Andersen AM. Advanced paternal age and stillbirth rate: A nationwide register-based cohort study of 944,031 pregnancies in Denmark. European Journal of Epidemiology. 2017;**32**(3):227-234

[96] Nybo Andersen AM, Urhoj SK. Is advanced paternal age a health risk for the offspring? Fertility and Sterility. 2017;**107**(2):312-318

[97] Dougherty CR, Jones AD. Obstetric management and outcome related to maternal characteristics. American Journal of Obstetrics and Gynecology. 1988;**158**(3 Pt 1):470-474

[98] Kenny LC, Lavender T, McNamee R, O'Neill SM, Mills T, Khashan AS. Advanced maternal age and adverse pregnancy outcome: Evidence from a large contemporary cohort. PLoS One. 2013;**8**(2):e56583

[99] Li G, Kong L, Li Z, Zhang L, Fan L, Zou L, et al. Prevalence of macrosomia and its risk factors in China: A multicentre survey based on birth data involving 101,723 singleton term infants. Paediatric and Perinatal Epidemiology. 2014;**28**(4):345-350

[100] Ganchimeg T, Morisaki N, Vogel JP, Cecatti JG, Barrett J, Jayaratne K, et al. Mode and timing of twin delivery and perinatal outcomes in low- and middle-income countries: A secondary analysis of the WHO Multicountry Survey on Maternal and Newborn Health. BJOG. 2014;**121**(Suppl 1):89-100

[101] Groenhof TKJ, van Rijn BB, Franx A, Roeters van Lennep JE, Bots ML, Lely AT. Preventing cardiovascular disease after hypertensive disorders of pregnancy: Searching for the how and when. European Journal of Preventive Cardiology. 2017;**24**(16):1735-1745

[102] Al-Safi Z, Imudia AN, Filetti LC, Hobson DT, Bahado-Singh RO, Awonuga AO. Delayed postpartum preeclampsia and eclampsia: Demographics, clinical course, and complications. Obstetrics and Gynecology. 2011;**118**(5):1102-1107

[103] Capula C, Chiefari E, Vero A, Foti DP, Brunetti A, Vero R. Prevalence and predictors of postpartum glucose intolerance in Italian women with gestational diabetes mellitus. Diabetes Research and Clinical Practice. 2014;**105**(2):223-230

[104] Huisman CM, Zwart JJ, Roos-Hesselink JW, Duvekot JJ, van Roosmalen J. Incidence and predictors of maternal cardiovascular mortality and severe morbidity in the Netherlands: A prospective cohort study. PLoS One. 2013;**8**(2):e56494

[105] Debost-Legrand A, Rivière O, Dossou M, Vendittelli F. Risk factors for severe secondary postpartum hemorrhages: A historical cohort study. Birth. 2015;**42**(3):235-241

[106] Waldman M, Sheiner E, Sergienko R, Shoham-Vardi I. Can we identify risk factors during pregnancy for thrombo-embolic events during the puerperium and later in life? The Journal of Maternal-Fetal & Neonatal Medicine. 2015;**28**(9):1005-1009

[107] Tepper NK, Boulet SL, Whiteman MK, Monsour M, Marchbanks PA, Hooper WC, et al. Postpartum venous thromboembolism: Incidence and risk factors. Obstetrics and Gynecology. 2014;**123**(5):987-996

[108] Groutz A, Helpman L, Gold R, Pauzner D, Lessing JB, Gordon D. First vaginal delivery at an older age: Does it carry an extra risk for the development of stress urinary incontinence? Neurourology and Urodynamics. 2007;**26**(6):779-782

[109] Hijaz A, Sadeghi Z, Byrne L, Hou JC, Daneshgari F. Advanced maternal age as a risk factor for stress urinary incontinence: A review of the literature. International Urogynecology Journal. 2012;**23**(4):395-401

[110] Fritel X, Ringa V, Quiboeuf E, Fauconnier A. Female urinary incontinence, from pregnancy to menopause: A review of epidemiological and pathophysiological findings. Acta Obstetricia et Gynecologica Scandinavica. 2012;**91**(8):901-910

[111] Kubotani JS, Araujo Júnior E, Zanetti MR, Passos JP, de Jármy Di Bella ZI, Júnior JE. Assessing the impact of twin pregnancies on the pelvic floor using 3-dimensional sonography: A pilot study. Journal of Ultrasound in Medicine. 2014;**33**(7):1179-1183

[112] Youn H, Lee S, Han SW, Kim LY, Lee TS, Oh MJ, et al. Obstetric risk factors for depression during the postpartum period in South Korea: A nationwide study. Journal of Psychosomatic Research. 2017;**102**:15-20

[113] Klock SC. Psychological adjustment to twins after infertility. Best Practice & Research. Clinical Obstetrics & Gynaecology. 2004;**18**(4):645-656

[114] Wenze SJ, Battle CL, Tezanos KM. Raising multiples: Mental health of mothers and fathers in early parenthood. Archives of Women's Mental Health. 2015;**18**(2):163-176

[115] Gulamani SS, Premji SS, Kanji Z, Azam SI. A review of postpartum depression, preterm birth, and culture. The Journal of Perinatal & Neonatal Nursing. 2013;**27**(1):52-59; quiz 60-1

[116] Wen SY, Ko YL, Jou HJ, Chien LY. Sleep quality at 3 months postpartum considering maternal age: A comparative study. Women and Birth. 2018. pii: S1871-5192(17)30591-7

[117] Durkin MV, Kaveggia EG, Pendleton E, Neuhaüser G, Opitz JM. Analysis of etiologic factors in cerebral palsy with severe mental retardation. I. European Journal of Pediatrics. 1976;**123**(2):67-81

[118] Schneider RE, Ng P, Zhang X, Andersen J, Buckley D, Fehlings D, et al. The association between maternal age and cerebral palsy risk factors. Pediatric Neurology. 2018;**82**:25-28

[119] Modabbernia A, Velthorst E, Reichenberg A. Environmental risk factors for autism: An evidence-based review of systematic reviews and meta-analyses. Molecular Autism. 2017;**8**:13

[120] Falster K, Hanly M, Banks E, Lynch J, Chambers G, Brownell M, et al. Maternal age and offspring developmental vulnerability at age five: A population-based cohort study of Australian children. PLoS Medicine. 2018;**15**(4):e1002558

[121] Saha S, Barnett AG, Foldi C, Burne TH, Eyles DW, Buka SL, et al. Advanced paternal age is associated with impaired neurocognitive outcomes during infancy and childhood. PLoS Medicine. 2009;**6**(3):e40

[122] Sutcliffe AG, Derom C. Follow-up of twins: Health, behaviour, speech, language outcomes and implications for parents. Early Human Development. 2006;**82**(6):379-386

[123] Ge ZJ, Schatten H, Zhang CL, Sun QY. Oocyte ageing and epigenetics. Reproduction. 2015;**149**(3):R103-R114

11

Twinning as an Evolved Age-Dependent Physiological Mechanism: Evidence from Large Brazilian Samples

Marco Varella, Eloisa Fernandes, Jonas Arantes, Tiziana Acquaviva, Tania Lucci, Rafael Hsu, Vinicius David, Vera Bussab, Jaroslava Valentova, Nancy Segal and Emma Otta

Abstract

Multiple pregnancies occur in humans and other primates, which indicate that the twinning propensity is phylogenetically old. Factors such as decreased sexual dimorphism and size, rich and diverse nutrition and paternal care are related to multiple pregnancies in other animals. In human populations, despite its costs, twinning has a genetic basis and in Europe, Africa, and America, it was found that it increases mothers' fitness. Here, we explore the hypothesis that twinning represents an evolved physiological mechanism, particularly in mothers of higher age, as an 'all-or-nothing' last chance strategy for reproduction just before menopause. We present decade-long, large-scale population data about maternities from the city of São Paulo and the entire country of Brazil that indicate a considerable main effect of advanced age in promoting twinning, particularly dizygotic (DZ) twinning, but also monozygotic (MZ) twinning and higher order maternities. We also show that socioeconomic status is an important contextual factor increasing twinning. Besides the theoretical implications, these datasets establish a Brazilian countrywide twinning rate of 9.39‰ and highlight an increasing historical trend. This chapter promotes the importance of integrating proximate patterns from human and nonhuman animals and evolutionary factors in order to reach a comprehensive view about twinning.

Keywords: twinning rates, age dependence, physiological mechanism, evolutionary theories, population data, socioeconomic status

1. Introduction

Multiple pregnancy, the gestation of two or more embryos at the same maternity, regularly occurs in humans and other primates, which indicates that the twinning propensity is phylogenetically old within the order of primates. Despite the general pattern within the primate order of having single infant litters, multiple births occur in a number of species. The occurrence of twinning has been described, for instance, in chimpanzees (*Pan troglodytes*) [1–3], gorillas (*Gorilla gorilla*) [4, 5], orangutans (*Pongo pygmaeus*) [6, 7], vervet monkeys (*Cercopithecus aethiops sabaeus*) [8], macaques (*Macaca fuscata*) [9] and (*Macaca thibetana*) [10], capuchins (*Cebus apella*) [11, 12], marmosets (*Callithrix jacchus*) [13, 14], and also in prosimians, such as pygmy loris (*Nycticebus pygmaeus*) [15], lemurs (*Lemur catta*), and galagos (*Galago crassicaudatus argentatus*) [16]. As the last common ancestor between prosimians and humans (and all other primates) lived approximately 75 million year ago [17], the tendency toward twinning in primates has deep-seated biological roots. Furthermore, the existence of higher order litter size in other mammals [18] suggests that phylogenetically speaking, twinning is an even older propensity.

Comparative studies have identified some general factors related to increased litter size. Carranza [18] analyzed 106 species of mammals and, controlling for body mass, he found that increased sexual dimorphism is linked with decreased number of offspring per litter. It was also found that higher body mass is related to reductions in litter size, but only among larger mammals. Within primates, multiple births are limited to the smallest species [19]. Chapman et al. [20] analyzed factors related to multiple births in 70 species of primates and found that twinning primates tend to be small, have short gestation periods and give birth to small infants that are weaned quickly, and mature rapidly. They also tend to be commonly insectivorous, which they argue would allow a relatively high metabolism facilitating large litters. The authors suggest that adopting a more diverse diet containing not only fruit, but also insects could ensure access to nutritional resources that are not restricted seasonally or by the presence of toxins. Finally, they determined that litter size among species with paternal care was significantly higher than that of species with no paternal care. This is especially true for marmosets which they claim have the best 'package deal' for twinning: small body size, monogamy (or polyandry), and paternal care. Aligned with this, Stockley and Hobson [21] analyzed 427 mammalian species and found that increases in offspring production follow the evolution of paternal care, specifically where males contribute with investments, such as food provisioning for young. Therefore, there is an overall pattern relating to decreased sexual dimorphism and size, rich and diverse nutrition, and higher paternal care to increase litter size in primates, and in mammals in general, which should be taken into account when focusing on humans.

In Brazil, two cases of twins in capuchin monkeys (*Sapajus libidinosus*) were observed in a free wildlife setting in *Fazenda Boa Vista*, south of Piauí State (Northeast, Brazil). Comparing these cases with two other populations of capuchin monkeys in Brazil (*Parque Estadual Carlos Botelho* located in São Paulo State and *Reserva Biológica de Una*, located in Bahia State), the one in Fazenda Boa Vista presented the lowest offspring interval, and was attributable to more food availability in this region (Izar, Fragaszy & Visalberghi, personal communication) [12]. Capuchin monkeys feed on fruits and invertebrates (**Figure 1**) and also help to care for the offspring of others (**Figure 2**).

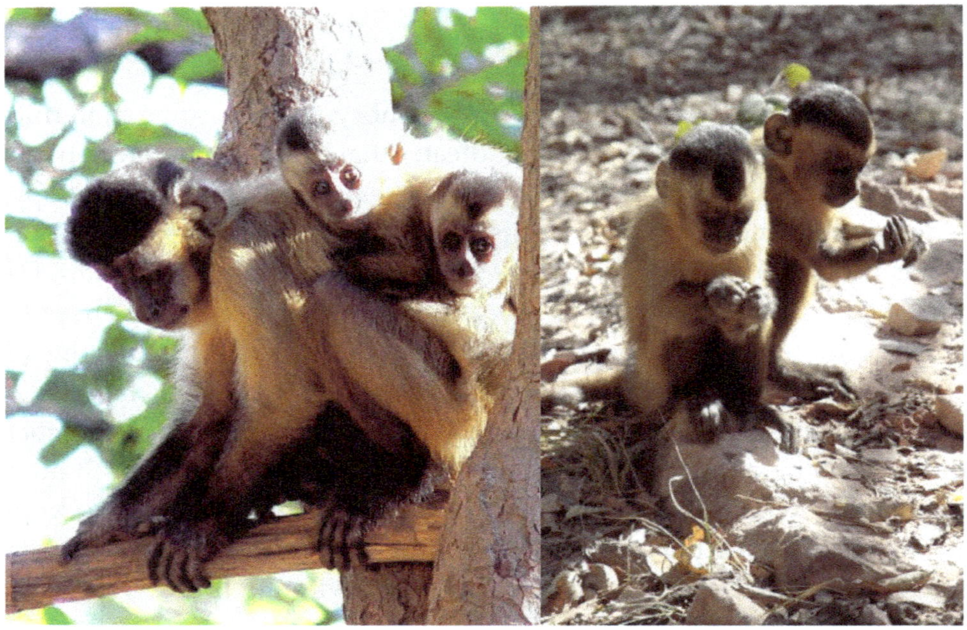

Figure 1. On the left, a female called 'Piaçava' carrying two female twin daughters: 'Paçoca' and 'Pamonha', 2009. On the right, the female twins Paçoca and Pamonha, from the 'Chicão' group. Photographed by Elisa Visalberghi.

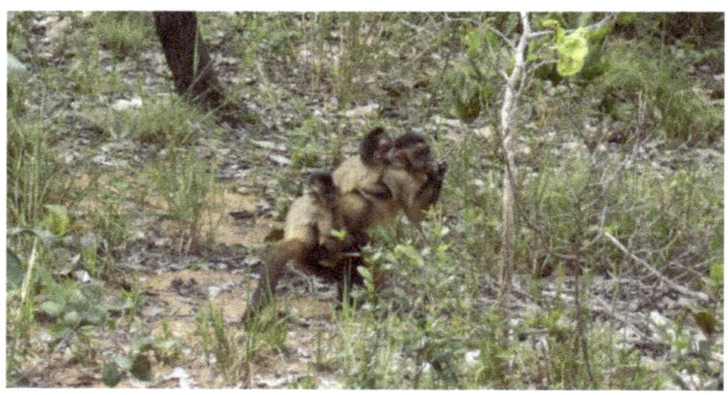

Figure 2. Twins carried by older female sister, *S. Libidinosus*, 2009, from 'Zangado' group. Photographed by Luiz Carlos M. Biondi.

1.1. Twin birth in the closest living relatives of humans

Chimpanzees are the closest living relatives of humans. The mean divergence estimation date between humans and chimpanzees is 7.65 ± 1.01 million years ago [17]. Therefore, from an evolutionary perspective, the comparison of humans with chimpanzees is especially interesting. Ely et al. [1] analyzed multiple births in chimpanzees using a database of 1,865 maternities recorded in the security, stability, and abundance of captivity (five different colonies) over a 76 years period from 1926 to 2002. When we compare the results from Ely et al. [1] to the corresponding Brazilian twinning rates from the city of Sao Paulo [22], we see that monozygotic (MZ) twinning rates were virtually the same comparing chimpanzees (4.3‰) and humans (4.42‰). However, dizygotic (DZ) twinning rates were more than three times higher in chimpanzees (23.6‰) than in humans (7.15‰). Similarly, higher order multiple birth rates were almost three times higher in chimpanzees (1.1‰) than in humans (0.36‰). Chimpanzee females that had given birth to twins were five times more likely to give birth to twins in a subsequent pregnancy in comparison with those who delivered singletons. Among humans, recurrence rates of twinning in a subsequent birth increase 2–3 times [23].

Among wild chimpanzees from 135 maternities recorded between 1965 and 1994 in the Mahale Mountains National Park, one birth of newborn twins was observed [24]. The twins' mother seemed overwhelmed and walked less than usual [2]. She stopped frequently to rest after walking 10–20 m. Whereas single newborn infants seldom vocalize, the twins exhibited a high frequency of vocalizations (5.8 per minute). During resting, both sometimes fell from her lap and uttered loud cries. The twins' mother had nursed her first single infant, but she did not nurse the newborn twins in spite of their nipple-rooting behavior. The explanatory hypothesis raised was insufficiency or absence of milk flow. After 1 week, the twins had disappeared. In the Gombe Stream National Park, one birth of newborn twins occurred in 59 recorded pregnancies [25, 26]. One of the twins gained weight and survived, but the other died when he was 10 months old. It is noted that even in captivity, 64% of the chimpanzees born as twins die during the first year of life. The mortality rate among singletons during the same period was only 23% [27].

At the Noichi Zoological Park, during a 1-year period, interesting observations of alloparenting behaviors toward a 2-year-old twin chimpanzee were made [28]. Alloparenting is defined as care provided by individuals other than the mother. Two adult females affiliated with the mother engaged in the same kinds of parenting behavior as the mother directed toward a female twin (walking, infant carriage, grooming, and physical contact). The father was mainly engaged in walking together, physical contact, and playing with the male co-twin. Alloparenting may have contributed to the successful rearing of these twins. Three years corresponds to the middle of infancy in the chimpanzee life cycle and the infants are still dependent on adults for transport during travels, but 2–3-year-olds already depart from their mother and make requests to other adults. Alloparenting in chimpanzees increases survival of the offspring, even twins, and decreases birth intervals [28]. Such results may explain coevolution of the relatively short birth intervals among humans and origins of human alloparenting institutions (e.g., nursery school).

Chimpanzees wean their single offspring at an average of approximately 5 years and the interbirth interval is about 4–5 years [29, 30]. Observations made at the Kibale National Park, Uganda showed a significant negative association between the speed at which chimpanzee females weaned their infants and the amount of alloparental care received [31]. The contribution of milk to infant diets, evaluated through fecal stable nitrogen isotopes, was lower when the infants received more alloparental care. This may benefit females enabling them to invest sooner in a subsequent offspring.

Alloparental care may have been significant in shaping human evolutionary history. Analysis of the dataset from the standard cross-cultural sample showed that the average age at weaning singletons for 58 traditional societies was 31 months [32]. Age at weaning tended to be about 6 months lower in societies in which allomothers helped with child care, compared with societies in which the burden of child care was on the mother alone. Alloparental care was also correlated with shorter birth intervals [33, 34]. It has been estimated that during their lifetime women reduce their child-care effort by 14–29%, in comparison with other mammals, due to the child care support they receive [35]. Menopause, which is present in humans and to some extent in nonhuman primates [36], is considered an adaptation that enables grandmaternal care, also contributing to a higher birth rate [37]. Sear and Mace [34] found that the death of the mother was clearly associated with high child mortality in 45 traditional societies they studied, especially when the mother died in the first year of the child's life. Examining whether the presence of kin affects child survival rates, they found that maternal grandmothers and siblings tended to improve child survival rates. Both fathers and paternal grandmothers showed somewhat more variation in their effects on child survival.

1.2. Twinning as an adapted propensity

In human populations, twinning is universal and a relevant part of cultural life, mythology, religion, and art [38–40]. There are documents on occurrences of twinning in historical populations, such as in seventeenth to eighteenth century French Canadian immigrants [41], or in eighteenth century Sweden [42]. Further, hereditary factors influence the propensity for twinning [39], typically DZ twinning [43, 44], although there is also some evidence for genetic influence on MZ twinning [45, 46]. For instance, in Brazil, one study found two genetic polymorphisms, TP53 Pro72Arg and MDM4 rs1563828, to be associated with twinning [47].

Twin pregnancies, especially monochorionic that are mostly MZ [39], are risky (e.g., adverse effects include twin-twin transfusion syndrome, twin anemia polycythemia sequence, selective intrauterine growth restriction, twin reversed arterial perfusion sequence), calling for increased medical and societal attention (e.g., [48, 49]). The chance of maternal mortality associated with multiple pregnancies is higher in comparison with singleton pregnancies. When one fetus dies, there is an increased risk of preterm delivery, neurological sequel, and co-twin death (Elito Jr., this volume).

Landy and Keith [50] used the expression *vanishing twin syndrome* (VTS) to refer to fetal resorption during the first months of gestation, thereby reducing a twin pregnancy to a singleton pregnancy, a phenomenon originally described by Stoeckel in 1945. In the past, this occurred without women's knowledge, but with the use of ultrasonography fetal resorption is more frequently diagnosed. Monitoring 228 twin pregnancies after natural conception, Márton et al. [51] reported an incidence of vanishing twin syndrome in 18.2% of twins, although it varies considerably, from 0 to 100% [39].

Despite all the costs and risks involved, the confluence of twinning's widespread occurrence, deep phylogenesis, universality, antiquity, and genetic basis point to the possibility of its important adaptive relevance in human evolution. Indeed, in contemporary Africa, Europe, and America, it was found that twinning increases mothers' fitness, that is, number of surviving offspring (e.g., [52–55]). Sear et al. [55] analyzed a database of 3,136 births, between 1950 and 1974, of a natural fertility population in rural Gambia, before the establishment of medical service. Fertility and mortality were also high in this population. The twinning rate was 15.9‰ (50 twin maternities). Twin mothers had higher fertility, shorter interbirth intervals, and later age at the last reproduction than their singleton-only bearing counterparts [55]. Therefore, the higher fertility of twin mothers outweighs the higher mortality of twins, indicating a fitness advantage of twin mothers in comparison with singleton mothers.

In the USA, Robson and Smith [54] accessed the Utah Population Database and compared the reproductive and survival events of 4,603 mothers who bore twins and 54,183 who bore singletons. These mothers were born between 1807 and 1899, lived at least to the age of 50 years and married once. They found that mothers of twins presented a robust phenotype, exhibited lower postmenopausal mortality, shorter average interbirth intervals, later ages at last birth and higher lifetime fertility than their singleton-only bearing counterparts. Beiguelman et al. [56] and Tagliani-Ribeiro et al. [47] also found that Brazilian twin mothers have a higher number of pregnancies than controls. Thus, because longevity and fecundity are increased in mothers of twins, the twinning propensity can offer some payoffs in terms of higher differential evolutionary fitness.

There are many evolutionary theories about twinning; however, here we outline two key hypotheses. The *insurance ova hypothesis,* proposed by Anderson [57], considers twinning as a by-product of selection for polyovulation, a mechanism which increases release of more than one oocyte per fertile phase of menstrual cycle due to multiple follicular development, promoting fertility and counterbalancing embryo defects and high spontaneous abortion rates. This event is associated with higher FSH concentrations induced by the decreased negative feedback mechanism reaching pituitary, which overshoots the threshold of ovarian follicle response in advancing maternal age [58]. In short, this hypothesis explains dizygotic twinning as an insurance mechanism against spontaneous abortion caused by both genetic and nongenetic defects. Apparently, the insurance ova hypothesis only explains higher rates of dizygotic twinning in older mothers. Ball and Hill [59] extended this hypothesis with their *insurance ova/pre-implantation selection model.* They agreed with Anderson that dizygotic twinning may be a by-product of selection for multiple ovulations. As such, multiple ovulations reduce the risk of embryo defects and conception failure. They went on to show that genetic defects covary with twinning rates across 24/25 countries; Nigeria, which has a unique biology when it comes to twinning, was the sole exception.

Forbes [60, 61] proposed an evolutionary explanation focused on relaxed maternal screening to eliminate genetically abnormal embryos—the *relaxed-screening hypothesis*. This screening system regulates both offspring quality and number; however, he argues that this system seems to falter in older mothers. He explains as a manifestation of this screening system the fact that twinning is two to four times more common at conception than at birth, hence the vanishing twin syndrome. The relaxed-screening hypothesis proposes an evolutionary framework in which the uterus of older mothers should become 'less selective' about offspring quality/quantity. He proposes two pathways for how this might happen. One is that as the mother approaches menopause, low quality offspring are better than no offspring at all. Another explanation is a maternal strategy to enhance the likelihood of carrying a normal pregnancy to term as a mother approaches menopause. This is plausible, given the conservative nature of the screening in which some healthy offspring are normally eliminated along with abnormal offspring. Thus, Forbes [60, 61] suggested that the maternal age increase in twinning rate arises not only from a greater frequency of poly-ovulation, but also from elevated embryo survival, in general, regardless of its origins from one or two zygotes, because of the relaxed screening. Therefore, even though initially not made explicit by Forbes [60], the relaxed-screening hypothesis explains higher rates of dizygotic and monozygotic twin births in some mothers approaching menopause. Interestingly, one MZ pair in a recent case of doubly exchanged MZ twins was born to a mother age 45 years [62]. It has been suggested that aging ova may lack certain sources of nutrition and energy, leading to delays in development and errors in the programming of some cells, which in turn result in the initial splitting of zygote that results in MZ twins [39, 62].

These two evolutionary hypotheses are not mutually exclusive as both take into account the shifts in conditions and prospects that affect women nearing menopause, which means the end of their reproductive career [60, 61]. The shifts in conditions that would enable twinning near the menopause relate to women's capacities, status, and context. During harsh ancestral times, women who were able to reach higher age probably successfully foraged, fought enemies, predators, parasites and disease, managed social alliances, acquired mate(s) and status, and survived the dangers of early childbirths [63–65]. This shows that women of a higher age in ancestral environments have stood the test of the time and, thus, had relatively better health and higher physical endurance, and social integration needed to successfully cope with multiple pregnancies. Moreover, older women would already have growing offspring that could act as 'helpers at the nest', alleviating part of the burden of twin childcare [66, 67]. The shifts in prospects that would enable twinning near the menopause related to the last chance for having own offspring, so having two or more babies at the same pregnancy would optimize and compensate for the later years without the possibility of new gestations.

However, considering the aforementioned risks of having a twin pregnancy, the pregnancies of mothers of higher age (≥35 years old), in general, are already associated with more chromosomal disease, complications, prematurity and low birth weight, and risks for abortion [68]. Thus, the fitness benefits of having twins in higher age must outweigh not only the costs of twinning, but also the costs of later age at conception.

1.3. Aim

In this chapter, we explore the general hypothesis that twinning represents an evolved physiological mechanism, particularly in mothers of higher age, as an 'all or nothing' last chance strategy for reproduction before menopause. We investigate twinning rates in representative data from São Paulo and the entire country of Brazil, and its distribution by age of the mother. We present decade-long, large-scale population data about maternities from the city of São Paulo and the entire country of Brazil. Moreover, by comparing the rates of dizygotic and monozygotic twinning among mothers of higher age in a São Paulo sample, we test both aforementioned hypotheses: the insurance ova hypothesis and the relaxed-screening hypothesis. If only dizygotic twinning rates increase maternal age, the insurance ova hypothesis would receive the most support. Alternatively, if both dizygotic and monozygotic twinning rates increase by the same amount with maternal age, the relaxed-screening hypothesis would receive the most support. Finally, if both dizygotic and monozygotic twinning rates increase with maternal age, but dizygotic twinning increases more than monozygotic twinning, then both hypotheses would receive support. However, both of these theories focus mostly on DZ twinning, which has a very different origin than MZ twinning. Therefore, while the MZ results may be consistent with what the theories predict, a causal interpretation in terms of their origin may not be warranted.

2. Twinning rates in São Paulo city

The USP Twin Panel (*Painel USP de Gêmeos*), based in the Institute of Psychology—University of Sao Paulo since 2015, has investigated the live birth twinning rate from São Paulo city (Brazil) using public data and additional information during the years 2003–2014 [22]. The public data on the singleton, twin, and higher order multiple live-born births were drawn from the Health Department database of Live Births Information System of São Paulo (SINASC) and included all deliveries registered between the years 2003 and 2014, from all 140 hospitals (56 public and 84 private) of the 31 districts of the city. We contacted SINASC and upon agreement from the Human Research Ethics Committee at the Institute of Psychology, University of São Paulo (Protocol Number 1,418,827), we received a more detailed database that included infants' sex, identification of the mother, date and hour of the delivery, place of the delivery, and register number. Based on these refined data, we determined the sex composition of twin maternities using Weinberg's differential method, which is a populational equation based on the sex ratio and the proportion of same-sex and opposite-sex twins. The validity of Weinberg's rule has been debated over the years. Using large samples and applying statistical assumptions may improve its utility; see [39]. As standard in the literature, we computed maternity rates per 1,000 (‰): individual twin births were divided by two and individual higher order multiple births were divided by three, assuming that the far majority of higher order multiple births were triplets. Mothers' age was recoded into eight classes (<15, 15–19, 20–24, 25–29, 30–34, 35–39, 40–44 and >45 years) (for details see, [22]).

For the first time in Brazil, we could establish live-birth rates in a decade-long, large-scale population sample encompassing 24,589 twin deliveries and 736 multiple deliveries out of a total of 2,056,016 deliveries during the studied time period. Precisely, the average rate of twin deliveries was 11.96‰, while the average of singletons was 987.42‰ and multiple births was 0.36‰. This was the largest study so far to calculate twinning rates in Brazil, which is in general in agreement with results from other countries [69], for example, Spain [70].

Interestingly, we found a strong positive correlation between the period (2003–2014) and twinning rate percentage and a strong negative correlation between the time period and both singleton rates and higher order multiple rates. This shows that while singletons and higher order multiple rates are diminishing, twinning rates are increasing. The twin birth rate rose 30.8% from 2003 to 2014, increasing from 10.19 to 13.33‰ [22]. Many factors may lead to this increase, such as increasing body mass index in women, improvement of quality of life, increase in social support, postponement of pregnancies until higher ages, use of assisted reproduction technologies and an increase in air pollution [22]. The pattern obtained in São Paulo city is aligned with the pattern in earlier decades in São Paulo [71] and with the worldwide increase in twinning rates (e.g., [42, 72, 73]), especially over the last several decades [68].

2.1. Twinning as a function of mothers' age in São Paulo

We documented a positive influence of mothers' age on twinning rates, in particular, women aged 25 years or more have more twins than younger women. The opposite pattern appeared to characterize the singleton mothers. Mothers' age was the strongest positive predictor, with the time period also positively, although weakly, predicting the twinning rates. Together, age of the mother and the time period explained 63% of the total variation. The model for higher order multiple rates was also significant, explaining 25% of the total variation, and mothers' age was its only positive predictor [22].

Furthermore, we used the Weinberg's differential method in order to estimate the average frequency of MZ and DZ twinning rates. We found that the average twinning rate for the whole period was 4.42‰ for MZ and 7.15‰ for DZ twins [22]. These rates were comparably increasing throughout the time period (2003–2014). The mothers' age positively and significantly correlated with both MZ and DZ birth rates. The model for DZ twinning rates was highly significant, explaining 61.3% of the total variation. Mothers' age was the strongest positive predictor, with the time period also positively, although weakly predicting the twinning rates. The model for MZ twinning rates was also significant, explaining 17.1% of the total variation. Mothers' age was the only positive predictor of the MZ twinning rates [22]. This general finding, regardless of the zygosity, agrees with the literature both in Brazil [56, 71] and in other countries [58].

We found that women aged 45 or more had almost three times more DZ twins than mothers aged between 40 and 44 years and seven times more DZ twins than women aged between 20 and 24 years [22] (see **Figure 3**). This finding agrees with the view that polyovulation is a major cause of twinning in older ages as predicted by the insurance ova hypothesis. Moreover, we found that women aged 45 or more had two times more MZ twins than mothers aged between 40 and 44 years, and women aged between 20 and 24 years. This increase in MZ twinning in older mothers was predicted by the relaxed-screening hypothesis. Both hypotheses and proposed mechanisms can, thus, explain higher rates of DZ twinning in older mothers. Thus, our data support both evolutionary hypotheses for higher twinning near menopause, but the specific reasons behind MZ and DZ twinning at older maternal ages most likely differ. Importantly, different countries around the world have already sparsely but consistently found that not only DZ but also to a smaller degree MZ twinning rates were higher in mothers closer to menopause, in the U.S.A. population [74], in a Jewish population [75], in a Jewish and Bedouin populations [76], in rural and urban Chinese populations [77], and also in Spanish populations [70]. This cross-cultural convergence adds support to both evolutionary hypotheses, particularly to the relaxed-screening hypothesis [60, 61].

2.2. Variation in twinning rates in different city districts of São Paulo

Additionally, we closely investigated how twinning rates are distributed within various subregions of the city of São Paulo, the biggest metropolis of Brazil. Considering mothers' home

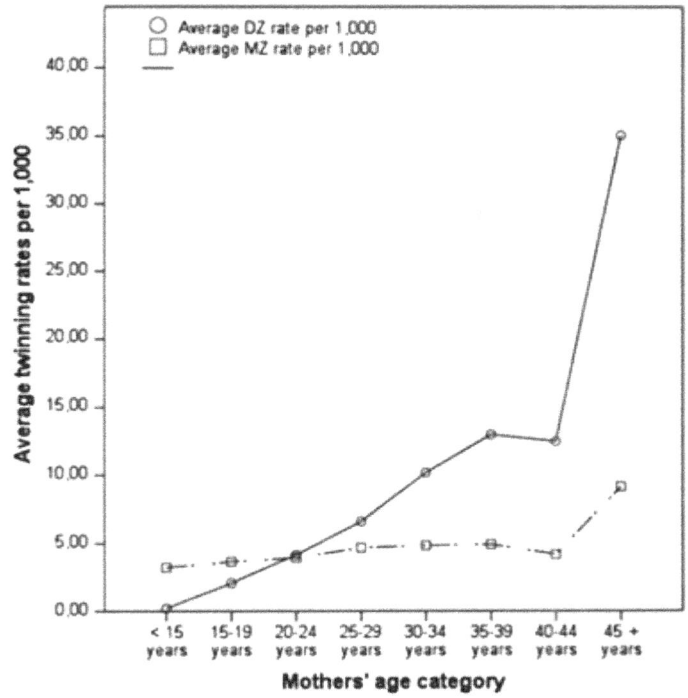

Figure 3. Dizygotic (DZ) and monozygotic (MZ) twin rates per 1,000 births as a function of mother's age; from [22].

addresses at the time of delivery, we found a large variance in the twinning rates among the 31 subregions of São Paulo: from 9.85 (district Itaim Paulista) to 24.32‰ (district Pinheiros). **Figure 4** shows the overall rate of twins' geographical distribution between 2003 and 2015 by the 31 subregions of the city. In **Figure 4**, we clearly show that in the central regions there are more twins born than in peripheral districts. This centralized distribution does not simply reflect the places where most hospitals are available, because we accessed the mothers' addresses and not the address of the maternity hospitals. Thus, this indicates that a real demographic factor is driving this distribution.

There was a pronounced positive correlation between the average income of each city district according to the 2010 Demographic census from Brazilian Institute of Geography and Statistics (IBGE) and the average twinning rates during the period from 2003 to 2015. The same result was found for the higher order multiple birth rates. This indicates that, in richer regions, there is a higher chance of twin and multiple births. This new finding from the USP Twin Panel can explain the centralized distribution of higher twinning rates shown in **Figure 4**. Many factors could be interacting to produce this result. Women with higher socioeconomic status tend to study longer and delay reproduction; thus, having offspring in higher age increases the chance of multiple pregnancies. Also those women can afford assisted reproduction technologies which increase the chance of multiple pregnancies. Moreover, those women have a richer and more diverse nutritional diet which, as found for nonhuman primates [1, 20], could increase the chance of multiple pregnancies. Colletto et al. [78] also found increased twinning rates as a function of women's higher socioeconomic

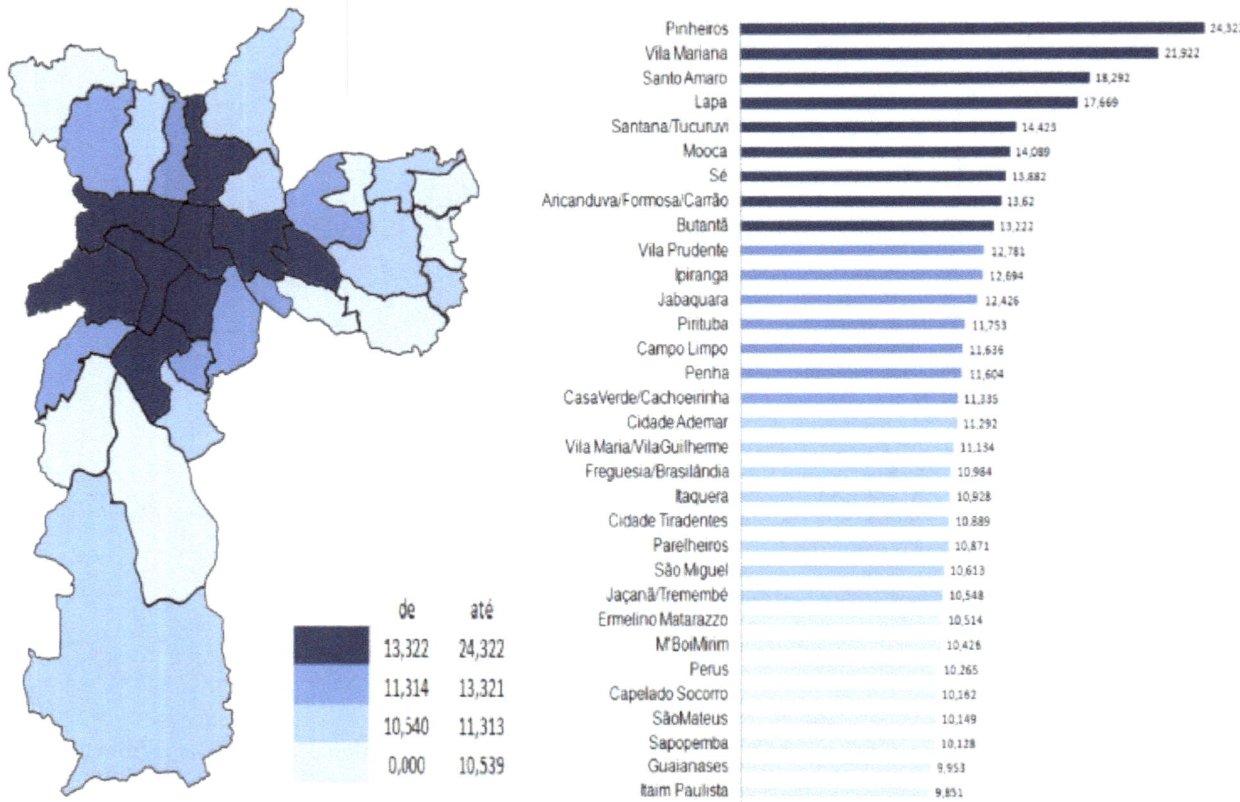

Figure 4. Overall geographical distribution of twinning rates between 2003 and 2015 by the 31 districts of the city. The darker the color, the higher the twinning rate. We used percentiles to create low, mid-low, mid-high, and high rates.

status. Further studies should attempt to disentangle the web of salient influential factors by accessing and integrating indicators such as nutrition, education, socioeconomic status, and assisted reproduction.

3. Twinning rates across the entire country of Brazil

Most recently, the USP Twin Panel (*Painel USP de Gêmeos*) has expanded the investigation of twinning rates to the entire country of Brazil between the years of 2002 and 2013. The data were drawn from TABNET within DATASUS, an official public governmental database and transformed into rates of maternities the same way it was done for the city of São Paulo [22]. A multivariate general linear model was used to explore the effects of region, maternal age, and time period on singleton, twin and higher order multiple birth rates. We obtained a total of 35,051,790 maternities between 2002 and 2013, 329,006 twinning maternities and 8,005 higher order maternities. Considering all regions of Brazil, the overall average rate of twins was 9.39‰ and higher order births were 0.23‰. These data show that the Brazilian countrywide twinning and multiple birth rates are lower than the twinning rates in the city of São Paulo (11.96 and 0.36‰) [22]. These rates are slightly lower than results from developed countries (e.g., [69]). The increase in the twinning rate over the years was 14.54%, from 8.80‰ in 2002 to 10.08‰ in 2013, a modest increase compared to the 30.8% in São Paulo [22]. The decade time period positively predicted, albeit weakly, twin birth rates, explaining 3% of the variance. It also negatively predicted singleton rates, explaining 2% of the variance, with no effect on multiple birth rates.

3.1. Twinning as a function of mothers' age in the entire country of Brazil

Our results showed that maternal age strongly and positively predicted twin and multiple birth rates, explaining 56 and 21% of the variances, respectively. It also negatively predicted singleton birth rates, explaining 62% of the variance. These results are in agreement with the results from São Paulo [22, 56, 71] and from other countries, such as Spain [70].

The finding that the higher maternal age predicts twin and multiple births corroborates the evolutionary hypotheses, the insurance ova hypothesis [57, 59] and the relaxed-screening hypothesis [60, 61], pointing to the existence of an age-dependent mechanism that leads to a strong increase in twinning and multiple births in women near menopause.

3.2. Variation in twinning rates in different regions of Brazil

Among the five major regions of Brazil (North, Northeast, Central-West, South, and Southeast), we found a small, but significant variation in twinning rates. **Table 1** presents maternity rates for singletons, twins, and higher order multiple births divided by Brazilian regions. In general, the developed areas (e.g., Southeast) presented higher twinning and multiple birth rates than developing ones (e.g., North). This is in line with the finding of the São Paulo city districts. Similarly to the possible effects of higher maternal age, higher access to assisted reproduction technologies, and higher nutritional diversity and abundance may contribute to the higher twinning rates in the Southeast and South developed regions, yielding regional discrepancy.

Furthermore, the ethnic composition may also play a role. In the North of Brazil, there is the highest proportion of indigenous intermixed individuals within the population (up to 32%), while in other regions it ranges from 11 to 16% [79]. Brazilian native Americans are closely

Mean	Singleton rates (‰)	Twins rates (‰)	Higher order rates (‰)
Southeast	988.08	10.34	0.25
South	989.32	10.06	0.23
Central-West	990.70	9.05	0.24
Northeast	988.54	8.68	0.23
North	991.30	7.32	0.14

Table 1. Maternity rates of singleton, twin and higher order births per Brazilian regions.

related to Asiatic populations [80] that have the lowest twin rates compared to other ethnicities [39, 81]. It is thus possible that Asian ancestry may underlie the relatively lower twinning rate in the northern region of Brazil. Future studies should further explore the influencing factors among the regions.

4. Conclusions

The overall observed pattern of results linking increased twinning in mothers near menopause, from both decade-long large-scale populational studies, is consistent across São Paulo and all of Brazil, and agrees with the literature from Brazil [56, 71] and from other countries, for example, the Netherlands [58], and even with reports from traditional societies with natural reproduction, such as agricultural areas of Costa Rica [72], Gambia [55], eighteenth century Sweden [42], and seventeenth to eighteenth century French Canadian immigrants [41]. This convergence of results supports both evolutionary hypotheses about twinning: it points to the existence of an age-dependent evolved mechanism of twinning as an 'all-or-nothing' last chance strategy for reproduction near menopause. The estimated twinning rate per zygosity allowed us to closely test both the insurance ova hypothesis and the relaxed-screening hypothesis. In at least seven different populations worldwide [22, 70, 74–77], both DZ and MZ twinning rates increased in mothers near menopause; thus, both evolutionary theories received support, because it identifies polyovulation and relaxed screening as possible underlying mechanisms of increased twin births in women of higher age. The appreciation that also MZ twin births cross-culturally increases with mothers' age is an underappreciated pattern in the literature. Again, as stated earlier, these results require additional examination with respect to MZ twinning which has its origins explained by biological events that do not apply to DZ twinning (e.g., zygotic division).

Additionally, our results showed that higher socioeconomic conditions are related to higher twinning rates. This was found in both São Paulo and the entire country of Brazil, and corroborates the literature that has already shown a link between higher socioeconomic status and increased twinning rates in Brazil [78, 82] and other countries, for example, in Greece [83]. This finding also agrees with the literature on nonhuman primates that shows relatively higher twinning in captive, safer, and abundant conditions [1] and in species with more diverse nutritional intake [20].

This chapter reflects the importance of integrating factors and patterns from studies conducted on nonhuman species, particularly primates, with the findings traditionally focused on humans. We have attempted the first step toward bringing the comparative approach into light in order to promote deeper understanding of demographic data on twinning and higher order maternities. The comparative approach can offer insights and increase our understanding of both commonalities and specificities of the human case. Along the same lines, we have stressed the importance of considering proximate factors, such as genetic, physiological, ontogenetic and contextual variables, and distal factors, such as ancestral selective pressures, and evolutionary reasoning. Both fields have a great deal to gain with a more integrated approach.

Acknowledgements

Grants: #2014/50282-5 and #2017/10501-8 of São Paulo Research Foundation (FAPESP) and Natura Cosméticos S.A.; #304740/2017-9 and #308597/2017-6 of National Council for Scientific and Technological Development (CNPq). We thank all members of the USP Twin Panel for the support (https://www.paineluspdegemeos.com.br/nossa-equipe).

Author details

Marco Varella[1*], Eloisa Fernandes[1], Jonas Arantes[2], Tiziana Acquaviva[1], Tania Lucci[1], Rafael Hsu[1], Vinicius David[1], Vera Bussab[1], Jaroslava Valentova[1], Nancy Segal[3] and Emma Otta[1]

*Address all correspondence to: macvarella@usp.br

1 Department of Experimental Psychology, Institute of Psychology, University de Sao Paulo, Sao Paulo, Brazil

2 Institute of Biosciences, University de Sao Paulo, Sao Paulo, Brazil

3 Department of Psychology, California State University, Fullerton, USA

References

[1] Ely JJ, Frels WI, Howell S, Izard MK, Keeling ME, Lee DR. Twinning and heteropaternity in chimpanzees (*Pan troglodytes*). American Journal of Physical Anthropology. 2006;**130**(1):96-102. DOI: 10.1002/ajpa.20310

[2] Matsumoto-Oda A. First record of a twin birth in chimpanzees of the Mahale Mountains National Park, Tanzania. African Study Monographs. 1995;**16**:159-164. DOI: 10.14989/68135

[3] Peacock LJ, Rogers MS. Gestation period and twinning in chimpanzees. Science. 1959; **129**:959. DOI: 10.1126/science.129.3354.959

[4] Langer S, Jurczynski K, Gessler A, Kaup FJ, Bleyer M, Mätz-Rensing K. Ischiopagus tripus conjoined twins in a western lowland gorilla (*Gorilla gorilla*). Journal of Comparative Pathology. 2014;**150**:469-473. DOI: 10.1016/j.jcpa.2013.12.002

[5] Rosen S. Twin gorilla fetuses. Folia Primatologica. 1972;**17**(1-2):132-141. DOI: 10.1159/000155420

[6] Goossens B, Kapar MD, Kahar S, Ancrenaz M. First sighting of Bornean orangutan twins in the wild. Asian Primates Journal. 2012;**2**(1):12-14

[7] Lang EM. Zwillinge bei unsern Orangutans. Zolli: Bulletin of Zoologischer Garten Basel. 1973;**31**:14-15

[8] Pollack DB, Raleigh MJ. Twinning in a colony of vervet monkeys (*Cercopithecus aethiops sabaeus*). American Journal of Primatology. 1994;**32**(1):57-60. DOI: 10.1002/ajp.1350320107

[9] Sugiyama Y, Kurita H, Matsui T, Shimomura T. Twinning frequency of Japanese macaques (*Macaca fuscata*) at Takasakiyama. Primates. 2011;**52**(1):19-23. DOI: 10.1007/s10329-010-0220-8

[10] Xia D, Li J, Matheson MD, Sun L, Sun B, Zhu Y. First occurrence of twins in provisioned free-ranging Tibetan macaques (*Macaca thibetana*) at Huangshan, China. Primates. 2012;**53**:1-5. DOI: 10.1007/s10329-011-0276-0

[11] Leighty KA, Byrne G, Fragaszy DM, Visalberghi E, Welker C, Lussier I. Twinning in tufted capuchins (*Cebus apella*): Rate, survivorship, and weight gain. Folia Primatologica. 2004;**75**(1):14-18. DOI: 10.1159/000073425

[12] Izar P. Análise socioecológica da diversidade social de macacos-prego [thesis]. São Paulo: Universidade de São Paulo; 2016

[13] Harris RA, Tardif SD, Vinar T, Wildman DE, Rutherford JN, Rogers J, Worley KC, Aagaard KM. Evolutionary genetics and implications of small size and twinning in callitrichine primates. Proceedings of the National Academy of Sciences. 2014;**111**(4):1467-1472. DOI: 10.1073/pnas.1316037111

[14] Tardif SD, Smucny DA, Abbott DH, Mansfield K, Schultz-Darken N, Yamamoto ME. Reproduction in captive common marmosets (*Callithrix jacchus*). Comparative Medicine. 2003;**53**:364-368

[15] Jurke MH, Czekala NM, Jurke S, Hagey LR, Lance VA, Conley AJ, Fitch-Snyder H. Monitoring pregnancy in twinning pygmy loris (*Nycticebus pygmaeus*) using fecal estrogen metabolites. American Journal of Primatology. 1998;**46**(2):173-183. DOI: 10.1002/(SICI)1098-2345(1998)46:2<173::AID-AJP7>3.0.CO;2-T

[16] Pasztor LM, Van Horn RN. Twinning in prosimians. Journal of Human Evolution. 1976;**5**(4):333-337. DOI: 10.1016/0047-2484(76)90037-3

[17] Pozzi L, Hodgson JA, Burrell AS, Sterner KN, Raaum RL, Disotell TR. Primate phylogenetic relationships and divergence dates inferred from complete mitochondrial genomes. Molecular Phylogenetics and Evolution. 2014;**75**:165-183. DOI: 10.1016/j.ympev.2014.02.023

[18] Carranza J. Sexual selection for male body mass and the evolution of litter size in mammals. The American Naturalist. 1996;**148**(1):81-100

[19] Leutenegger W. Evolution of litter size in primates. The American Naturalist. 1979;**114**(4):525-531

[20] Chapman CA, Walker S, Lefebvre L. Reproductive strategies of primates: The influence of body size and diet on litter size. Primates. 1990;**31**(1):1-13. DOI: 10.1007/BF02381026

[21] Stockley P, Hobson L. Paternal care and litter size coevolution in mammals. Proceedings of the Royal Society B. 2016;**283**(1829):20160140. DOI: 10.1098/rspb.2016.0140

[22] Otta E, Fernandes E, Acquaviva T, Lucci T, Kiehl L, Varella M, Segal N, Valentova J. Twinning and multiple birth rates according to maternal age in the city of São Paulo, Brazil: 2003-2014. Twin Research and Human Genetics. 2016;**19**(6):679-686. DOI: 10.1017/thg.2016.75

[23] Rydhstroem H. Twinning in Sweden between 1973 and 1990. The recurrence rate. Early Human Development. 1998;**51**(1):7-12. DOI: 10.1016/S0378-3782(97)00068-6

[24] Nishida T, Takasaki H, Takahata Y. Demography and reproductive profiles. In: Mat-sumoto-Oda A, Nishida T, editors. The Chimpanzees of the Mahale Mountains. Tokyo: University of Tokyo Press; 1990. pp. 63-98

[25] Goodall J. The Chimpanzees of Gombe: Patterns of Behavior. Cambridge: Belknap Press of Harvard University Press; 1986. 673 p

[26] Goodall J. Through a Window: My Thirty Years with the Chimpanzees of Gombe. Boston: Houghton Mifflin Company; 1990. p. 337

[27] Seal US, Flesness N, Foose T. Neonatal and infant mortality in captive-born great apes. In: Graham CE, Bowen JA, editors. Clinical Management of Infant Great Apes. New York: Alan R. Liss Inc; 1985. pp. 193-203

[28] Kishimoto T, Ando J, Tatara S, Yamada N, Konishi K, Kimura N, Fukumori A, Tomonaga M. Alloparenting for chimpanzee twins. Scientific Reports. 2014;**4**:6306

[29] Galdikas BM, Wood JW. Birth spacing patterns in humans and apes. American Journal of Physical Anthropology. 1990;**83**(2):185-191. DOI: 10.1002/ajpa.1330830207

[30] Kennedy GE. From the ape's dilemma to the weanling's dilemma: Early weaning and its evolutionary context. Journal of Human Evolution. 2005;**48**(2):123-145. DOI: 10.1016/j.jhevol.2004.09.005

[31] Bădescu J, Watts DP, Katzenberg MA, Sellen DW. Alloparenting is associated with reduced maternal lactation effort and faster weaning in wild chimpanzees. Royal Society Open Science. 2016;**3**(11):160577. DOI: 10.1098/rsos.160577

[32] Quinlan RJ, Quinlan MB. Human lactation, pair-bonds, and alloparents. Human Nature. 2008;**19**:87-102. DOI: 10.1007/s12110-007-9026-9

[33] Lahdenperä M, Lummaa V, Helle S, Tremblay M, Russell AF. Fitness benefits of prolonged post-reproductive lifespan in women. Nature. 2004;**428**(6979):178-181. DOI: 10.1038/nature02367

[34] Sear R, Mace R. Who keeps children alive? A review of the effects of kin on child survival. Evolution and Human Behavior. 2008;**29**:1-18. DOI: 10.1016/j.evolhumbehav.2007.10.001

[35] Bogin B, Bragg J, Kuzawa C. Humans are not cooperative breeders but practice biocultural reproduction. Annals of Human Biology. 2014;**41**:368-380. DOI: 10.3109/03014460.2014.923938

[36] Rovirosa-Hernández MJ, González MH, Guevara-Pérez MÁ, García-Orduña F, de los Ángeles Aguilar-Tirado A, Puga-Olguín A, Vásquez-Domínguez BP. Menopause in nonhuman primates: A comparative study with humans. In: Rodríguez-Landa JF, editor. A Multidisciplinary Look at Menopause. Croatia: IntechOpen; 2017. pp. 25-48. DOI: 10.5772/66558

[37] Hawkes K, O'Connell JF, Jones NB, Alvarez H, Charnov EL. Grandmothering, menopause, and the evolution of human life histories. Proceedings of the National Academy of Sciences. 1998;**95**(3):1336-1339. DOI: 10.1073/pnas.95.3.1336

[38] Fava JL, Guerzet EA, Mattar R, Souza E, Camano L. Twins in the mythology and religion. Femina. 2002;**30**(2):137-140

[39] Segal NL. Twin Mythconceptions: False Beliefs, Fables, and Facts about Twins. Cambridge, MA: Academic Press; 2017. 334 p

[40] Wright L. Twins: And What They Tell Us About Who We Are. New York: John Wiley & Sons, Inc; 1997. 202 p

[41] Nonaka K, Desjardins B, Charbonneau H, Légaré J, Miura T. Slow twin conception at first birth and subsequent maternal twin proneness in a natural fertility population. Acta Geneticae Medicae et Gemellologiae: Twin Research. 1995;**44**:215-222. DOI: 10.1017/S000156600000163X

[42] Fellman J, Eriksson AW. Demographic analysis of the variation in the rates of multiple maternities in Sweden since 1751. Human Biology. 2004;**76**:343-359. DOI: 10.1353/hub.2004.0044

[43] Mbarek H, Steinberg S, Nyholt DR, Gordon SD, Miller MB, McRae AF, Hottenga JJ, Day FR, Willemsen G, de Geus EJ, Davies GE, Martin HC, Penninx BW, Jansen R, McAloney K, Vink JM, Kaprio J, Plomin R, Spector TD, Magnusson PK, Reversade B, Harris RA, Aagaard K, Kristiansson RP, Olafsson I, Eyjolfsson GI, Sigurdardottir O, Iacono WG, Lambalk CB, Montgomery GW, McGue M, Ong KK, Perry JRB, Martin NG, Stefánsson H, Stefánsson K, Boomsma DI. Identification of common genetic variants influencing spontaneous dizygotic twinning and female fertility. The American Journal of Human Genetics. 2016;**98**(5):898-908. DOI: 10.1016/j.ajhg.2016.03.008

[44] Painter JN, Willemsen G, Nyholt D, Hoekstra C, Duffy DL, Henders AK, Wallace L, Healey S, Cannon-Albright LA, Skolnick M, Martin NG, Boomsma DI, Montgomey GW. A genome wide linkage scan for dizygotic twinning in 525 families of mothers of dizygotic twins. Human Reproduction. 2010;**25**(6):1569-1580. DOI: 10.1093/humrep/deq084

[45] Machin G. Familial monozygotic twinning: A report of seven pedigrees. American Journal of Medical Genetics Part C: Seminars in Medical Genetics. 2009;**151**(2):152-154. DOI: 10.1002/ajmg.c.30211

[46] Shur N. The genetics of twinning: From splitting eggs to breaking paradigms. American Journal of Medical Genetics Part C: Seminars in Medical Genetics. 2009;**151**(2):105-109. DOI: 10.1002/ajmg.c.30204

[47] Tagliani-Ribeiro A, Paskulin DD, Oliveira M, Zagonel-Oliveira M, Longo D, Ramallo V, Ashton-Prolla P, Saraiva-Pereira ML, Fagundes NJ, Schuler-Faccini L, Matte U. High twinning rate in Cândido Godói: A new role for p53 in human fertility. Human Reproduction. 2012;**27**(9):2866-2871. DOI: 10.1093/humrep/des217

[48] Elito Jr J, Santana EFM, Cecchino GN. Monochorionic twin pregnancy—Potential risks and perinatal outcomes. In: Darwish A, editor. Contemporary Gynecologic Practice. 1st ed. Croatia: IntechOpen; 2015. pp. 203-234. DOI: 10.5772/58951

[49] Suzuki S. Perinatal outcomes of monochorionic-diamniotic twin pregnancies uncomplicated at 28 weeks of gestation. Japanese Clinical Medicine. 2016;**7**:15-17. DOI: 10.4137/JCM.S38895

[50] Landy HJ, Keith LG. The vanishing twin: A review. Human Reproduction Update. 1998;**4**(2):177-183

[51] Márton V, Zádori J, Kozinszky Z, Keresztúri A. Prevalences and pregnancy outcome of vanishing twin pregnancies achieved by in vitro fertilization versus natural conception. Fertility and Sterility. 2016;**106**(6):1399-1406. DOI: 10.1016/j.fertnstert.2016.07.1098

[52] Gabler S, Voland E. Fitness of twinning. Human Biology. 1994;**66**:699-713

[53] Helle S, Lummaa V, Jokela J. Selection for increased brood size in historical human populations. Evolution. 2004;**58**:430-436. DOI: 10.1554/03-307

[54] Robson SL, Smith KR. Twinning in humans: Maternal heterogeneity in reproduction and survival. Proceedings of the Royal Society B: Biological Sciences. 2011;**278**(1725):3755-3761. DOI: 10.1098/rspb.2011.0573

[55] Sear R, Mace R, Shanley D, McGregor IA. The fitness of twin mothers: Evidence from rural Gambia. Journal of Evolutionary Biology. 2001;**14**:433-443. DOI: 10.1046/j.1420-9101.2001.00287.x

[56] Beiguelman B, Franchi-Pinto C, Magna LA. Biological and social traits associated with twinning among Caucasoids and Negroids. Brazilian Journal of Genetics. 1997;**20**(2):311-318

[57] Anderson DJ. On the evolution of human brood size. Evolution. 1990;**44**(2):438-440

[58] Beemsterboer SN, Homburg R, Gorter NA, Schats R, Hompes PGA, Lambalk CB. The paradox of declining fertility but increasing twinning rates with advancing maternal age. Human Reproduction. 2006;**21**(6):1531-1532. DOI: 10.1093/humrep/del009

[59] Ball HL, Hill CM. Insurance ovulation, embryo mortality and twinning. Journal of Biosocial Science. 1999;**31**(2):245-255

[60] Forbes LS. The evolutionary biology of spontaneous abortion in humans. Trends in Ecology and Evolution. 1997;**12**(11):446-450. DOI: 10.1016/S0169-5347(97)01179-8

[61] Forbes S. A Natural History of Families. Princeton NJ: Princeton University Press; 2005. 231 p

[62] Segal NL, Montoya YM. Accidental Brothers: The Story of Twins Exchanged at Birth and the Power of Nature and Nurture. New York: St. Martin's Press; 2018. 352 p

[63] Adovasio JM, Soffer O, Page J. The Invisible Sex: Uncovering the True Roles of Women in Prehistory. New York: Routledge; 2016. 320 p

[64] Hrdy SB. Mother Nature: Maternal Instincts and How They Shape the Human Species. New York: Ballantine Books; 2000. 752 p

[65] Hrdy SB. The Woman That Never Evolved. Revised Ed. Cambridge: Harvard University Press; 2009. 422 p

[66] Gosso Y, Otta E, Morais MLS, Ribeiro FJL, Bussab VSR. Play in hunter-gatherer society. In: Pellegrini AD, Smith P, editors. The Nature of Play: Great Apes and Humans. 1st ed. New York: The Guilford Press; 2005. pp. 213-253

[67] Kramer KL, Veile A. Infant allocare in traditional societies. Physiology and Behavior. 2018;**193**:117-126. DOI: 10.1016/j.physbeh.2018.02.054

[68] Petkova R, Dimitrova V, Zhelev N, Chakarov S. An old wives' tale. Reproductive outcomes in pregnant women aged 35 or older: The role of individual repair capacity. BioDiscovery. 2015;**18**:e8970. DOI: 10.7750/BioDiscovery.2015.18.2

[69] Pison G, D'Addato AV. Frequency of twin births in developed countries. Twin Research and Human Genetics. 2006;**9**:250-259. DOI: 10.1375/twin.9.2.250

[70] Luna F, Alonso V. Factores reguladores de la monocigocia y dicigocia en España (2006). Revista Española de. Antropología Física. 2016;**37**:55-61

[71] Colletto GMDD. Twinning rate trend in a population sample from the city of São Paulo, Brazil. Genetics and Molecular Biology. 2003;**26**(3):245-248. DOI: 10.1590/S1415-47572003000300005

[72] Madrigal L. Twinning trend in Escazú, Costa Rica, 1851-1901. Human Biology. 1997;**69**(2):269-276

[73] Razzaque A, Ahmed K, Wai L. Twinning rates in a rural area of Bangladesh. Human Biology. 1990;**62**:505-514

[74] Myrianthopoulos NC. An epidemiologic survey of twins in a large prospectively studied population. American Journal Human Genetics. 1970;**22**(6):611-629

[75] Harlap S. Multiple births in former oral contraceptive users. BJOG: An International Journal of Obstetrics and Gynaecology. 1979;**86**(7):557-562. DOI: 10.1111/j.1471-0528.1979.tb10809.x

[76] Picard R, Fraser D, Hagay ZJ, Leiberman JR. Twinning in southern Israel; secular trends, ethnic variation and effects of maternal age and parity. European Journal of Obstetrics and Gynecology and Reproductive Biology. 1989;**33**(2):131-139. DOI: 10.1016/0028-2243(89)90205-0

[77] Gan JP, Wu ZH, Tu ZM, Zheng J. The comparison of twinning rates between urban and rural areas in China. Twin Research and Human Genetics. 2007;**10**(4):633-637. DOI: 10.1375/twin.10.4.633

[78] Colletto GMDD, Segre CA, Rielli ST, Rosário H. Multiple birth rates according to different socioeconomic levels: An analysis of four hospitals from the city of Sao Paulo, Brazil. Twin Research and Human Genetics. 2003;**6**:177-182. DOI: 10.1375/twin.6.3.177

[79] Saloum de Neves Manta F, Pereira R, Vianna R, Rodolfo Beuttenmüller de Araújo A, Leite Góes Gitaí D, et al. Revisiting the genetic ancestry of brazilians using autosomal AIM-indels. PLoS One. 2013;**8**(9):e75145. DOI: 10.1371/journal.pone.0075145

[80] Bailliet G, Rothhammer F, Carnese FR, Bravi CM, Bianchi NO. Founder mitochondrial haplotypes in Amerindian populations. American Journal of Human Genetics. 1994; **55**(1):27-33

[81] Saldanha PH. Gêmeos: Hereditariedade versus Ambiência. São Paulo: HUCITEC-Edusp; 1980. 92 p

[82] Colletto GMDD, Segre CADM, Beiguelman B. Twinning rate in a sample from a Brazilian hospital with a high standard of reproductive care. Sao Paulo Medical Journal. 2001;**119**:216-219. DOI: 10.1590/S1516-31802001000600007

[83] Malamitsi-Puchner A, Voulgaris K, Sdona E, Christou C, Briana DD. Twins and socioeconomic factors: changes in the last 20 years. The Journal of Maternal-Fetal and Neonatal Medicine. 2017;**119**:1-6. DOI: 10.1080/14767058.2017.1382469

12

Prenatal Attachment in Twin Pregnancy

Chiara Ionio, Eleonora Mascheroni,
Caterina Colombo and Gianluca Lista

Abstract

Twin births are associated with several medical, healthcare, socio-emotional, psychological and developmental consequences for families. Parents generally describe twin pregnancies as physically and emotionally difficult. Moreover, compared to singleton pregnancies, twin pregnancies are reported to carry higher maternal as well as perinatal morbidity and mortality. The aim of this chapter is to review literature on twin pregnancy and to give a comprehensive framework about parents' experience of expecting twins. An important issue related to the psychological adjustment during twin pregnancies is prenatal attachment. During pregnancy, mothers use to think about their child-to-be, and they start to create representation of themselves as mothers. Prenatal attachment in twin pregnancies may differ from that in singleton ones. During a twin pregnancy, the mother-to-be has to deal with an identification process with two children at the same time and have to create a mental space that allow her to make representation of both children. The monitoring of these pregnancies is important for the creation and the consolidation of these maternal representations: ultrasound examinations revealed the fetal gender that facilitates naming the unborn twins and thinking to them as individuals and this is particularly important in the case of complicated twin pregnancies.

Keywords: twins, twin pregnancy, prenatal attachment, maternal-fetal relationship

1. Introduction

Currently, twin pregnancies account approximately for 3% of all live births [1]. The number of twin pregnancies has dramatically increased over the last four decades in all of the countries where we have information from vital statistics [2]. One of the main reasons for this recent increase of twin pregnancies is associated to the fact that mean maternal age at childbearing has considerably raised. The responsible factors are socio-economic contingencies and the increase in the female employment rate. There is evidence indicating that the incidence of twin pregnancies is known to rise with mother's age [3]. This pattern has been attributed both to an increase in the level of gonadotropins with the age and to the rise of medically assisted reproductive technologies (ART) among older women.

This extraordinary growth in twinning rates in different developed countries must be considered as an important public health issue since twin pregnancies are generally associated with greater risk for both infants and mothers. Twin babies are more fragile, have lower birth weight and born preterm more often than singleton babies. In addition, many of the risks to the mother are also risks to the child-to-be, since they can lead to premature labor, complications or, in the worst cases, fetal death. For these reasons, twin babies are more frequently admitted to neonatal intensive care units (NICUs) and subjected to more prolonged hospitalization with potential negative effects both on infants and parental behavior. Other complications for the mother are gestational diabetes, hypertension, preeclampsia and acute polyhydramnios.

Moreover, twin births can have negative effects on parents' adjustment as well. In fact, although it is possible to identify similarities in pregnancy and parenthood for twin and singleton births, the experience of expecting and parenting twins seems to be very different [4]. The responses to a multiple pregnancy and parenthood by most of the parents may be associated with ambivalence and surprise, even if the pregnancy resulted from infertility treatment [5], as well as with higher levels of anxiety, distress and higher risk of depression in the postpartum period both in the case of twins conceived naturally and in the case of twins conceived with ART [4, 6]. In addition, due to the medical risk associated, twin pregnancies need to be closely monitored [7, 8]. On one hand, this frequent and intensive monitoring could reassure parents, but, on the other, it constantly reminds them that their pregnancies could be associated with serious risks for the babies and the mothers. Different researches tried to evaluate the association between the presence of mood disorders and stress in parents and twin pregnancies. Researchers that focused on parental experience associated to twin pregnancy that occurs both naturally or with ART investigated either the joint experience of mothers and fathers [9–12] or of mothers alone [13–16]. It was observed that the risks usually associated to twin pregnancy lead to higher level of stress [17] and seemed to increase the incidence of depression and anxiety in parents of twins and especially in mothers [6, 9–11, 16, 18]. In addition, it was also observed that the presence of medical risk as well as psychological suffering in mothers during twin pregnancy is generally associated to higher level of fatigue, loss of energy, depressed mood and feelings of worthlessness and guilt [14].

Another important aspect related to the mothers' psychological adjustment during twin pregnancies is related to the building process of the relationship between the mother and the child-to-be [19]. During pregnancy, mothers use to think about their child-to-be, and they start to create representation of themselves as mothers. During twin pregnancies, the mother-to-be has to deal with an identification process with two children at the same time and have to create a mental space that allow her to make representation of both children. These processes include representations of physical and emotional characteristics of two different fetuses and of the interactions between the mother and her future babies, as well as dreams and expectations about both the children-to-be. For these reasons, it is possible to infer that the building process of this relationship between the mother and the child-to-be may differ among woman who are expecting twins and those who are expecting singleton [19].

2. Medical issues associated to twin pregnancy and twin birth

2.1. Twin pregnancy: fertilization, intrauterine growth and associated fetal risk factors

Twin pregnancy can be the result of multiple ovulations with fertilization of any oocyte by a sperm and in that case we have dizygotic twins (DZ) or a consequence of the fertilization of an oocyte by a sperm with subsequent division of the single zygotes and in this case we will have monozygotic twins (MZ). All DZ pregnancies are dichorionic (two placentas) and diamniotic (two amniotic cavities). MZ pregnancies, in relation to the gestational age in which the division into two embryos occurs, may be dichorionic and diamniotic (about 1/3 of the cases) if the division takes place between the first and the third day of gestation or monochorionic (single placenta) and diamniotic (about 2/3 of cases) if the division takes place between the fourth and the eighth day of gestation. Finally, the division could rarely occur between the ninth and the thirteenth day of gestation, resulting in monochorionic monoamniotic pregnancy (about 1% of the MZ pregnancies). Overall, DZ twins represent 70% of twin pregnancies and MZ twins represent 30% [20, 21]. From the genetic point of view, DZ twins (fraternal twins) can be assimilated to natural brothers, while MZ twins (identical twins) have always been thought to have the same genetic heritage. However, epigenetic alterations and environmental factors may be responsible for different phenotypic expressions at physical, neuropsychological and behavioral levels, in the absence of variations in the genetic sequence.

In twin pregnancies, it is essential to define if twins share or not placenta as soon as possible. Chorionicity determination in the first trimester is almost 100% accurate [20]. The most reliable signs to determine chorionicity are the number of gestational sacs between 7 and 10 weeks of gestation and the presence of lambda sign (a subtle triangular strip of cortical tissue separating the two placenta) between 11 and 14 weeks of gestation [21, 22]. The determination of chorionicity is particularly important from a clinical and prognostic point of view, since monochorionic (MC) twin pregnancies are complicated by an incidence of 10–15% of twin-to-twin transfusion syndrome (TTTS). TTTS is a chronic midtrimester complication of MC twin pregnancies that causes significantly higher perinatal mortality and morbidity rates in monochorionic than in dichorionic twins [23]. MC twins share their placenta and their blood circulation is connected by vascular anastomoses at the placenta surface. Placenta vascular anastomoses allow acute or chronic inter-twin blood transfusions between the circulations of the two fetuses. Imbalanced inter-twin blood flow can lead to a severe complication such as TTTS. In TTTS, imbalanced blood flow from one twin (the donor) to the other twin (the recipient) results in hypovolemia and oligohydramnios in the donor and hypervolemia and polyhydramnios in the recipient twins with transient or persistent right ventricular hypertrophy [24].

Another important issue related to twin pregnancy concerns fetal growth. In single pregnancies, progressive and linear fetal growth is observed until the 37th week of gestation, whereas in twin pregnancies the overlap is observed with single pregnancy only in the first two trimesters. Recent data from an Italian sample compared the twin birth weight curves with those of single birth ones, indicating differences in 3, 50 and 97° percentiles, starting from 32 weeks of gestational age and increasing according to gestational age: at 37 weeks, twins' weight differs by about 9% compared to single babies' weight. Similar differences were observed for length, whereas for the cranial circumference differences occur later, around the 36 weeks of gestation [25]. Fetal growth depends on fetal genetic inheritance and on factors related to the uterine-placental development environment that can impair placental circulation with fetal hypoperfusion. The anomalies in placental circulation establish a high risk of fetal hypoxia and reduced amount of nutrients (e.g. glucose and amino acids) essential for fetal growth. In the case of twin pregnancies and in the absence of genetic-metabolic fetal abnormalities, a proper maternal nutritional input is crucial for proper development. From a physiological point of view, twin pregnancy provides, compared to single pregnancy, an estimated weight gain of 3.5 kg higher. Although the weight is different, the feeding regime to follow is similar in both types of pregnancy. Neonatal weight of twins also depends on their zygosis and chorionicity. MZ twins weigh less than DZ twins and MC twins weigh less than dichorionic twins (DC). Intrauterine growth is also negatively influenced by IVF with multiple embryo transfer. Also during TTTS, it is common that the donor twin weighs 25% less than the other twin. Another situation defined as selective intrauterine growth restriction (sIUGR) could lead to a high risk of intrauterine death or extreme prematurity [24, 26].

The presence of discordant anomalies, which occur more frequently in elderly women with twins, is another important risk factor. In fact, it is well documented that, if discordant anomaly is noted, the likelihood of adverse outcomes both for the discordant twin and for the normal twin is increased [27, 28]. Particularly, it was observed that the presence of discordant anomalies is significantly associated with preterm birth, lower birth weight, IUGR and neonatal and infant death. Moreover, it was observed that discordant twins showed higher physiological and behavioral dysregulation [29, 30].

Finally, an additional factor for fetal risk concerns the phenomenon of the "vanishing twin." Early prenatal ultrasound for fetal monitoring has shown that at 8 weeks of gestation the incidence of multiple pregnancies is 3.3–4.5% that spontaneously evolves in single pregnancy in 21–30% of cases, after the reabsorption of an embryo by the placenta or of the other twin. This event is a potential risk factor for the development of complications in the surviving fetus [31]. Data from the Danish nationwide registers have demonstrated that IVF singleton babies born from vanished twin pregnancies had higher rates of small for gestational age (SGA) and term low birth weight (LBW) compared with IVF singleton pregnancies [32]. Furthermore, studies have noted an association with cerebral palsy in IVF children when the number of gestations at delivery was less than the number of embryos transferred compared with pregnancies in which the number of gestations at delivery was the same as the number of embryos transferred [33].

2.2. Twin delivery and perinatal risk factors

In twin pregnancies, antenatal care involves more intensive monitoring and protocols that are usually different to those for a singleton pregnancy. Ultrasound assessment of fetal biometry, anatomy and Doppler velocimetry is used to monthly monitor dichorionic twin pregnancies

[7] while, since risks are significantly higher in monochorionic compared with dichorionic pregnancy [8], antenatal assessment should be scheduled more often, usually every 15 days or less when decided by the gynecologists, in order to prevent adverse perinatal outcomes associated to this type of twin pregnancy.

Moreover, since twin pregnancies are associated with an increase in mortality and morbidity rates, a careful planning of delivery and adequate neonatal care in the delivery room are needed [21]. It has long been recognized that the timing of delivering twins constitutes a significant issue [34]. Despite in high-risk pregnancies there is the temptation to be reassured by increasing gestational age as the potential complications of prematurity, different studies suggest that the offspring of a twin gestation may benefit from delivering prior to their expected date of delivery [35, 36]. Several studies have focused on the "prospective risk of foetal death" to help determine by which gestational age a twin pregnancy should be delivered [37]. For twins, the prospective risk of fetal death appears to be equivalent to that of post-term singletons at about 37–38 weeks of gestation [35, 37]. The prospective risk of fetal death for twins intersects with neonatal death at about 39 week of gestation, showing that it may be reasonable to consider delivery of uncomplicated twins before 40 weeks of gestation [36]. These studies, however, did not address the impact of chorionicity on the decision to deliver a twin pregnancy. Other research focused on this aspect, indicating that in the case of dichorionic and diamniotic twin pregnancies, delivery should be scheduled from 38 weeks, while in uncomplicated monochorionic twins delivery should be scheduled from 36 weeks of gestation [22, 38].

Additionally, obstetrics and gynecologists broadly recognized that the delivery of twins constitutes an area of significant risk [34]. Perinatal mortality is five times higher in twins than in singletons [39]. In fact, the conduct of a twin delivery remains one of the most challenging events in the daily practice of obstetrics [34]. In particular, an important issue related to twin birth is associated with the choice of the mode of delivery. Although approximately 60% of twins are delivered by cesarean section [40], choosing the mode of delivery, spontaneous or cesarean, depends on multiple factors linked to both maternal and fetal characteristics [21]. Spontaneous delivery is generally used when both twins are vertex at the moment of childbirth. However, in this case, ultrasonographic examination is a useful adjunct after delivery of the first twin in order to establish the presentation of the second twin. In fact, after the delivery of the first twin, up to 20% of the second baby spontaneously changes presentation [41]. This emphasizes that, in case of a vaginal delivery in twin pregnancy, it is necessary to monitor all the process since the situation can rapidly change from a relatively low-risk delivery to one fraught with complications for mother and baby [34]. As regards the choice of cesarean delivery, there are few absolute indications to planned cesarean section. It seems that cesarean section without a trial of labor should be performed in cases of monoamniotic twins. The other indications are not dissimilar to those of a singleton pregnancy and include placenta previa and antenatal evidence of significant fetal compromise (e.g. severe selective IUGR) likely to worsen during labor. In addition, Cesarean section is generally the recommended method of delivery in twin gestations when one twin is non-vertex [42].

Twin delivery constitutes a challenge in daily obstetric practice, which becomes even more difficult in cases with preterm birth, the main perinatal risk factors associated with twin pregnancy [43]. Advancement of gestational age is crucial to achieve acceptable fetal growth rates and better perinatal conditions after birth [44]. Compared to term twin pregnancies, preterm twin pregnancies increase the risk of complications such as neonatal mortality, respiratory distress syndrome (RDS), sepsis, periventricular leukomalacia (PVL) and intraventricular hemorrhage (IVH). In addition, population-based studies from large databases have shown a higher risk of cerebral palsy in twins than in singletons. Studies found different risk profiles in relation to gestational age at birth. In particular, it was found that the presence of one or more of the above complications is present in 30% of moderately preterm infants (born between 32 and 33 + 6 weeks of GA), in 13% of late preterm infants (born between 34 and 36 + 6 weeks of GA) and only in 0.5% of twins born at term [21]. Therefore, all the complicated twin pregnancies have to be managed in tertiary level perinatal centers with both skilled gynecologists and neonatologists in this field.

Finally, another relevant aspect that needs to be taken into account is breastfeeding. Mothers of risk infants, as some twins are, may not have the opportunity to experience breastfeeding. Additionally, also in the case of healthy twins, breastfeeding can result a challenge for mothers. It is documented that a mother's feelings and attitudes on breastfeeding can considerably influence on its initiation [45]. For mothers of twins, breastfeeding may be physically uncomfortable; some of them are not able to establish an adequate milk support for two babies [46]. Moreover, several mothers of twins find that their experience of breastfeeding two children is stressful and fraught. Additionally, Mitra et al. [47] observed that those mothers who were well prepared for the realities of breastfeeding had a more successful experience in terms of its duration. Mothers of twins usually feel ill-prepared for breastfeed their twins and reported a lack of information and support during pregnancy [4, 48].

3. Psychological issues associated with twin pregnancy: the building of prenatal attachment

3.1. What is prenatal attachment?

Research on the mother-infant relationship has its origins in Bowlby's attachment theory [49]. This theory is raised from different disciplines such as ethology, cybernetics, information processing, developmental psychology and psychoanalysis, and it originally focused both on the infant's biological need for a secure early attachment to the mother and on the mother's response [49, 50]. Starting from Bowlby's theory, Mary Ainsworth added to the attachment theory the emotional component, based on the idea that the infant's contribution to the attachment process was more than biological and included baby's affective evaluation of the mother's behaviors [51]. Starting from this theoretical framework, many researches investigated mother-infant attachment during infancy [52], adolescence and adulthood [53–55], focusing both on behavioral and emotional markers to measure attachment.

Attachment has been described as "the innate tendency of children to create privileged affective bonds with at least one adult person (the caregiver) who takes care of them from birth" [50]. The study of how children develop this bond with their caregiver has identified two main types: secure and insecure [51]. The first would be those children who could use their mother (the caregiver) as a "safe base" that allow the children to explore the environment. These children usually cry at the time of separation, but they are capable to comfort themselves at the time of the reunion with the mother, returning to play. On the other hand, children with insecure attachment explore the environment less and are anxious when a stranger stays with them in the same room, even if the caregiver is near them; moreover, they become anxious also at the moment of separation from their caregiver and they usually cannot be consoled at the moment of the reunion with their caregiver. On the basis of the attachment relationship experienced, children would build a sort of primary mental "representations," the Internal Working Models (IWMs), that will regulate their peculiar interactive patterns [56]. The IWMs develop from the internalization of recurring interactive experiences between the children and their caregiver and the quality of their organization depends on the quality of care received during childhood. In the secure attachment pattern, IWMs would consist of representing the attachment figure as available to respond positively and consistently to requests for help and comfort, while in insecure attachment patterns, the IWMs would be organized starting from the representation of the caregiver as not available to respond properly at the requests of help and comfort, an attachment figure that is not attuned to the needs of the child, that are usually distant and, sometimes, even hostile. In reality, further studies pointed out that IWMs does not depend exclusively on the quality of the care received, but in a more complex way on the meanings that the caregiver communicate to the child with their behavior and conduct.

While the theory of neonatal attachment places the emphasis on the child, the theory of prenatal attachment emphasized the type of affective investment that parents, and especially mothers, have towards the child-to-be, an investment that begins and developed during the different stages of pregnancy. In fact, it was observed that the very early relationship between the mother and her babies does not start at birth [57], but it was recognized that it begins while the child is still a fetus [58]. With the perception of the fetal movements, the pregnant woman starts a process of psychological separation from the fetus and begins to view herself as a "mother" [59]. In particular, the concept of prenatal attachment is defined as "*the unique relationship that develops between a woman and her fetus*" [60] and "*the emotional tie or bond which normally develops between the pregnant parent and her unborn infant*" [61].

Different studies on prenatal attachment investigated its intensity during different period of gestation. Research that used a longitudinal design demonstrated a significant increase in terms of level of prenatal attachment measures during the entire course of the pregnancy [60, 62–64]. It was observed that immediately after the beginning of pregnancy, the level of prenatal attachment may depend on some situational factors, for example, if the woman has perceived fetal movement or if has seen an ultrasound image of the fetus [63]. It was also found that prenatal attachment develops in an orderly sequential way during the course of pregnancy [57, 58, 65]. In the first trimester, relatively low levels of prenatal attachment were observed, while with the increasing of gestational age, mothers start talking to the fetus, call the child-to-be per name [63] and, in the second and third trimesters, increase "nesting" behaviors. Also in a recent literature review on maternal-fetal attachment, Yarcheski et al. [66] suggested that the magnitude of this relationship is strongest during the third trimester of pregnancy.

Moreover, in recent years, different researches started to deeply investigate prenatal attachment, with particular attention to the link between the nature of this early mother-fetus relationship and the mother's early parenting experiences and attachment style in the postpartum period [67]. In fact, pregnancy could be considered a developmental process in which pregnant women start their transition into parenthood. This process implies different psychological changes and challenges that play an important role in the establishment of a successful parent-child relationship. Different researches showed that prenatal attachment could play an important role in identifying as soon as possible parents who found difficulties in developing a close and positive parent-child interaction during infancy [68].

Other studies focused on the examination of potential risk or protective factors that could influence prenatal attachment. It was observed that fetal movement and increased gestational age were positively related with attachment [62, 64]. There are also pieces of evidence that some demographic variables, such as maternal age and education, may correlate with attachment [19]. Positive correlations have also been found between prenatal attachment and the quality of marital status [58, 61, 68], as well as between prenatal attachment and perceived social support during pregnancy. In addition, other researches identified other situational risk factors that could modify the quality and the intensity of expression of prenatal attachment [63] as loss or stillbirth in a previous pregnancy [69, 70], medical risk during pregnancy [71], physical symptoms [72, 73], depression and anxiety [74] and twin pregnancies [19, 75, 76].

3.2. Prenatal attachment in twin pregnancy: a review of existing literature

Focusing on prenatal attachment in twin pregnancy, it is possible to observe that it may be different from singleton ones [18]. In fact, during a twin pregnancy, the mother-to-be has to deal with an identification process with two babies simultaneously and has to build a space that allows her to make representation of both children. This process includes representations of physical and emotional characteristics of two different fetuses and of the interactions between the mother and her child-to-be, as well as dreams and expectations about both the babies.

Despite previous works on prenatal attachment in mother of twins observed that it may be a risk factor for the development of a close and positive relationship between the mother and the babies, as far as we know, only six studies explored prenatal attachment in twin pregnancies [13, 19, 48, 75–77].

In a descriptive study of 10 women using grounded theory methodology, Van der Zalm observed that the process of prenatal attachment depends on *zygosity*. In particular, in the case of identical twin, mothers used to view their babies as a pair with similar characteristics, while in the case of fraternal twin mothers used to think about their babies as individuals with different characteristics [77].

A second study conducted by Colpin and colleagues aimed to evaluate the quality of prenatal attachment in a sample of 61 mothers expecting twins at the beginning of the last trimester of pregnancy. Higher quality of prenatal attachment was predicted by higher maternal psychosocial well-being and by higher marital satisfaction. However, it was observed that these variables explained only a small portion of variance of the quality of maternal attachment [48].

A third descriptive correlational study by Damato investigated through an online survey the level of prenatal attachment for each twin in a sample of 202 expectant mothers. It was found that the mother experience a significant higher level of prenatal attachment for the twin that later has been born for second. In addition, it was also observed a small but significant correlation between prenatal attachment and both gestational age and fetal movement [75].

The same author conducted two other studies on prenatal attachment during twin pregnancy [19, 76]. In the first study, a predictive correlational descriptive design was used to evaluate the role played by demographic and biological factors, as well as personal resources in predicting the level of prenatal attachment during twin pregnancy in a sample of 241 women expecting twins. It was demonstrated that history of infertility treatment, older age and lower family income predicted lower level of prenatal attachment, while the presence of fetal movement, higher gestational age and higher self-esteem predicted higher level of prenatal attachment. However, it was observed that only a small portion of variance was explained by the predictors considered in the study.

The other study by Damato investigated the influence of prenatal attachment and other relevant perinatal variables such as method of delivery, mother's health and depression, infant birth weight and neonatal intensive care unit (NICU) admission, on postnatal attachment in a sample of 139 mothers of twins. A modest but significant relationship between prenatal and postnatal attachment was observed. Moreover, it was found that also maternal characteristics, such as depression, and the context of the perinatal experience, such as delivery method and the NICU admission of the babies, influence the attachment process [76].

Finally, the most recent study that investigated prenatal attachment during twin pregnancy aimed at exploring the level of prenatal attachment in a sample of 83 expectant mothers during dichorionic pregnancies, uncomplicated monochorionic pregnancies and monochorionic pregnancies complicated by twin-to-twin transfusion syndrome (TTTS). In particular, it was showed that the increase of prenatal attachment in the last trimester of pregnancy, usually described in singleton pregnancies [78], was observed both in dichorionic and uncomplicated monochorionic pregnancies, while this intensification was not observed in pregnancies complicated by TTTS. The fear represented by the high risk associated to TTTS pregnancies, the uncertainty for the pregnancy outcome and the doubt for the health of the fetus seemed to reduce prenatal attachment [13].

3.3. Risk and protective factors for prenatal attachment in twin pregnancy

Starting from the existing literature on prenatal attachment both in singleton and in twin pregnancies and from those studies that investigate possible threat associated to twin pregnancies considering both medical and psychological risks factors, it is possible to suppose and infer which further variables may play a relevant role during twin pregnancy in impairing the building process of prenatal attachment or, on the contrary, in promoting the building of a close positive mother-fetus relationship.

Previous studies showed that the presence of medical risk and the higher prevalence of complication during pregnancy are generally associated to psychological suffering in mothers [14]. It

Multiple Pregnancy - New Challenges was observed that the presence of medical risk may impair the process of the building of representation of the child-to-be as well as the of themselves as mothers [79]. In twin pregnancies, antenatal care involves more intensive monitoring and protocols that are usually different to those for a singleton pregnancy. Ultrasound assessment of fetal biometry, anatomy and Doppler velocimetry is used to monthly monitor dichorionic twin pregnancies [7], while, since risks are significantly higher in monochorionic compared with dichorionic pregnancy [8], antenatal assessment should be scheduled more often in order to prevent adverse perinatal outcomes associated to this type of twin pregnancy. This frequent and intensive monitoring constantly remind to the mother that twin pregnancies could be associated with serious risks for the babies and the mothers [4], such as preterm delivery, low birth weight, IUGR, presence of discordant anomalies, increased risk of mortality and morbidity, preeclampsia, gestational diabetes and placental abruption [80]. When pregnancy is diagnosed as MC twin pregnancy, these could be even amplified for parents. The announcement of monochorionicity and its specific risks influences how parents deal with pregnancy [13]. Morbidity and mortality rates are higher than in DC pregnancies, and parents have to face concepts related to different complications associated with this kind of pregnancies as twin-to-twin transfusion syndrome (TTTS) or severe sIUGR.

As the presence of medical complication during pregnancy, also the loss of a baby in a previous pregnancy may have an impact on maternal well-being as well as on prenatal attachment in the subsequent pregnancy. Fetal loss may represent the breaking of a preexisting attachment bond [61] to someone who would eventually have contributed to the bereaved individual's life [70]. For mothers who experience fetal loss, the sufferance could be linked to their experience of being pregnant and this may worry them in a subsequent pregnancy [81]. As seen before, a concerning factor for fetal risk in twin pregnancy is the phenomenon of the "vanishing twin." This event is not only a potential risk factor for the development of complications in the surviving fetus [31]. In fact, the possible loss of a fetus during pregnancy usually triggers considerable negative feelings and thoughts in mothers, and this may be an obstacle for the building process of the babies' representations.

Moreover, it was also observed that higher level of negative mood states during pregnancy may be an obstacle for prenatal attachment. The risks usually associated to twin pregnancy could lead to higher level of negative mood states in mothers of twins [9–11, 16, 18]. The risks usually associated to twin pregnancy lead to higher level of stress [17] and increased the incidence of depression and anxiety in mothers of twins during pregnancy [6, 9–11, 16, 18]. It was observed that during twin pregnancy 33.3% of mothers-to-be suffer from major depression and experience higher level of stress and greater emotional and social fragilities. Moreover, the presence of medical risk as well as psychological suffering in mothers during twin pregnancy is generally associated to higher level of fatigue, loss of energy and feelings of worthlessness and guilt [14]. Worried, depressed and stressed mothers may not be able to start to create a mental space for the representation of the child-to-be, and this could be a disadvantage for the construction of mother-fetus relationship.

Despite most of the studies focused on risks factors for prenatal attachment, previous works observed that higher level of perceived social support as well as a positive relationship with the partner positively influences the mother-fetus relationship building during pregnancy [82]. Inevitably, fathers of twins will be more involved than a father of a singleton both during pregnancy and then with the babies' care. The earlier the partner is helped to recognize this need and is positively encouraged and supported to participate, the better. In addition, as previously seen, during pregnancy women are generally more exposed to emotional distress and depressive reactions related not only to the physical and hormonal changes but also to changes in their status, especially. Previous studies on singleton pregnancies indicated that fathers play an important role in helping mothers-to-be facing these difficulties, providing them emotional support, protecting from excessive psychological suffering and, consequently, promoting prenatal attachment [83].

4. Conclusions

Given the current "epidemic of multiple pregnancies" in much of the Western countries, it is surprising that still few studies examined the psychological impact of twin pregnancy and twin birth on parents' experience.

This chapter underlined that twin babies are generally more fragile and more at risks of born preterm and with lower birth than singleton babies. The medical risks associated to twin pregnancies may influence both twins' developmental outcomes [84] and the building of a close and positive mother-child relationship [85]. It was also pointed out that medical risks, usually associated to twin pregnancy, may be linked to negative effects on parents' and especially mothers' experiences.

In particular, it was observed that despite it is possible to identify some similarities to singleton pregnancy, the experience of expecting twins may be very different. Parents and in particular mothers of twins have unique needs and have to face unique challenges. Risks usually associated to twin pregnancy may lead to higher level of stress and negative mood states in parents. In fact, mothers of twins seem to be less psychological adjusted to their pregnancy in terms of lower level of prenatal attachment.

In reviewing the research that investigated prenatal attachment, it was observed that the quality of the relationship established by the mother-to-be with their fetus could be an important diagnostic information to identify as soon as possible women who may have difficulties during the interaction with their babies mostly because prenatal attachment is usually associated to the quality of mother-infant interaction in the postpartum period [68, 76].

Healthcare practitioners should be aware of the unique experience and challenges associated to expecting and parenting twins, which are often underestimated by society and even by other new mothers. In addition, it is known that perinatal period until the first 3 months postpartum has been demonstrated to be the most vulnerable period for mothers of twin [86]. Paying attention to the issues involved in expecting and parenting twins, starting from pregnancy, may support mothers in their transition to motherhood. This may be accomplished by the implementation of target peer support group prenatally and/or postnatally (both during hospitalization and then after discharge at home), so that women can gain from the experience of others with a similar life event.

Conflict of interest

The authors (Chiara Ionio, Eleonora Mascheroni, Caterina Colombo, Gianluca Lista) certify that they have NO affiliations with or involvement in any organization or entity with any financial interest (such as honoraria; educational grants; participation in speakers' bureaus; membership, employment, consultancies, stock ownership or other equity interest and expert testimony or patent-licensing arrangements) or non-financial interest (such as personal or professional relationships, affiliations, knowledge or beliefs) in the subject matter or materials discussed in this manuscript.

Author details

Chiara Ionio[1]*, Eleonora Mascheroni[2], Caterina Colombo[3] and Gianluca Lista[4]

*Address all correspondence to: chiara.ionio@unicatt.it

1 Department of Psychology, CRIdee, Catholic University, Milan, Italy

2 CRIdee, Catholic University, Milan, Italy

3 Department of Obstetrics and Gynaecology and NICU, Buzzi Children's Hospital, ASST Fatebenefratelli-Sacco, Milan, Italy

4 Pediatric Department, Buzzi Children's Hospital, ASST Fatebenefratelli-Sacco, Milan, Italy

References

[1] Long E, Ferriman E. Twin pregnancy. Obstetrics, Gynaecology and Reproductive Medicine. 2016;**26**(2):38-45

[2] Hoekstra C, Zhao ZZ, Lambalk CB, Willemsen G, Martin NG, Boomsma DI, Montgomery GW. Dizygotic twinning. Human Reproduction Update. 2007;**14**(1):37-47

[3] Bulmer MG. The Biology of Twinning in Man. Oxford: Clarendon Press; 1970. 205 p. DOI: 10.1002/tera.1420040214

[4] Leonard L, Denton J. Preparation for parenting multiple birth children. Early Human Development. 2006;**82**(6):371-378. DOI: 10.1016/j.earlhumdev.2006.03.009

[5] Gromada KK. Mothering Multiples: Breastfeeding & Caring for Twins or More!!! Rev ed. Schaumburg, IL: La Leche League International; 1999. p. 429

[6] Choi Y, Bishai D, Minkovitz CS. Multiple births are a risk factor for postpartum maternal depressive symptoms. Pediatrics. 2009;**123**(4):1147-1154. DOI: 10.1542/peds.2008-1619

[7] Khalil A, Rodgers M, Baschat A, Bhide A, Gratacos E, Hecher K, et al. ISUOG practice guidelines: Role of ultrasound in twin pregnancy. Ultrasound in Obstetrics and Gynecology. 2016;**47**(2):247-263. DOI: 10.1002/uog.15821

[8] Hack KEA, Derks JB, Elias SG, Franx A, Roos EJ, Voerman SK, et al. Increased perinatal mortality and morbidity in monochorionic versus dichorionic twin pregnancies: Clinical implications of a large Dutch cohort study. BJOG: An International Journal of Obstetrics and Gynaecology. 2008;**115**(1):58-67. DOI: 10.1111/j.1471-0528.2007.01556.x

[9] Baor L, Blickstein I. En route to an "instant family": Psychosocial considerations. Obstetrics and Gynecology Clinics of North America. 2005;**32**(1):127-139

[10] Ellison MA, Hall JE. Social stigma and compounded losses: Quality-of-life issues for multiple-birth families. Fertility and Sterility. 2003;**80**(2):405-414

[11] Kalra SK, Milad MP, Klock SC, Grobman WA. Infertility patients and their partners: Differences in the desire for twin gestations. Obstetrics and Gynecology. 2003;**102**(1):152-155

[12] Vilska S, Unkila-Kallio L, Punamäki RL, Poikkeus P, Repokari L, Sinkkonen J, et al. Mental health of mothers and fathers of twins conceived via assisted reproduction treatment: A 1-year prospective study. Human Reproduction. 2008;**24**(2):367-377. DOI: 10.1093/humrep/den427

[13] Beauquier-Maccotta B, Chalouhi GE, Picquet AL, Carrier A, Bussières L, Golse B, Ville Y. Impact of monochorionicity and twin to twin transfusion syndrome on prenatal attachment, post-traumatic stress disorder, anxiety and depressive symptoms. PLoS One. 2016;**11**(1):e0145649. DOI: 10.1371/journal.pone.0145649

[14] Benute GR, Nozzella DC, Prohaska C, Liao A, de Lucia MC, Zugaib M. Twin pregnancies: Evaluation of major depression, stress, and social support. Twin Research and Human Genetics. 2013;**16**(2):629-633. DOI: 10.1017/thg.2012.153

[15] Fisher J, Stocky A. Maternal perinatal mental health and multiple births: Implications for practice. Twin Research and Human Genetics. 2003;**6**(6):506-513. DOI: 10.1375/136905203322686509

[16] Yokoyama Y. Comparison of child-rearing problems between mothers with multiple children who conceived after infertility treatment and mothers with multiple children who conceived spontaneously. Twin Research and Human Genetics. 2003;**6**(2):89-96. DOI: 10.1375/136905203321536218

[17] Cataldo NA, Gauer G, Furtado NR. Psiquiatria para Estudantes de Medicina. EDIPUCRS: Porto Alegre; 2003. 944 p

[18] Campbell D, van Teijlingen ER, Yip L. Economic and social implications of multiple birth. Best Practice and Research Clinical Obstetrics and Gynaecology. 2004;**18**(4):657-668. DOI: 10.1016/j.bpobgyn.2004.04.016

[19] Damato EG. Predictors of prenatal attachment in mothers of twins. Journal of Obstetric, Gynecologic, and Neonatal Nursing. 2004;**33**(4):436-445. DOI: 10.1177/0884217504266894

[20] Fox TB. Multiple pregnancies: Determining chorionicity and amnionicity. Journal of Diagnostic Medical Sonography. 2006;**22**(1):59-65. DOI: 10.1177/8756479305284101

[21] Piro E, Corsello G. Gemellarità e prematurità. In: Sansavini A, Faldella G, editors. Lo sviluppo dei bambini nati pretermine: Aspetti neuropsicologici, metodi di valutazione e interventi. Milano: Franco Angeli; 2013. pp. 27-39

[22] Vayssière C, Beucher G, Dupuis O, Feraud O, Simon-Toulza C, Sentilhes L, et al. Instrumental delivery: Clinical practice guidelines from the French College of Gynaecologists and Obstetricians. European Journal of Obstetrics and Gynecology and Reproductive Biology. 2011;**159**(1):43-48. DOI: 10.1016/j.ejogrb.2011.06.043

[23] Umur A, van Gemert MJ, Nikkels PG. Monoamniotic-versus diamniotic-monochorionic twin placentas: Anastomoses and twin-twin transfusion syndrome. American Journal of Obstetrics and Gynecology. 2003;**189**(5):1325-1329

[24] van Klink JM, Koopman HM, van Zwet EW, Middeldorp JM, Walther FJ, Oepkes D, Lopriore E. Improvement in neurodevelopmental outcome in survivors of twin–twin transfusion syndrome treated with laser surgery. American Journal of Obstetric Gynecology. 2014;**210**:540.e1-540.e7

[25] Bertino E, Spada E, Occhi L, Coscia A, Giuliani F, Gagliardi L, et al. Neonatal anthropometric charts: The Italian neonatal study compared with other European studies. Journal of Pediatric Gastroenterology and Nutrition. 2010;**51**(3):353-361. DOI: 10.1097/MPG.0b013e3181da213e

[26] Bennasar M, Eixarch E, Martinez JM, Gratacós E. Selective restriction of intrauterine growth in twin singletonic twin pregnancies. Neonatal Medicine. 2017;**22**(6):376-382. DOI: 10.1016/j.siny.2017.05.001

[27] Blickstein I. Normal and abnormal growth of multiples. Seminars in Neonatology. 2002; **7**(3):177-185. DOI: 10.1053/siny.2002.0105

[28] Chauhan SP, Scardo JA, Hayes E, Abuhamad AZ, Berghella V. Twins: Prevalence, problems, and preterm births. American Journal of Obstetrics and Gynecology. 2010;**203**(4): 305-315. DOI: 10.1016/j.ajog.2010.04.031

[29] Minde K, Corter C, Goldberg S, Jeffers D. Maternal preference between premature twins up to age four. Journal of the American Academy of Child and Adolescent Psychiatry. 1990;**29**(3):367-374. DOI: 10.1097/00004583-199005000-00006

[30] Zeskind PS, Goff DM, Marshall TR. Rhythmic organization of neonatal heart rate and its relation to atypical fetal growth. Developmental Psychobiology. 1991;**24**(6):413-429. DOI: 10.1002/dev.420240604

[31] Landy HJ, Keith LG. The vanishing twin: A review. Human Reproduction Update. 1998; **4**(2):177-183. DOI: 10.1093/humupd/4.2.177

[32] Pinborg A, Lidegaard Ø, la Cour FN, Andersen AN. Vanishing twins: A predictor of small-for-gestational age in IVF singletons. Human Reproduction. 2007;**22**(10):2707-2714. DOI: 10.1093/humrep/dem225

[33] Barton SE, Missmer SA, Hornstein MD. Twin pregnancies with a 'vanished' embryo: A higher risk multiple gestation group? Human Reproduction. 2011;**26**(10):2750-2753. DOI: 10.1093/humrep/der221

[34] Barrett JFR, Ritchie WK. Twin delivery. Best Practice and Research Clinical Obstetrics and Gynaecology. 2003;**16**(1):43-56. DOI: 10.1053/beog.2002.0254

[35] Cleary-Goldman J, D'Alton ME. Uncomplicated monochorionic diamniotic twins and the timing of delivery. PLoS Medicine. 2005;**2**(6):e180. DOI: 10.1371/journal.pmed.0020180

[36] Sairam S, Costeloe K, Thilaganathan B. Prospective risk of stillbirth in multiple-gestation pregnancies: A population-based analysis. Obstetrics and Gynecology. 2002;**100**(4):638-641. DOI: 10.1016/S0029-7844(02)02174-9

[37] Kahn B, Lumey LH, Zybert PA, Lorenz JM, Cleary-Goldman J, D'alton ME, Robinson JN. Prospective risk of fetal death in singleton, twin, and triplet gestations: Implications for practice. Obstetrics and Gynecology. 2003;**102**(4):685-692. DOI: 10.1016/S0029-7844(03)00616-1

[38] Cheong-See F, Schuit E, Arroyo-Manzano D, Khalil A, Barrett J, Joseph KS, et al. Prospective risk of stillbirth and neonatal complications in twin pregnancies: Systematic review and meta-analysis. British Medical Journal. 2016;**354**:i4353. DOI: 10.1136/bmj.i4353

[39] Imaizumi Y. Perinatal mortality in twins and factors influencing mortality in Japan, 1980–98. Paediatric and Perinatal Epidemiology. 2001;**15**(3):298-305

[40] Breeze AC, Smith G. Mode of delivery of twins. The Obstetrician and Gynaecologist. 2004;**6**(4):222-226. DOI: 10.1576/toag.6.4.222.27019

[41] Houlihan C, Knuppel RA. Intrapartum management of multiple gestations. Clinics in Perinatology. 1996;**23**(1):91-116. DOI: 10.1016/S0146-0005(05)80019-9

[42] Adams DM, Chervenak FA. Intrapartum management of twin gestation. Clinical Obstetrics and Gynecology. 1990;**33**(1):52-60. DOI: 10.1016/S0146-0005(05)80019-9

[43] Santolaya J, Faro R. Twins-twice more trouble? Clinical Obstetrics and Gynecology. 2012;**55**(1):296-306. DOI: 10.1097/GRF.0b013e3182446f51

[44] Dolgun ZN, Inan C, Altintas AS, Okten SB, Sayin NC. Preterm birth in twin pregnancies: Clinical outcomes and predictive parameters. Pakistan Journal of Medical Sciences. 2016;**32**(4):922. DOI: 10.12669/pjms.324.10409

[45] Bentovim A. Shame and other anxieties associated with breast-feeding: A systems theory and psychodynamic approach. In: Elliott K, Fitzsimons DW, editors. Breastfeeding and the Mother. Chichester, UK: John Wiley & Sons, Ltd; 1976. pp. 159-178

[46] Neifert M, Thorpe J. Twins: Family adjustment, parenting, and infant feeding in the fourth trimester. Clinical Obstetrics and Gynecology. 1990;**33**(1):102-113

[47] Mitra A, Khoury A, Hinton A, Carothers C. Predictors of breastfeeding intention among low income women. Maternal and Child Health Journal. 2004;**8**(2):65-70. DOI: 10.1023/B: MACI.0000025728.54271.27

[48] Colpin H, De Munter A, Nys K, Vandemeulebroecke L. Prenatal attachment in future parents of twins. Infant and Child Development. 1998;**7**(4):223-227. DOI: 10.1002/(SICI) 1099-0917(199812)7:4<223::AID-EDP184>3.0.CO;2-7

[49] Bowlby J. Attachment and Loss, Volume I Attachment. 1st ed. London: Chatto & Windus; 1969. 448 p

[50] Fonagy P, Target M. Attaccamento e Funzione Riflessiva Selected Papers of Peter Fonagy and Mary Target. Raffaello Cortina: Milano; 2001. p. 464

[51] Ainsworth MDS, Blehar MC, Waters E, Wall SN. Patterns of Attachment: A Psychological Study of the Strange Situation. Psychology Press; 2015. 446 p

[52] Main M, Kaplan N, Cassidy J. Security in infancy, childhood, and adulthood: A move to the level of representation. Monographs of the Society for Research in Child Development. 1985:66-104. DOI: 10.2307/3333827

[53] Bartholomew K, Horowitz LM. Attachment styles among young adults: A test of a four-category model. Journal of Personality and Social Psychology. 1991;**61**(2):226. DOI: 10.1037//0022-3514.61.2.226

[54] Hazan C, Shaver P. Romantic love conceptualized as an attachment process. Journal of Personality and Social Psychology. 1987;**52**(3):511

[55] Kobak RR, Sceery A. Attachment in late adolescence: Working models, affect regulation, and representations of self and others. Child Development. 1988:135-146

[56] Della Vedova AM, Dabrassi F, Imbasciati A. Assessing prenatal attachment in a sample of Italian women. Journal of Reproductive and Infant Psychology. 2008;**26**(2):86-98. DOI: 10.1080/02646830701805349

[57] DiPietro JA. Psychological and psychophysiological considerations regarding the maternal–fetal relationship. Infant and Child Development. 2010;**19**(1):27-38. DOI: 10.1002/icd.651

[58] Alhusen JL. A literature update on maternal-fetal attachment. Journal of Obstetric, Gynecologic, and Neonatal Nursing. 2008;**37**(3):315-328. DOI: 10.1111/j.1552-6909.2008.00241.x

[59] Attrill B. The assumption of the maternal role: A developmental process. The Australian Journal of Midwifery. 2002;**15**(1):21-25. DOI: 10.1016/S1445-4386(02)80019-2

[60] Muller ME, Mercer RT. Development of the prenatal attachment inventory. Western Journal of Nursing Research. 1993;**15**(2):199-215. DOI: 10.1177/019394599301500205

[61] Condon JT, Corkindale C. The correlates of antenatal attachment in pregnant women. Psychology and Psychotherapy: Theory, Research and Practice. 1997;**70**(4):359-372. DOI: 10.1111/j.2044-8341.1997.tb01912.x

[62] Bloom KC. The development of attachment behaviors in pregnant adolescents. Nursing Research. 1995;**44**(5):284-289. DOI: 10.1097/00006199-199509000-00005

[63] Doan HM, Zimerman A. Prenatal attachment: A developmental model. International Journal Prenatal and Perinatal Psychology and Medicine. 2008;**20**:20-28

[64] Wayland J, Tate S. Maternal-fetal attachment and perceived relationships with important others in adolescents. Birth. 1993;**20**(4):198-203. DOI: 10.1111/j.1523-536X.1993.tb00227.x

[65] Habib C, Lancaster S. Changes in identity and paternal–foetal attachment across a first pregnancy. Journal of Reproductive and Infant Psychology. 2010;**28**(2):128-142. DOI: 10.1080/02646830903298723

[66] Yarcheski A, Mahon NE, Yarcheski TJ, Hanks MM, Cannella BL. A meta-analytic study of predictors of maternal-fetal attachment. International Journal of Nursing Studies. 2009; **46**(5):708-715. DOI: 10.1016/j.ijnurstu.2008.10.013

[67] Cannella BL. Maternal–fetal attachment: An integrative review. Journal of Advanced Nursing. 2005;**50**(1):60-68. DOI: 10.1111/j.1365-2648.2004.03349.x

[68] Siddiqui A, Hägglöf B. Does maternal prenatal attachment predict postnatal mother–infant interaction? Early Human Development. 2000;**59**(1):13-25. DOI: 10.1016/S0378-3782(00)00076-1

[69] Armstrong D, Hutti M. Pregnancy after perinatal loss: The relationship between anxiety and prenatal attachment. Journal of Obstetric, Gynecologic, and Neonatal Nursing. 1998; **27**(2):183-189. DOI: 10.1111/j.1552-6909.1998.tb02609.x

[70] O'Leary J. Grief and its impact on prenatal attachment in the subsequent pregnancy. Archives of Women's Mental Health. 2004;**7**(1):7-18. DOI: 10.1007/s00737-003-0037-1

[71] Feldman R, Weller A, Leckman JF, Kuint J, Eidelman AI. The nature of the mother's tie to her infant: Maternal bonding under conditions of proximity, separation, and potential loss. Journal of Child Psychology and Psychiatry and Allied Disciplines. 1999;**40**(6):929-939. DOI: 10.1111/1469-7610.00510

[72] Huang HC, Wang SY, Chen CH. Body image, maternal-fetal attachment, and choice of infant feeding method: A study in Taiwan. Birth. 2004;**31**(3):183-188. DOI: 10.1111/j.0730-7659.2004.00303.x

[73] Lai BPY, Tang CSK, Tse WKL. A longitudinal study investigating disordered eating during the transition to motherhood among Chinese women in Hong Kong. International Journal of Eating Disorders. 2006;**39**(4):303-311. DOI: 10.1002/eat.20266

[74] Hart R, McMahon CA. Mood state and psychological adjustment to pregnancy. Archives of Women's Mental Health. 2006;**9**(6):329-337. DOI: 10.1007/s00737-006-0141-0

[75] Damato EG. Maternal-fetal attachment in twin pregnancies. Journal of Obstetric, Gynecologic, and Neonatal Nursing. 2000;**29**(6):598-605. DOI: 10.1111/j.1552-6909.2000.tb02073.x

[76] Damato EG. Prenatal attachment and other correlates of postnatal maternal attachment to twins. Advances in Neonatal Care. 2004;**4**(5):274-291. DOI: 10.1177/0884217504266894

[77] Van der Zalm JE. The perinatal death of a twin Karla's story of attaching and detaching. Journal of Nurse-Midwifery. 1995;**40**(4):335-341. DOI: 10.1016/0091-2182(95)00017-E

[78] Narita S, Maehara S. The development of maternal-fetal attachment during pregnancy. Nihon Kango Kagakkai shi = Journal of Japan Academy of Nursing Science. 1993;**13**(2):1-9

[79] Brandon AR, Pitts S, Denton WH, Stringer CA, Evans HM. A history of the theory of prenatal attachment. Journal of Prenatal and Perinatal Psychology and Health: APPPAH. 2009;**23**(4):201

[80] Bryan E. The impact of multiple preterm births on the family. BJOG: An International Journal of Obstetrics and Gynaecology. 2003;**110**(s20):24-28. DOI: 10.1046/j.1471-0528.2003.00014.x

[81] Klass D. The inner representation of the dead child in the psychic and social narratives of bereaved parents. In: Neimeyer R, editor. Meaning Reconstruction and the Experience of Loss. Washington DC: American Psychological Association; 2001. pp. 77-94

[82] Anderson A, Anderson B. Toward a substantive theory of mother-twin attachment. MCN: The American Journal of Maternal/Child Nursing. 1990;**15**(6):373-378

[83] Baldoni F. Funzione paterna e attaccamento di coppia: l'importanza di una base sicura. In: Bertozzi N, Hamon C, editors. Padri & paternità. Bergamo: Edizioni Junior; 2005. pp. 79-102

[84] Stanton-Chapman TL, Chapman DA, Bainbridge NL, Scott KG. Identification of early risk factors for language impairment. Research in Developmental Disabilities. 2002;**23**(6):390-405. DOI: 10.1016/S0891-4222(02)00141-5

[85] Müller-Nix C, Forcada-Guex M, Pierrehumbert B, Jaunin L, Borghini A, Ansermet F. Prematurity, maternal stress and mother-child interactions. Early Human Development. 2004;**79**:145-158. DOI: 10.1016/j.earlhumdev.2004.05.002

[86] Beck CT. Releasing the pause button: Mothering twins during the first year of life. Qualitative Health Research. 2002;**12**(5):593-608. DOI: 10.1177/104973202129120124

Permissions

All chapters in this book were first published in MPNC, by InTech Open; hereby published with permission under the Creative Commons Attribution License or equivalent. Every chapter published in this book has been scrutinized by our experts. Their significance has been extensively debated. The topics covered herein carry significant findings which will fuel the growth of the discipline. They may even be implemented as practical applications or may be referred to as a beginning point for another development.

The contributors of this book come from diverse backgrounds, making this book a truly international effort. This book will bring forth new frontiers with its revolutionizing research information and detailed analysis of the nascent developments around the world.

We would like to thank all the contributing authors for lending their expertise to make the book truly unique. They have played a crucial role in the development of this book. Without their invaluable contributions this book wouldn't have been possible. They have made vital efforts to compile up to date information on the varied aspects of this subject to make this book a valuable addition to the collection of many professionals and students.

This book was conceptualized with the vision of imparting up-to-date information and advanced data in this field. To ensure the same, a matchless editorial board was set up. Every individual on the board went through rigorous rounds of assessment to prove their worth. After which they invested a large part of their time researching and compiling the most relevant data for our readers.

The editorial board has been involved in producing this book since its inception. They have spent rigorous hours researching and exploring the diverse topics which have resulted in the successful publishing of this book. They have passed on their knowledge of decades through this book. To expedite this challenging task, the publisher supported the team at every step. A small team of assistant editors was also appointed to further simplify the editing procedure and attain best results for the readers.

Apart from the editorial board, the designing team has also invested a significant amount of their time in understanding the subject and creating the most relevant covers. They scrutinized every image to scout for the most suitable representation of the subject and create an appropriate cover for the book.

The publishing team has been an ardent support to the editorial, designing and production team. Their endless efforts to recruit the best for this project, has resulted in the accomplishment of this book. They are a veteran in the field of academics and their pool of knowledge is as vast as their experience in printing. Their expertise and guidance has proved useful at every step. Their uncompromising quality standards have made this book an exceptional effort. Their encouragement from time to time has been an inspiration for everyone.

The publisher and the editorial board hope that this book will prove to be a valuable piece of knowledge for researchers, students, practitioners and scholars across the globe.

List of Contributors

Panagiotis Antsaklis, Marianna Theodora and George Daskalakis
Alexandra Maternity Hospital, University of Athens, Athens, Greece

Maria Papamichail
University of Athens, Athens, Greece

Michael Syndos
Obstetrics and Gynecology, Alexandra Maternity Hospital, Athens, Greece

Melinda Mátyás and Gabriela Zaharie
Department of Neonatology, University of Medicine and Pharmacy, Cluj-Napoca, Romania

Vivian Melo Corrêa
Department of Obstetrics, Paulista School of Medicine, Federal University of São Paulo (EPM-UNIFESP), São Paulo, SP, Brazil

Isabela Bottura and José Pedro Parise Filho
Department of Perinatology, Albert Einstein Hospital, São Paulo, SP, Brazil

Eduardo Félix Martins Santana
Department of Obstetrics, Paulista School of Medicine, Federal University of São Paulo (EPM-UNIFESP), São Paulo, SP, Brazil
Department of Perinatology, Albert Einstein Hospital, São Paulo, SP, Brazil

Johan Fellman
Hanken School of Economics, Helsinki, Finland

Fiona Langdon
King Edward Memorial Hospital, Subiaco, WA, Australia
Fertility Specialists of Western Australia, Bethesda Hospital, Claremont, WA, Australia
Division of Obstetrics and Gynaecology, University of Western Australia, Perth, WA, Australia

Roger Hart
Fertility Specialists of Western Australia, Bethesda Hospital, Claremont, WA, Australia
Division of Obstetrics and Gynaecology, University of Western Australia, Perth, WA, Australia

Bruno Rodrigues Toneto
Federal University of São Paulo, São Paulo, Brazil

Marcelo Santucci Franca and Tatiana E. N. K. Hamamoto
Discipline of Fetal Medicine, Obstetrics Department, Federal University of São Paulo—UNIFESP, São Paulo, Brazil

Antônio Fernandes Moron
Institute of Tropical Medicine, University of São Paulo (USP), São Paulo, Brazil

Diego Hernández Molina, Jessica L. Barajas Vega, Sylvia E. Totsuka Sutto, Fernando Grover Paéz, Francisco J. Hernández Mora, Ernesto J. Ramírez Lizardo, Sara Pascoe Gonzalez, David Cardona Müller and Ernesto G. Cardona Muñoz
INTEC, Centro Universitario de Ciencias de la Salud, Universidad de Guadalajara, México

Hernández Mora
Hospital Civil de Guadalajara "Fray Antonio Alcalde", Guadalajara, Jalisco, México

Leonel García Benavides
INTEC, Centro Universitario de Ciencias de la Salud, Universidad de Guadalajara, México
Hospital Civil de Guadalajara "Fray Antonio Alcalde", Guadalajara, Jalisco, México

Stelios Fiorentzis
Agios Nikolaos Crete, Greece

Styliani Salta
Cancer Biology and Therapeutics, Centre de Recherche Saint-Antoine, Institut National de la Santé et de la Recherche Médicale (INSERM) U938 and Institut Universitaire de Cancérologie, Faculté de Médecine, Sorbonne Université, Paris, France
Service d'Hématologie Biologique Hôpital Tenon, Hôpitaux Universitaires Est Parisien, Assistance Publique Hôpitaux de Paris (AP-HP), Paris, France

Michail Pargianas
Medical School, University of Ioannina, Obstetrics and Gynecology, Ioannina, Greece

Artemis Pontikaki
Department of Obstetrics and Gynecology, University Hospital of Heraklion, Greece

Dimitrios P. Koutsoulis
General Panarcadian of Tripolis, Greece

Christodoulos Akrivis, Dimitrios Akrivis and Ioannis Kosmas
Department of Obstetrics and Gynecology, Ioannina State General Hospital G. Chatzikosta, Ioannina, Greece

Laura Pérez Martín
HM Fertility Center Puerta del Sur, Móstoles, Spain

Duna Trobo Marina
Gregorio Marañón University Hospital, Madrid, Spain

Marco Varella, Eloisa Fernandes, Tiziana Acquaviva, Tania Lucci, Rafael Hsu, Vinicius David, Vera Bussab, Jaroslava Valentova and Emma Otta
Department of Experimental Psychology, Institute of Psychology, University de Sao Paulo,Sao Paulo, Brazil

Jonas Arantes
Institute of Biosciences, University de Sao Paulo, Sao Paulo, Brazil

Nancy Segal
Department of Psychology, California State University, Fullerton, USA

Chiara Ionio
Department of Psychology, CRIdee, Catholic University, Milan, Italy

Eleonora Mascheroni
CRIdee, Catholic University, Milan, Italy

Caterina Colombo
Department of Obstetrics and Gynaecology and NICU, Buzzi Children's Hospital, ASST Fatebenefratelli-Sacco, Milan, Italy

Gianluca Lista
Pediatric Department, Buzzi Children's Hospital, ASST Fatebenefratelli-Sacco, Milan, Italy

Index

www.ingramcontent.com/pod-product-compliance
Lightning Source LLC
LaVergne TN
LVHW060517210926
848485LV00005B/1097